CAREER
DEVELOPMENT
for HEALTH PROFESSIONALS

Withdrawn

Fourth Edition

CAREER DEVELOPMENT

for HEALTH PROFESSIONALS

Success in School & On the Job

Lee Haroun

MA (Education), MBA, EdD

Educator and Health Care Writer
Sunriver, Oregon

ELSEVIER

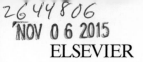

ELSEVIER

3251 Riverport Lane
St. Louis, Missouri 63043

CAREER DEVELOPMENT FOR HEALTH PROFESSIONALS:
SUCCESS IN SCHOOL & ON THE JOB, FOURTH EDITION

ISBN: 978-0-323-31126-7

Notices

Knowledge and best practice in this field are constantly changing. As new research and experience broaden our understanding, changes in research methods, professional practices, or medical treatment may become necessary.

Practitioners and researchers must always rely on their own experience and knowledge in evaluating and using any information, methods, compounds, or experiments described herein. In using such information or methods they should be mindful of their own safety and the safety of others, including parties for whom they have a professional responsibility.

With respect to any drug or pharmaceutical products identified, readers are advised to check the most current information provided (i) on procedures featured or (ii) by the manufacturer of each product to be administered, to verify the recommended dose or formula, the method and duration of administration, and contraindications. It is the responsibility of practitioners, relying on their own experience and knowledge of their patients, to make diagnoses, to determine dosages and the best treatment for each individual patient, and to take all appropriate safety precautions.

To the fullest extent of the law, neither the Publisher nor the authors, contributors, or editors, assume any liability for any injury and/or damage to persons or property as a matter of product liability, negligence or otherwise, or from any use or operation of any methods, products, instructions, or ideas contained in the material herein.

Previous editions copyrighted 2011, 2006, 2001.
Library of Congress Cataloging-in-Publication Data

Haroun, Lee, author.
  Career development for health professionals : success in school & on the job / Lee Haroun. -- Fourth edition.
     p. ; cm.
  Includes bibliographical references and index.
  ISBN 978-0-323-31126-7 (pbk. : alk. paper)
  I. Title.
  [DNLM: 1. Health Personnel. 2. Career Choice. 3. Vocational Guidance. W 21]
  R690
  610.69--dc23
                                                                    2015007444

Executive Content Strategist: Jennifer Janson
Content Development Manager: Ellen Wurm-Cutter
Associate Content Development Specialist: Kelly Skelton
Publishing Services Manager: Jeff Patterson
Senior Project Manager: Anne Konopka
Senior Book Designer: Amy Buxton

Printed in China

Last digit is the print number: 9 8 7 6 5 4 3 2 1

Working together
to grow libraries in
developing countries

www.elsevier.com • www.bookaid.org

**To David, whose spirit and optimism remind me
daily that all things are possible.**

Reviewers

Lori King, NRCMA
Medical Program Instructor
Great Lakes Institute of Technology
Erie, Pennsylvania

Dana Kullman, LMT, BSM, M.ED
Sr. Academic Chair
Blue Cliff College
Lafayette, Louisiana

Colene Melson, CPC, CPC-H, CMBS
Instructor
Buffalo Center for Arts and Technology
Buffalo, New York

Carrie Ann Mozdy, BS in Education
Instructor
Great Lakes Institute of Technology
Erie, Pennsylvania

Kristen Sexton, Certified Health Information Technologist
Instructor
Great Lakes Institute of Technology
Erie, Pennsylvania

Gail Winkler, MHIIM, RHIA
Director HIT Programs
Walters State Community College
Morristown, Tennessee

Preface

This book is intended to help students in allied health care programs improve the quality of their own lives, get the most from their education, and make meaningful contributions to the lives of others. Specifically, the purpose in writing this book is to help students achieve the following four goals:

1. Successfully complete their educational programs
2. Think and act professionally
3. Find the right jobs
4. Attain long-term career success

Many students who begin health care studies with great enthusiasm drop out when they discover they lack some of the study, personal, and organizational skills necessary for academic and career success. This book shows students that becoming a health care professional begins *as soon as they start school*. In truth, many of the skills needed for academic success are the same as those needed on the job.

During my years working with postsecondary students, I learned that they want to begin their occupational studies as soon as possible. Showing students how study and other school success skills are directly related to job success in health care makes learning organizational and study skills more meaningful.

Who Will Benefit from this Book?

Students enrolled in all types of postsecondary health care programs, such as medical assisting, dental assisting, nursing, physical therapy assisting, x-ray technology, and health information technology, will benefit. The study, life, and professional skills covered are applicable to all health care occupations, and the on-the-job examples presented throughout the book are drawn from a variety of health care settings.

This book is designed to be flexible and can meet a variety of needs. It can be used in a number of courses and learning contexts, such as the following:

- Orientation and study skills classes for new students
- Introductory health care courses
- Professional development courses
- Job search courses
- Academic refresher and review classes for math, writing, and communication
- A supplement to health care specialty courses to expand the coverage of oral and written communication skills; to provide a math review; to teach note taking, research, and test-taking strategies; to enhance personal organization and problem-solving skills; and to teach soft skills (professionalism)

- Independent study in which students are assigned to work on developing specific skills
- A reference book for students to use, as needed, for help with their study, organizational, and job search needs
- To help adult students and students with learning disabilities to succeed in school

Why Is this Book Important to the Profession?

The need for competent, thinking health care professionals continues to grow as health care remains one of the fastest growing industries in the United States. Helping students succeed in their educational programs has the greater benefit of providing society with the competent, caring employees needed to fill the growing number of positions available today … and tomorrow.

Organization

Career development for health professionals is divided into two major sections. The first section, consisting of chapters 1 through 11, introduces students to the world of health care and presents the life-management, study, and professional skills essential for both learning in school and working successfully in a health care occupation. These include the following:

- Understanding what it takes to be a competent and caring health care professional
- Planning and preparing ahead for employment success
- Developing a positive attitude and effective personal organizational skills
- Taking care of personal health
- Succeeding as an adult student
- Improving English language skills when English is the student's second language
- Developing strategies to overcome learning disabilities
- Taking good notes in class
- Reading for understanding and learning
- Conducting useful research
- Improving writing skills
- Preparing to take tests successfully
- Getting the most from lab classes and clinical experience
- Communicating and working effectively with others
- Applying problem-solving techniques
- Overcoming math anxiety
- Developing professional skills and habits

Chapters 3 through 11 may be presented and studied in any order depending on the needs of the students. Chapter 2 introduces the concept of the resume as a tool that can be used to encourage success in school. Students are encouraged to begin building their resumes early in their educational programs. Some instructors prefer to teach this chapter later as part of the job search process. This can be done without disrupting the flow of the book; however, students should not be assigned the "Building Your Resume" activities in the subsequent chapters.

The second section, consisting of Chapters 12 through 17, focuses on job search skills and how to achieve and maintain career success. These skills include the following:

- Locating job leads
- Creating an appealing resume
- Taking advantage of new trends, such as using the Internet and preparing a scannable resume
- Presenting oneself effectively and confidently at interviews
- Increasing the chances of being hired
- Becoming a valued employee
- Keeping career progress on course

Note that Chapters 11 through 15 focus on the job search and would be best presented in order. Chapters 16 and 17 apply to success on the job and are appropriate for use at any point in a professional development class or unit.

Distinctive Features of this Book

Emphasis on Connecting School and Health Care Careers

Examples are given throughout the text that show students how they will use personal management and study skills on the job.

Connecting School and Career

The process of becoming a health care professional began the day you started classes. In addition to providing you with opportunities to learn important technical skills, this process involves acquiring the **attitudes**, personal characteristics, and habits of a successful professional. What you think and do while in school will determine, to a great extent, the quality of the professional you will become. Students who demonstrate good work habits in school generally carry the same habits into the workplace. The opposite is true, too. Students who practice poor conduct in school tend to struggle on the job. You are faced with a great opportunity to determine your future. Your career has indeed started now.

The organizational and study skills presented in the first 10 chapters of this book are designed to help you succeed in school. But they can also be applied to your professional and personal life. In fact, the term "study skills" is misleading, because these skills are not isolated sets of activities restricted to school situations. "Study skills" have many applications on the job. Let's look at four skills that will be discussed more fully in future chapters. Each one can be applied to your studies, your job search, and your future work in health care. The four skills, along with examples, are summarized in Table 1-1.

TABLE 1–1
Examples of Skill Applications

School	Job Search	Career
Applications of Time Management Skills		
Plan study schedule	Pursue job leads without delay	Balance work, family, and personal needs
Attend classes on time	Schedule interviews	
Meet deadlines for assignments	Arrive on time for appointments and interviews	Schedule and track patient appointments
Prepare for exams	Send thank-you notes promptly	Allocate time for patient treatments
Balance school and job schedules	Follow up with prospective employers in a timely way	Follow facility schedules
Allocate time for family		Schedule time for continuing education activities
Applications of Oral Communication Skills		
Ask questions in class	Make telephone inquiries about job openings	Participate in staff meetings
Answer questions in class	Introduce yourself to potential employers	Give instructions to patients
Present oral reports	Ask questions of potential employers	Relay information to co-workers
Share information with classmates	Present your qualifications at interviews	Give reports to supervisor
Applications of Note-Taking Skills		
Take notes during lectures	Write down facts about job openings	Take notes at staff meetings
Write instructions during lab demonstrations	Find and write down information about the organizations with which you have interviews	Fill out medical history forms
List important ideas when reading	Note times, directions, and other information about interviews	Accurately record telephone messages
Develop review outlines	List facts learned during interviews	Make notes on patient charts
Applications of Test-Taking Skills		
Take daily quizzes	Prepare for national and/or professional exams	Perform daily work accurately and completely
Review and take final exams	Present self successfully at interviews	Participate in annual performance evaluation with supervisor
Demonstrate practical skills	Answer interviewer's questions effectively	It's all a test!

On the Job

Using Abbreviations on the Job Abbreviations are used in health care work, so learning to apply them is an important skill. The following is an example of notes on a patient history form.[3]

Chief complaint: Ⓛ shoulder pain p̄ playing basketball this AM.

Present illness: Soreness and immobility Ⓛ shoulder × 8 hours; strained on collision w/another player.

Important note: Abbreviations used on medical records *must be standardized* (the same for everyone who adds information), so be sure to use only those that are approved by the facility in which you work. Also, some abbreviations are no longer allowed because they lead to confusion and medical errors. The Joint Commission and the Institute for Safe Medication Practices have both published lists of abbreviations that should not be used on the job.

Information and Skills to Encourage and Empower Students to Succeed

The book is written in a conversational, reader-friendly style. Each major skill, such as test taking, contains many suggestions from which students can choose what they think will work best for them. Specific examples are given so students can see how to apply what is presented in the book.

Tests can turn otherwise sensible individuals into quivering masses of anxiety. For many students, the grades earned on tests influence their feeling of self-worth. You may be worried about appearing stupid and wonder if you have the ability to learn. Or you may feel insecure about your test-taking skills. Although there is no denying that tests are used as indicators of progress by both instructors and students, understanding more about tests and their purpose can help you control them rather than letting them control you.

Understanding Your Instructors

Instructors are individuals who have their own ideas about education, teaching methods, and the proper roles of teachers and students. Understanding what is important to your instructors will help you benefit fully from your classes. You will use the same skills to identify the characteristics of your future supervisors so you can work with them more effectively.

Specific Suggestions and Tips for Success

Suggestions for applying the information in the chapters are consolidated into lists called "Success Tips For …" to help students focus on finding methods that will work for them.

Positive Self-Talk for This Chapter

- I have many qualities that will be of value to my future employers.
- I have a plan for preparing to become a successful health care professional.
- I am on my way to a great future.

BOX 3-2   Greg's Plan for Mastering a List of Medical Terms

- *Goal:* Over the next 10 weeks, I will learn the meaning, pronunciation, and correct spelling of 300 new medical terms.
- *Plan:* Learn 30 new terms each week. Study terminology 4 hours per week using flash cards, the workbook, CDs, and self-quizzes. Quiz myself at the end of each week.
- *Deadline:* 30 terms each week. Achieve goal of 300 words at the end of 10 weeks on (date).
- *Resources:* Text and workbook; CD that came with the textbook; additional tapes and CDs from the library; suggestions from instructors on the best way to learn; the medical dictionary.
- *Visualization:* I see myself in class receiving 100% on the medical terminology test. I see myself using medical terms correctly when talking with a co-worker on the job.
- *Affirmation:* "I, Greg, am mastering medical language easily and on schedule."

Success Tips for Managing Your Time

- Consider your priorities and goals when you plan your schedule and decide how to spend your time.
- Write out a weekly schedule. Take a few minutes every week to plan ahead. This allows you to coordinate your activities with family members, plan ahead for important days (to avoid trying to find just the right birthday present on the way to the party), combine errands to save time, and plan your study time to avoid last-minute cramming.
- Write a to-do list each day. List the activities in their order of importance.
- Schedule study time every day. This is a high priority! Give yourself a chance to succeed. Arrange not to be disturbed, and let friends and family members know that when you are at your desk, the time is yours.
- Schedule around your peak times. We all have individual body rhythms, specific times of the day when we feel most alert and energetic. Some people do their best work late at night. Others accomplish the most between 5:00 AM and 9:00 AM. Class and work schedules cannot always accommodate your needs, but when you have a choice, do the most challenging tasks during your best hours.
- Do the hardest thing first. When you have a number of things to do or subjects to study, try tackling the most difficult one first, when you are freshest. Completing unpleasant tasks gives you a surge of energy by removing a source of worry and distraction from your mind and rewarding you with a sense of accomplishment.

- Be realistic about what you can accomplish and how much time tasks will take to complete. For example, thinking you can complete a research paper in one weekend can be a serious mistake because you may run into difficulties and end up with no time to spare. You will learn more about your work speed as you progress through your program. At the beginning, it is best to plan more time than you think you will need.
- Prevent feeling overwhelmed by breaking work into small segments. (The thought of writing this book was overwhelming until I broke it down into chapters, topics, and pages.) Plan deadlines for each segment, and put them on your calendar.
- Learn to say "no." Your schedule cannot always accommodate the requests of other people. It's difficult, but sometimes necessary, to turn down demands on our time such as an invitation to a party or a request to help at the church rummage sale. An instructor who reviewed this book said the following response works very well: "I'm really sorry but I won't be able to help. I wish you the best in finding someone who can."
- Use down time to your advantage. There are many pockets of time that usually go to waste, such as when waiting for an appointment or using public transportation. Use this time to study flash cards, write lists, review class notes, brainstorm topics for a research paper, review the steps involved in a lab procedure, or summarize the major points of a class lecture. (I did about half the work toward my last college degree while sitting in airports and on airplanes.)

Assignments Targeted to Meet Specific Student Needs

Many of the exercises in the text ask the students to apply what they have learned to their own situation.

Prescription for Success: 8-8 Studying for a Test

1. Choose at least three study techniques to use when you prepare for your next test.
2. Create a plan for using these ideas, including the actions you will take and a study schedule.
3. After you have taken the test, describe how the techniques worked for you.

Prescription for Success: 9-3 Try Something!

Choose a real problem you would like to solve and go through the six-step process.
1. Define the problem.
2. Gather information. List your sources, and the facts, ideas, and opinions you find.
3. Brainstorm alternative solutions.
4. Consider the possible results and consequences. Do you have questions or need information about any of these results or consequences?
5. Describe the solution you chose and the action you took.
6. Describe and evaluate the results, and describe any necessary revisions.

Resume Building Block #10 Languages Spoken

Complete the "To Do Now" section as you proceed through your classes. Complete the "Writing Your Resume" section as you read Chapter 13, "Finalizing Your Employment Presentation Materials."

To Do Now
1. List the languages you speak other than English.
2. List the languages spoken by the patients in your geographic area.
3. Name any opportunities there may be to learn another language (even a few phrases are useful in the health care setting).

Writing Your Resume
1. What languages do you speak?

New to this Edition

New Chapter

A new chapter entitled "Becoming a Professional" has been added to this edition. The chapter contains applications of the skills presented in previous chapters specific to the workplace, along with new topics. For example, the section on communication which was introduced in Chapter 10, "Developing Your People Skills," is presented in terms of therapeutic skills; that is, communication skills specific to working with patients.

This chapter was added in response to requests for more coverage of "soft skills:" the non-technical skills essential for success in health care work.

Topics in this chapter include:
- The meaning and importance of professionalism in health care
- A professional attitude
- A professional appearance
- The business of health care (customer service)
- The professional's effect on patients
- Therapeutic communication
- Consideration for co-workers
- Adapting to change
- Mastering technical skills

Topics Added

Chapter 3: Nutrition and Physical Activity
Chapter 8: Writing Effective E-mails
Chapter 9: Critical Thinking, Online Courses, and Simulated Externships
Chapter 10: Effective Telephone Technique
Chapter 14: Group and Telephone Job Interviews
Chapter 15: Understanding Work Schedules

Reformatting of Material

The math tables in Chapter 9 and the grammar topics for ESL students in Chapter 5 have been reformatted to make them easier for students to understand.

New Features

Case studies and "Trouble Ahead?" boxes were added throughout the chapters to provide students with real-world examples of problems or issues they may encounter in their programs and careers.

Learning Aids

- **Objectives** that help students focus on the most important chapter topics. They provide direction and serve as a checklist for students to assess their mastery of chapter material.
- **Key Terms and Concepts** that include definitions to ensure understanding of important concepts and ideas.

- **Quotes** to inspire, motivate, and promote thinking.
- **Boxes** to provide additional information or applications of chapter material. These include specific examples of how the skills presented are used on the job and interviews with health care professionals.
- **Tables** to present facts in an easy-to-read and an easy-to-understand format.
- **Personal Reflection** questions that are opportunities for students to reflect on how the chapter content applies to them.
- **Prescription for Success** exercises that provide a wide variety of assignments for students to apply the ideas presented, collect additional information, and develop practical skills.
- **To Learn More**, at the end of each chapter, that lists books, articles, and websites that contain further information about the chapter topics.
- **Positive Self-Talk** that encourages students to use affirmations and keep an optimistic attitude.
- **Summary of Key Ideas** that reviews important points from the chapter.
- **Building Your Resume** exercises that enable students to use resume writing to positively guide their actions while in school and create a resume over time.
- **Internet Activities** that build research skills while taking advantage of student interest in the Internet and the vast number of resources available.

Ancillaries

Evolve Resources for the Student

- Chapter quizzes in which students apply what they have learned to themselves
- Internet activities to apply research skills and learn more about each chapter's content

Evolve Resources for the Instructor

- TEACH Instructor's Resource, including:
  - Lesson plans that include learning objectives; background information about the chapter; references to the book and other instructional materials; and ideas for discussion and critical thinking, class activities, and assessments.
  - Lecture outlines for each chapter to guide the presentation of major topics to students.
  - PowerPoint slides that include major topics and are coordinated with the lecture outlines.
  - Instructor's Resource with additional learning activities for students.
- ExamView test bank with a variety of questions for each chapter to be used for student performance evaluation

For Students

DEAR STUDENT,

I have devoted my professional life to working in education and helping students achieve their education and life goals. The purpose of this book is to provide you with tools to become your best and realize your dreams. It is filled with information and practical tips to help you succeed not only in school, but also on the job. It is not simply a book you will use in class but a useful self-help reference you can use in the years to come.

To make the best use of this book and the tools it contains, I suggest you try the following:

1. Trust yourself. You have the power and ability to succeed.
2. Be willing to try new ideas. If something in the book looks like "too much trouble" or even a little crazy, give it a try and see if it works for you.
3. Don't be overwhelmed by the number of ideas and suggestions in each chapter. They are intended to appeal to a wide range of learning styles, personal preferences, and student needs. You are not expected to do all of them, but rather to choose the ones you think will work best for you.
4. Put forth your best efforts when doing the Prescription for Success exercises. Use them as opportunities to learn, not as "must-dos" to complete an assignment and get a grade.
5. Apply the ideas to your own life. The material is meant to be practical, not simply topics to read and discuss in class.

Start now to become a competent, caring health care professional who will enjoy a satisfying career while making a positive contribution to the lives of others.

Wishing you success,
Lee Haroun

Acknowledgments

I would like to thank Patrick Wenrick, RHIA, Director of the Institute of Technology, Inc., and Director of the Coastal Education Institute in Tampa, Florida, for reviewing this text.

Contents

CHAPTER 1

Your Career Starts Now

OBJECTIVES

1. Explain the meaning of the concept: "Study skills are job skills."
2. Give four examples of study skills that can help you succeed in school, obtain the job you want, and increase your value as a health care professional.
3. List four ways you can maximize your school experience.
4. Understand your responsibilities as a student.
5. Describe how the principles of marketing can be applied to career preparation and the job search.
6. Describe what employers and patients expect from health care professionals and identify the skills and attitudes you need to develop more fully.
7. Develop a personal philosophy of work, identify your work preferences, and realize the importance of realistic expectations when it comes to choosing your employer and your profession.

KEY TERMS AND CONCEPTS

Attitude Your mental approach to any situation. It is under your control and can be either positive or negative.

Career Ladder The organization of occupations or positions in a related field that requires progressively higher levels of skill and responsibility. Additional education or training is often needed to move up the ladder.

Certification Recognition from a professional organization or government agency that you have specific knowledge and skills. Certification usually requires taking written and/or hands-on tests.

Charting Making notes on patient medical records.

Commitment Dedication to something, such as an idea, a relationship, or an organization.

Competency Mastery of a skill; performance of a skill in a manner that meets predetermined standards.

Confidentiality The act of keeping something, such as medical records, absolutely private.

Consequence The result, either positive or negative, of taking a certain action.

Empathy An understanding of the experiences and feelings of another person gained by considering a situation from the other person's point of view.

Ethical Morally good and correct.

Ethnic Referring to the customs and behaviors practiced by a specific racial or national group of people as distinguished from other groups.

Externship The term used in this book to describe supervised, unpaid work experiences performed by students in health facilities or offices to gain hands-on, practical experience. Other names for this experience include "clinical," "fieldwork," "internship," "practicum," and "preceptorship."

Habits Ways of acting or thinking that are developed over time and become automatic, with little awareness.

Informational Interview A meeting with a professional to learn about his or her career field, job duties, etc. The purpose is not to obtain a job but to ask questions and learn as much as possible about the nature of the work.

Integrity Behavior based on honesty, sincerity, and good intentions.

Job shadowing Spending time with a professional as he or she works and performs typical duties.

License Legal approval given to professionals to ensure that only those who are properly trained can perform certain duties. Licenses are granted by governmental bodies and require applicants to meet specific educational requirements and to pass tests.

Per Diem Work performed on an on-call basis.

Philosophy The system of beliefs that forms the foundation of a person's view of the world and ideas about the meaning of life.

Prioritize To rank a group of items or tasks in order of importance.

Reasoning Organizing facts so they make sense and/or help you draw correct conclusions.

Self-Esteem The way people see themselves and the opinions they have about their appearance, competence, intelligence, and other personal characteristics.

Standard Precautions Practices that prevent the transmission of disease through the micro-organisms (germs) present in blood and other body fluids.

Sterile Technique Special procedures used to create an environment that is free of all living microorganisms.

Vulnerable Being physically and/or emotionally weakened and possibly dependent on others.

Your First Step on the Road to Success

"Today is the first day of the rest of your life."

Congratulations! By choosing to study for a career in health care, you have taken the first step toward achieving a productive and satisfying future. You have made a significant **commitment** to yourself and your community. By enrolling in an educational program, you have demonstrated your ability to set your sights on the future, make important decisions, and follow through with action. You have proved you have the strong personal foundation on which you can build the skills and **habits** needed to ensure your success in school and in your career.

The purpose of this book is to help you succeed in this building process by sharing the knowledge and techniques that have helped other students achieve their goals. It is written with the hope that you will apply what you learn here to maximize your investment in education, secure the job that you want after graduation, and find satisfaction in your career as a competent and caring health care professional like the young woman in Figure 1-1.

Connecting School and Career

The process of becoming a health care professional began the day you started classes. In addition to providing you with opportunities to learn important technical skills, this process involves acquiring the **attitudes**, personal characteristics, and habits of a successful professional. What you think and do while in school will determine, to a great extent, the quality of the professional you will become. Students who demonstrate good work habits in school generally carry the same habits into the workplace. The opposite is true, too. Students who practice poor conduct in school tend to struggle on the job. You are faced with a great opportunity to determine your future. Your career has indeed started now.

The organizational and study skills presented in the first 10 chapters of this book are designed to help you succeed in school. But they can also be applied to your professional and personal life. In fact, the term "study skills" is misleading, because these skills are not isolated sets of activities restricted to school situations. "Study skills" have many applications on

the job. Let's look at four skills that will be discussed more fully in future chapters. Each one can be applied to your studies, your job search, and your future work in health care. The four skills, along with examples, are summarized in Table 1-1.

1. **Time management.** For busy people, time is one of their most precious possessions. Juggling class attendance and study time with family responsibilities, work, and personal time involves **prioritizing** and careful planning. Your success in school depends heavily on how well you organize your time.

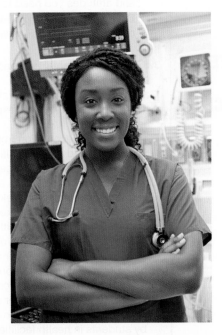

FIGURE 1-1 What you do now while in school will influence your future. While studying for your career, act as you would on a job. Develop good work habits by dressing professionally, arriving in class on time, and completing all homework. Having good references, such as instructors and school personnel, who will vouch for you to potential employers is especially important today. Be sure to conduct yourself in a way that enables them to recommend you. *What are five additional positive workplace behaviors you can practice while pursuing your education?* (Copyright monkeybusinessimages/iStock/Thinkstock)

TABLE 1–1

Examples of Skill Applications

School	Job Search	Career
Applications of Time Management Skills		
Plan study schedule	Pursue job leads without delay	Balance work, family, and personal needs
Attend classes on time	Schedule interviews	
Meet deadlines for assignments	Arrive on time for appointments and interviews	Schedule and track patient appointments
Prepare for exams	Send thank-you notes promptly	Allocate time for patient treatments
Balance school and job schedules	Follow up with prospective employers in a timely way	
Allocate time for family		Follow facility schedules
		Schedule time for continuing education activities
Applications of Oral Communication Skills		
Ask questions in class	Make telephone inquiries about job openings	Participate in staff meetings
Answer questions in class	Introduce yourself to potential employers	Give instructions to patients
Present oral reports	Ask questions of potential employers	Relay information to co-workers
Share information with classmates	Present your qualifications at interviews	Give reports to supervisor
Applications of Note-Taking Skills		
Take notes during lectures	Write down facts about job openings	Take notes at staff meetings
Write instructions during lab demonstrations	Find and write down information about the organizations with which you have interviews	Fill out medical history forms
List important ideas when reading	Note times, directions, and other information about interviews	Accurately record telephone messages
Develop review outlines	List facts learned during interviews	Make notes on patient charts
Applications of Test-Taking Skills		
Take daily quizzes	Prepare for national and/or professional exams	Perform daily work accurately and completely
Review and take final exams	Present self successfully at interviews	Participate in annual performance evaluation with supervisor
Demonstrate practical skills	Answer interviewer's questions effectively	It's all a test!

An effective job search typically requires you to devote time each day to identifying leads, making appointments, attending interviews, and completing follow-up activities. You must allocate adequate amounts of time for these efforts and organize your time to avoid delays that could cost you employment opportunities.

Once you are on the job, the effective use of time is critical in health care work. Many health care professionals are responsible not only for their own time but also for planning other people's time. Medical assistants, for example, are often in charge of the physician's daily appointment scheduling, a task that can affect the profitability of the practice. Insurance coders and billers must submit claims on time to avoid rejections and financial losses. Nurses who have patient care responsibilities must plan a schedule that permits them to complete these during their shifts.

2. **Oral communication.** Strong communication skills are essential for success. Expressing yourself clearly is important for giving presentations, as well as for asking and answering questions in class. It is also necessary for establishing and maintaining satisfactory relationships with your instructors and classmates.

A critical part of the job search process is the interview, in which you combine your ability to think clearly and use verbal skills effectively. Feeling confident about expressing yourself will enable you to present your qualifications in a convincing way.

All jobs today require good communication skills. This is especially true in health care because many positions involve constant interaction with others, including patients, co-workers, supervisors, and the general public. Interaction with a patient is illustrated in Figure 1-2. Physical and occupational therapy assistants are examples of the many health professionals who provide extensive patient education. The effectiveness of their explanations of exercises and self-care techniques influences the rehabilitation progress of their clients.

3. **Taking notes.** You may think of note-taking as being limited to use in lectures but this skill is used extensively outside the classroom. During the job search, it is important to accurately record information about job openings, as well as interview appointment dates, and times and directions to facilities. After interviews, you may want to make notes about the job requirements, additional information you need to send to the prospective employer, and other important facts.

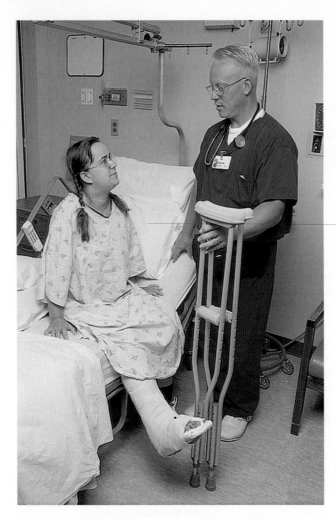

FIGURE 1-2 Trustworthiness, technical competence, concern for the welfare of others, and good communication skills are necessary characteristics of a health care professional. *What would be potential consequences for this patient if the nurse lacked one or more of these characteristics? Why is effective communication especially important in the situation illustrated in this photo?* (From deWit S, O'Neill P: *Fundamental concepts and skills for nursing*, ed 4, St Louis, 2014, Saunders.)

When you become employed, you will be expected to absorb a lot of new information about your facility's rules and procedures, the location of supplies and equipment, people's names, and many other details. You can use your note-taking skills to create a personal reference notebook, a resource that will increase your efficiency on the job. Note-taking is also an important health care job skill. Many professionals are responsible for interviewing patients and taking notes on special forms called patient histories. Another specialized form of medical note-taking is called **charting**, which means making notes on patient medical records, either in written or electronic form. The notes include information about symptoms, treatments, and medications prescribed. These medical records not only affect patient care, they are also legal documents. They must be clear, accurate, and complete.

4. **Taking tests.** You may think you have escaped the dreaded test once you leave school, but testing is not limited

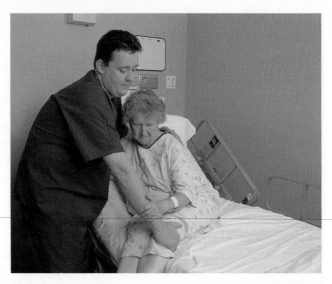

FIGURE 1-3 It cannot be emphasized enough that studying for a career in health care requires more than merely passing classes. It requires *mastering* subjects to become highly competent. Today's health care professionals are likely to work with many elderly patients. *How can you best prepare to help patients such as the woman in this photo? If you are in administrative work, why is it important that you code and bill properly for her care?* (From deWit S, O'Neill P: *Fundamental concepts and skills for nursing*, ed 4, St Louis, 2014, Saunders.)

to the classroom. The truth is that life is full of tests. Job interviews are a form of test designed to assess your ability to present yourself and your qualifications. To legally work in many health care occupations, such as a licensed practical nurse, radiologic technologist, or physical therapist, you must pass a professional exam. Other occupations, such as medical assistant, have voluntary tests to obtain the certification that improves your chances of getting a job. In fact, many employers hire only certified medical assistants. (More about tests in Chapter 8.)

Once on the job, you are, in a sense, being tested every day. Although you may not think of your everyday tasks as tests, they are applications of what you have learned, and your ability to perform them correctly will be noted by your patients, co-workers, and supervisor. The annual employee performance evaluation, discussed in Chapter 17, may be considered a type of test in which your supervisor writes a report about your work and then meets with you to discuss it. Learning to perform "when it counts" is a valuable skill and represents the ultimate ability to take and successfully pass a test. The patient in Figure 1-3 wants to know that the health care professional helping her has "passed the test" and is qualified to help her get out of bed safely.

From these four examples, you can see that skills traditionally labeled as personal or school skills have valuable applications during the job search and on the job. Throughout this book you will continue to see how "school skills" are also valuable job skills.

Maximizing Your Education

You are making a significant investment of time, effort, and money in your education. You can simply get by, doing only what is required to pass your classes, or you can benefit fully from this investment. A worthy personal goal is to do everything possible to become the best health care professional possible. Both you and your school have responsibilities to ensure that this happens.

Your Rights as a Student

"Making mistakes is inevitable. Not learning from them is inexcusable."

1. **Make mistakes.** You may think this sounds a little strange. After all, aren't you supposed to do the best you can, earning the highest grades possible? Yes, but many students see grades as ends in themselves, rather than as signs of having mastered the skills they will need in the future. Good grades do not guarantee mastery, nor will you receive grades for all the skills that will determine your future success.

   Many students want to know "what's on the test" so they can focus their efforts on learning only what they will be tested on. But think about it—can you possibly be tested on everything you will need to know and do to perform your future job in health care? If you were, all class time would have to be devoted to testing, leaving little or no time for learning! Studying only what you need to pass tests and earn grades may make you a "good student" but a good student is not necessarily a good health care professional.

   Compare your educational experience with learning to ride a bike. First, you use training wheels, go slowly, and tip over once in a while. Eventually you become a proficient cyclist, ready for the big race. School offers you a rehearsal for professional life, providing you with opportunities to learn from mistakes that would be unacceptable if you were to make them on the job. If you do not score 100% on an exam, it has still served you by allowing you to make mistakes and learn from them so you avoid making them on the job when the **consequences** are more serious. The massage therapist in Figure 1-4 may have made mistakes when she practiced working with a classmate but she learned from them and is now able to use correct techniques to help her clients.

2. **Ask questions.** You are attending school to benefit from the knowledge and experience of your instructors. Take advantage of this opportunity by being an active participant in

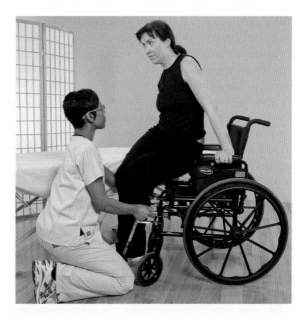

FIGURE 1-4 The time to learn—and even make a few mistakes—is while you are in school. You want to be competent when performing the requirements of your job, such as working with patients, processing their paperwork, or assisting the dentist. This massage therapist practiced transfer skills many times during her training in order to become proficient. *What is your plan for profiting from your mistakes?* (From Fritz S: *Mosby's Fundamentals of Therapeutic Massage*, ed 5, St Louis, 2013, Mosby.)

your classes. Don't be an invisible student. Even if the textbooks and lectures are excellent, you may still need to ask for explanations, examples, and additional resources. If there is anything you don't understand, ask questions. Students aren't expected to understand everything the first time they hear or read it—maybe not even the second time. Consider this: there would be no need for you to attend school at all if you already knew the information presented in your program.

Some students are afraid of "looking stupid" and hesitate to admit they don't understand or are confused. However, failing to ask questions not only decreases the chances of maximizing your education, it prevents you from learning a critical health care skill—asking questions. Consider the serious consequences for professionals who are not sure of drug dosages or the steps in a procedure but are afraid to ask their supervisors for direction. In these situations, risking the well-being of patients is indeed stupid, whereas asking questions demonstrates intelligence. Start learning now to be comfortable asking questions. If it is too difficult for you to speak up in class the first few times you have questions, start out by speaking with your instructor at the break, after class, or during office hours.

Of course, you should not use questions to substitute for reading your textbook or studying assigned material before each class meeting. This results in the misuse of class time and is unfair to students who have prepared. A related on-the-job example is employees who arrive late and unprepared for meetings, thus wasting their co-workers' time. Develop habits that show consideration for others and will contribute now to the efficiency of the classroom and later to that of the workplace.

3. **Take advantage of school resources.** Every school wants every student who enrolls to graduate and considerable resources are spent on services to support this effort. Find out now what services are available to you, the hours they can be accessed, and whether appointments are necessary. Two of the most important services that all students should become familiar with are the library (or resource center) and career services (sometimes called *job placement*).

If you are having personal problems or academic difficulties, ask whether your school provides counseling and/or tutoring. Some schools refer their students to outside agencies that offer assistance for difficulties such as dealing with domestic abuse and finding reliable child care. Asking for help when you need it can make the difference between dropping out and graduating and becoming successfully employed.

The school catalog is an often overlooked information resource that can help you succeed in school. Many students never take the time to read it and as a result are unaware of available resources. Even worse, they risk unknowingly breaking rules or missing important deadlines. Spend a few minutes becoming an informed student by reading the catalog and other printed information. On the job, you will likely be expected to read employee handbooks and procedure manuals. Getting into the habit of reading informational literature is a good job skill.

4. **Have your privacy protected.** The Family Educational Rights and Privacy Act restricts access to student educational records. It does allow students to inspect their own records, request inaccurate information to be corrected, and add written explanations about information they believe to be incorrect.

Prescription for Success: 1-2 Resource Treasure Hunt

When you need help, school services can seem like treasures. But to take advantage of everything your school has to offer, you must know about it. Take a tour of your school and keep track of the services provided and how to access them for each resource. If your school does not offer all these services, find out if they are available elsewhere in the community.

What Resources are Available at Your School?

Advising or Counseling: Academic, personal
Career Services: Job search assistance, school job fairs, part-time jobs, résumé preparation, interviewing skills, employer contacts, classes, or workshops

Financial Aid

Information Sources and Referrals: Child care, financial help, transportation, other
Learning Assistance: Learning center, study skills, instructors, tutors, other students, study groups, refresher, and basic skills classes
Library: Books, periodicals, Internet access, journals, reference assistance, other

Professional Organizations (student chapters)

School Organizations: Special interest groups, social clubs, service clubs
Special Needs and Referrals: Alcohol abuse, drug dependency, family planning, domestic abuse, other
Volunteer Opportunities

Case Study 1-1

Getting Help to Overcome Obstacles

Kyle had always been very close to his Grandpa Ed. His mother's father, Ed, took the place of Kyle's father who left the family when Kyle was 2 years old. Ed served as a role model, taking Kyle on summer camping trips in the woods of Michigan, teaching him how to fish and appreciate the outdoors. During the cold winters, they played chess and talked about Ed's experiences growing up on a farm, serving in the army, and working for General Motors.

When Ed was diagnosed with stage IV lung cancer, Kyle was devastated. But determined to be supportive, he spent as much time as possible with Ed, even arranging to work the night shift at his factory job so he could visit his grandfather during the day.

Kyle was surprised to see that several of the nurses who cared for his grandfather were male. He had always thought of nursing as a "girl thing." He also didn't realize that RNs were highly trained technical experts, many with supervisory duties. Spending a lot of time with his grandfather allowed him to talk with the nurses and learn more about why they chose this profession.

Once his grandfather was released from the hospital, he went to live with Kyle and his mother. Hospice services were called in and nurses visited daily to monitor Ed's pain medications; certified nursing assistants helped with bathing and hygiene; and a chaplain came weekly to provide comfort to the family. The care provided by the hospice team furthered Kyle's respect for health care professionals.

After Ed's death, Kyle did a lot of thinking about his life. What did he really want to do? His job at the factory had seemed his best option following high school, but now he thought he would rather do something more satisfying—something more important. He reflected on what he had observed during his grandfather's illness and decided to look into nursing. The hospice group had continued to provide support for him and his mother as they grieved over his grandfather's death, and Kyle decided to ask if he could talk to the nurses about their work. He also contacted the local community college to learn about the requirements for their nursing program.

Kyle enrolled in the RN program that started the following fall. He had to work hard in the general education

Getting Help to Overcome Obstacles

courses but was determined to pass them and start the nursing courses. Not long into his program, however, he found himself overcome by grief and had difficulty focusing on his studies. He felt sad and lonely and began to have trouble getting himself to class. He was at the point of giving up school, but decided to talk with his mother, explaining that suddenly he just couldn't seem to keep it together.

"Kyle," she said, "let's think about what Grandpa would want you to do."

Kyle thought about this for a moment. "Well, I imagine he'd want me to buck up and move along with my life. But I just don't seem to have it in me."

His mother had read the literature from hospice and knew that grief affects people in different ways. It looked as if Kyle was having an episode of delayed grief that was interfering with his daily life. She decided to contact the folks at hospice to ask for their advice. Learning that they offered counseling to family members, even months following a death, she suggested that Kyle get in touch with them.

Kyle followed his mother's advice and joined a support group for young people who had experienced the loss of a family member or friend. He learned that his grief was normal and learned helpful coping techniques. He also decided to speak with his instructors and let them know what he was going through. He didn't ask for special treatment, but wanted them to know that in spite of his recent poor performance, he was serious about pursuing a career in nursing and was doing his best to cope with his situation and get back on track with his studies.

Questions for Thought and Reflection

1. Did Kyle make a good career choice? Why or why not?
2. Do you think it was a good idea for Kyle to confide in his instructors? Why or why not?
3. Why do you think Kyle waited to seek help with his problems at school?
4. Do you think he will successfully complete his program and become a nurse? Why or why not?

Your Responsibilities as a Student

1. **Attend all scheduled learning activities.** Health care educational programs feature a variety of learning opportunities that include lectures, lab sessions, guest speakers, field trips, and hands-on experiences in health care facilities. Your instructor may also recommend additional activities outside of those organized by the school, such as watching a television documentary, attending a professional meeting, or visiting a medical supply company. These activities are designed to help you understand and master all the knowledge and skills necessary for your future work, as well as provide exposure to your future work environment. You cannot afford to miss them. They are opportunities to develop the **competencies** essential for working in health care. Learning to perform essential tasks, such as giving injections, requires you to spend time and effort under the guidance of your instructors. Some day you will be performing tasks that affect the well-being of others, so it is essential that you fully participate in every learning activity offered in your program.

Employers routinely request information about a student's attendance record. Good attendance is considered a valuable job skill because health care services are driven by time requirements. The success of a private physician's practice depends heavily on efficient patient scheduling and service. Hospitals have daily responsibilities for performing hundreds of treatments, procedures, and surgeries that must be completed in a timely way. In both settings, effective care can be provided only if the staff is available to do the work. Patients who need help should not have to wait because someone didn't show up. Start now to develop the habit of consistent and punctual attendance.

> **Prescription for Success: 1-3 Overcoming Obstacles**
> 1. What obstacles might interfere with your school attendance (e.g., problems with child care)?
> 2. What can you do now to overcome these obstacles (e.g., find backup for child care)?

2. **Apply your best efforts to learning.** As a student, you have the right to ask questions and make mistakes. At the same time, it is your responsibility to complete all reading, writing, and lab assignments and to participate actively in class. Instructors cannot cover everything you are expected to know. Learning will require effort on your part. The study techniques and suggestions for learning presented in the following chapters are intended to help you succeed as a student.

In performing your work as a health care professional, you will encounter new situations in which you will apply what you learned in school. To be successful in those situations, you must now focus on your studies, work hard, and be persistent. Your willingness to do the "shoulds" when you would rather be doing the "wants" will be a major determinant of your success. You will not always feel like studying after a day that may include classes, a few hours on the job, and family responsibilities. Being a college student is not always easy. Keeping your long-term career goals clearly in mind will help you find the self-discipline to stick with it.

3. **Ask for help when you need it.** Instructors and administrators want to see their students succeed. Educators are interested in helping students complete their programs and graduate. At the same time, you must take responsibility for requesting assistance. Ignoring problems will not solve them; they usually only get worse. Don't wait

until you are hopelessly lost in a class and cannot possibly be ready for the upcoming final exam before asking for help. Take charge of your learning and at the first sign of trouble, ask about tutoring, study groups, computer labs, and other resources available at your school.

If you experience problems of a personal or financial nature, refer to the list of school resources you prepared in Prescription for Success 1-2. Remember that asking for help when you need it is a sign of strength, not weakness, and it is one of the main actions that distinguish a graduate from a dropout.

The flip side of asking for help is being willing to give it. Offer your assistance to others in the school community. Volunteer to hand out papers for the instructor. Give a student who lives in your area a ride to school. Tutor a classmate who is struggling with a subject you find easy. (This doesn't mean sharing your work; it means helping the other person understand and learn.) You have chosen a profession that is based on giving service and this is a habit you can start practicing now, in all areas of your life. Students who give of themselves are the type of people who become indispensable employees.

Case Study 1-2

Fed Up

Karolyn has just about had it. She is tired of her friend and classmate, Julie, asking for help. It started with their anatomy homework. At first, Karolyn didn't mind. She enjoyed learning about the body and was doing well in the class. She liked Julie and wanted to help her succeed.

But after finishing their anatomy class, with Julie just scraping by, the request came for help with medical terminology. More than just tutoring this time.

"Karolyn," Julie begged, "if you could just let me see your homework. Jimmy was sick last night and I just didn't have a chance to do the assignment."

Karolyn felt sorry for Julie. She was a single mom and there always seemed to be problems with her kids—the baby sitter didn't show up, someone was sick, the kids bothered her when she was trying to study. So the first few times, she gave her a copy of the medical terminology homework. After all, the purpose was just to memorize a list of terms. What harm was there if Julie learned them in a way other than doing the fill-in exercises that comprised most of the homework?

It was when they got to the hands-on courses that Karolyn started to wonder if she was doing Julie any favors. Or doing *anyone* any favors. If Julie didn't master the material and understand exactly why and how they were doing certain procedures, would she be safe in the workplace? Would Karolyn want to be in the hands of a medical assistant who gives an injection without knowing something about the underlying muscles? Or why this drug was being given?

These questions bothered Karolyn and she decided to discuss the situation with her friend, Stephanie, a nurse at St. Francis.

"I see what you mean, Karolyn," said Stephanie. "And frankly, you're right. Someone who performs patient procedures, especially invasive ones like injections, and doesn't really understand what they're doing ... that could be dangerous. I really wouldn't want someone like that on my team."

"I know," said Karolyn, "this is really a tough one. Julie seems to want this so much, but she just isn't doing the work."

"It's hard when it's a friend, I know," responded Stephanie. "But you've got to take a broader view. What does it mean to the community if our health care professionals just get by in school without really knowing what they are doing? It could be dangerous."

Karolyn sighed. "You're right. I'm just going to have to do the right thing."

The next day, Karolyn told Julie she could no longer share her homework assignments and "help" her with tests. Julie was upset and accused Karolyn of not being her friend. Karolyn tried to explain why she had decided that Julie must study and do her own work, but Julie was not interested in hearing what Karolyn had to say. They both completed their medical assisting program, but they were no longer friends.

Questions for Thought and Reflection
1. Did Stephanie give Karolyn good advice?
2. Do you think Karolyn was right in refusing to continue helping Julie?
3. Was it worth losing Julie's friendship for Karolyn to be honest with her?
4. What kind of medical assistant do you think Julie will be?

Trouble Ahead? 1-1

Julie, who we met in the previous case study, did not give up. She found another student to befriend and started with her requests for help with class, "help" with the homework, and "help" with the tests. She did finish her program, just barely passing her finals. And she did okay on her externship by being friendly with the supervisor.

Julie was able to find a job at a local clinic and things went well for the first few days. However, Julie realized

that there was much she didn't know. In school, she had depended on others rather than figuring out how to learn for herself. She tried the same strategy at work, frequently interrupting her co-workers with questions about how to do this or that; where to find information she needed; how to determine proper drug dosages; and so on.

It was the drug dosage requests that drew the attention of her physician, Dr. Kent. He was concerned that she didn't seem to have mastered this important skill. In fact, it was Karolyn back in school who did the computations that got Julie through that portion of the class. Dr. Kent called Julie into his office.

"Julie, I've been told that you seem to always be unsure of the drug dosages you are to administer to patients. Tell me about this."

Julie responded, "Well, Dr. Kent, I'm only a recent graduate and I really need more time to master all the details of this job."

Dr. Kent said, "Julie, this knowledge is part of the medical assisting program at your college. This is something you should have learned about in school and practiced during your externship. When I hired you, I knew you were just starting out, but I expected you to have mastered certain skills. And this was one of them."

"Well," said Julie, "I think your expectations may have been a bit unreasonable."

"I will say that drug dosages can be confusing and I understand that you might be nervous about making mistakes

with pharmaceuticals," said Dr. Kent. "But this isn't the only thing. I've received a lot of complaints from my staff about your constant questions when they are working. It seems to have gotten out of control and is affecting some of their work."

"You know what, Dr. Kent?" Julie said. "If this is the kind of unfriendly atmosphere you've got in this office, I don't think it's a place I want to work." And she stomped out the door. Dr. Kent sighed and called in his office manager. "Louise," he said, "I think we're going to have to look for another medical assistant."

Questions for Thought and Reflection

1. How did the "favors" from Karolyn and others contribute to Julie's failure on the job?
2. Was Dr. Kent right in being concerned about Julie's lack of knowledge? Why or why not?
3. Was Julie's response to Dr. Kent appropriate? Explain.
4. What must Julie do if she wants to have a career in health care?

Personal Reflection

1. What are some other ways I can take responsibility for my own learning so that I succeed in my health care program?

Planning for Career Success

The time to start thinking about your first job in health care is now, as you are starting your educational program. In the following pages, we look at how you can use job search tools, such as a résumé, to help guide you to a successful career.

And the Product Is…You!

Marketing is a multi-step process that begins with an idea for a new product and ends with the sale of that product. Successful marketing is similar to successfully starting a new career. You—the combination of your skills, characteristics, and talents—are the product. To make sure you have the skills and qualities needed by employers, you must prepare appropriately for the workplace and learn to present yourself effectively during the job search.

The marketing process can be organized into a five-part plan called the "Five Ps of Marketing," as follows:
1. Planning
2. Production
3. Packaging
4. Presentation
5. Promotion

You can use the 5 Ps to develop your own personal marketing plan now, as you begin your health care studies, to help

ensure future career success. We will discuss the first P, planning, in this chapter, and the remaining four Ps in Chapter 2.

Planning: The First "P" of Marketing

"Give yourself a running start."

Studying the needs of customers is called *market research*, and its purpose is to find out what customers want. Your customers include your future employers and patients. Waiting until the end of your educational program to think about getting a job is like creating a product without doing any market research. Designing and manufacturing a product that no one wants or needs doesn't make sense. Just like a business, you are investing time, effort, and money in the development of yourself as a product.

What Do Employers Want?

In recent years, employers in all industries have expressed concern that entry-level workers are not adequately prepared for the modern workplace. Employers are looking for job candidates who are not only qualified technically, but also bring essential supporting skills such as the ability to communicate effectively, work cooperatively with others, accept responsibility, and solve problems. These skills are especially critical in the health care industry because it is service-based and depends heavily on the quality of its personnel. This is even truer today as health care facilities strive to provide higher quality care and control costs. See Box 1-1 for a sample of the skills requested in 2014 job posts.

SCANS Report

In the late 1980s, a commission appointed by the U.S. Secretary of Labor conducted a nationwide employer survey to determine the competencies required of all entry-level workers. The resulting report, called *A SCANS Report for America 2000*, was published in 1991. It organized lists of competencies that have become known as the SCANS Skills. (*SCANS* stands for Secretary's Commission for Achieving Necessary Skills). Even though this report has been out for a number of years, the skills listed are still relevant today. For example, "being responsible" remains an essential characteristic for an employee, especially in health care.

Earlier in this chapter, you read about how the sets of skills commonly referred to as "study skills" can be applied to all areas of your life. Take a look at the SCANS Competencies in Box 1-2 and note that the same is true for them. For example, demonstrating **integrity** and honesty as a student means you set high standards for yourself and do your own work to complete assignments and take exams; as a job applicant, it means you present yourself honestly in

job interviews and apply for only those positions for which you are competent; and as an employee, it means you never cut corners when working with patients and fellow staff members.

National Healthcare Foundation Standards and Accountability Criteria

A project of special interest to future health care professionals is the list of entry-level competencies developed by the National Consortium for Health Science Education. Box 1-3 contains examples that apply to all health care occupations.[1] You can see that they are not limited to technical skills, such as taking blood pressure, but include the ability to communicate and dress appropriately. Some employers report that these so-called "soft skills" are as important as technical skills in providing good health care.

Prescription for Success: 1-5 The Ideal Candidate

Imagine yourself as a busy pediatrician who runs a clinic in a low-income neighborhood. You need to hire a medical assistant. You have found a candidate who appears to have the necessary technical skills and experience.
1. Name five other characteristics you would want the candidate to have.
2. Why did you choose these five characteristics?
3. Now answer the following questions for yourself:
   a. How does understanding the needs of employers help you to better prepare for your future career?
   b. Which of your own personal qualities do you believe will be most valuable to future employers?

What Do Patients Want?

"Patients do not care how much you know until they know how much you care."

Patients want to receive competent care delivered with consideration and respect. When seeking health care, people are often at their most **vulnerable**. They fear what might be discovered during a diagnostic test or that they will experience pain during a necessary treatment. The **self-esteem** of patients can be threatened by the feeling of powerlessness that often accompanies illness and injury.

At the same time, many patients want to participate in making decisions about their care. They have the right, both **ethically** and legally, to be fully informed about their condition, the treatment options, and possible outcomes. Health care professionals must give clear explanations in everyday language and give patients the opportunity to ask questions and receive honest answers. Patients also want and have the legal right to **confidentiality**. As a health care professional, you must guard the privacy of your patients. Without the patient's permission, nothing can be discussed with anyone other than the health care team members directly involved with that patient's care, and all files and paperwork must be securely stored and electronic records protected.

Changes in American society and the increasing costs of providing medical care have brought special challenges for patients and for health care professionals. In the past, many people had the same physician throughout their lives. Doctor and patient belonged to the same community and a sense of trust developed over the years. Patients today may see a different physician each time they visit their health care facility. They may face a serious illness or life-threatening situation in the care of a stranger, adding to the stress of an already difficult situation. Studies have shown that patients who belong to a caring, supportive community recover more successfully than patients who don't. As a health care professional, you can demonstrate a caring attitude that helps develop a bond of trust with patients by being attentive, listening carefully, and practicing **empathy**.

Health care professionals today face the challenge of working with patients from many different **ethnic** backgrounds, some of whom have beliefs about health care practices that differ from those of traditional Western medicine. Patients also come from many different economic and social groups. They may have lifestyles or personal beliefs with which you disagree. But all patients have the right to be respected and to receive appropriate, high-level care, regardless of your personal opinions about them. Every patient deserves your best efforts.

Patients seek help in solving their health problems but your responsibilities in meeting their needs go beyond performing a painless blood draw, giving effective breathing treatments, or sending out accurate bills for payment. You must be willing to combine a caring attitude with technical competence by treating each patient as worthy of your full attention. Studies have found that even if a health professional excels in one area, poor communication skills or the appearance of not caring can cause patients to view that person negatively.[2] Box 1-4 contains a list of important characteristics that patients seek in their health care providers.

The Patient Care Partnership

Health care organizations have formally recognized the rights of patients to receive proper care. The American Hospital Association (AHA) has written a brochure for patients, entitled "The Patient Care Partnership: Understanding Expectations, Rights and Responsibilities," which is used by many health care facilities nationwide. These include, among others, the rights of patients to the following:
- Be treated with compassion and respect
- Receive information about the benefits and risks of treatments
- Have their privacy protected
- Participate in making decisions regarding their care, including the right to refuse treatment
- Have their health goals and values taken into account as much as possible

Many other health organizations, as well as governmental agencies and the new Patient Protection and Affordable Care Act, recognize the importance of patients having more control over their health care. They have also created their own statements of patient rights.

- Competent care
- Someone who listens
- Clear communication
- Courtesy
- Compassion
- Empathy
- Understanding
- Sincerity
- Respect

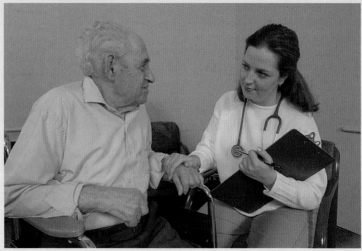

(From Klieger D: *Saunders essentials of medical assisting*, ed 2, 2010, Saunders.)

Prescription for Success: 1-6 And the Patient Is...You

Imagine you have just arrived at an urgent care facility with a suspected broken arm. You were out for an enjoyable Sunday afternoon, skating with friends, when you hit a hole in the pavement and fell. Your arm is very painful, and you are worried about your ability to work if you end up in a cast.

1. Describe how you would feel if you found yourself in this situation.
2. How would you hope to be treated by the health care professionals at the urgent care facility?
3. What would be most important to you?
4. What would be least important to you?
5. Did you learn anything from this exercise that might influence your approach to working with future patients?

What Do You Want?

"If you don't know where you're going, chances are you'll end up somewhere else."

In addition to exploring the needs of your "customers"—your employers and patients—an important part of planning is to identify what *you* want. You must consider your own needs and desires as you create your professional self. The clearer you are about your career goals and expectations, the greater your chance of achieving them.

Beginning now to think about your specific career goals and workplace priorities will keep you alert to appropriate employment possibilities as you go through your educational program. Take every opportunity during your studies to observe, ask questions, and read about your field. Then compare your findings with your own interests. Many fields in health care today feature newly created positions and expanded responsibilities for traditional jobs. A wide variety of choices is available for new graduates.

Developing a Philosophy of Work

Most of us spend a significant number of our waking hours on the job. How we spend that time determines, to a large degree, the quality of our lives. It makes sense, then, to think about what work means to you. Exploring your personal beliefs will help you increase the amount of satisfaction you get from your career. There are many reasons why people work, including the desire to[3]:

- Survive financially
- Define self
- Gain self-respect demonstrate competence
- Gain power
- Help others
- Learn
- Experience variety
- Contribute to the community
- Experience enjoyment
- Fill time

People are generally happiest and most productive when their work provides them with more than material rewards. Some people are motivated by continual challenges, others value consistency, and still others are content with either condition as long as their work allows them to help others.

Health care is a complex, ever-changing field that offers both opportunities and challenges for those who choose to work in it. Here are some of the major sources of satisfaction you can expect.

1. **Meaningful work.** Good health is a basic need for human survival and happiness. Working in a field that promotes

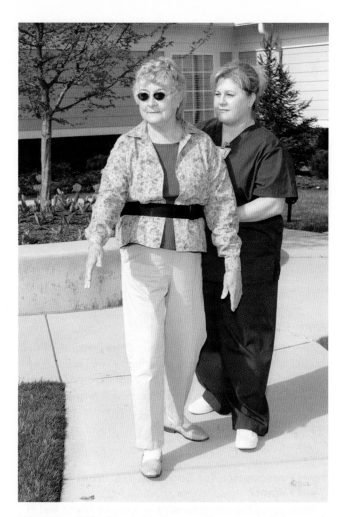

FIGURE 1-5 Working in health care allows you to help people improve their quality of life. This health care worker is helping a patient recover her mobility. *Write a list of the ways you will be able to help others when working in your future career.* (From Sorrentino S, Remmert L: *Mosby's textbook for nursing assistants*, ed 8, St Louis, 2012, Mosby.)

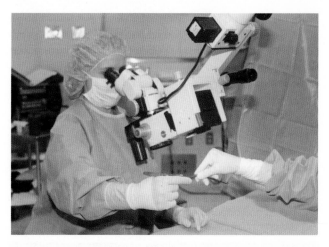

FIGURE 1-6 Advances in medical science and health care are occurring at an astonishing rate. Life-saving drugs, the use of DNA to develop more effective cancer treatments, and sophisticated computer software are only a few examples. *What changes do you think will affect your work? Why is it important for you to stay current?* (From Fuller JK: *Surgical technology: Principles and practice*, ed 6, St Louis, 2013, Saunders.)

health gives you the opportunity to make meaningful contributions to the well-being of others. Whether you provide direct patient care or perform supporting activities, your work directly affects patients and the quality of your work can truly make a difference in their lives. A career in health care has purpose and value.

2. **Opportunity to serve.** People seek the services of health care professionals when they need help. They come with the hope that you can help them solve their problems and they entrust themselves to your care. You have the opportunity to enter both the physical and emotional space of others, sharing close personal contact. People who are ill or injured are often afraid and anxious. You, like the health care professional assisting the patient in Figure 1-5, are in a position to influence their safety and well-being.

3. **Career stability.** The need for health care will always exist, even if job titles change over time. The reorganization taking place in today's health care delivery systems is causing continual shifts in the need for specific occupational positions. A decrease in the number of job openings for one position is often balanced by an increase in another. You may need to redefine your job in the future, but you will always have a solid knowledge base to which you can add the experience or training required to qualify for new positions.

4. **Interesting work environment.** The world of health care is changing at a rapid rate, both scientifically and organizationally. Advances in our understanding of how the body works, along with discoveries about the causes and treatments of diseases, are reported almost daily. Computers have increased our capacity to collect and organize information and the software than runs them is constantly being upgraded. New technology, such as the surgical equipment shown in Figure 1-6, is being developed at an astonishing rate. You will witness advances in knowledge that extend and improve the quality of human life. The health care environment is never boring. There will be a steady stream of interesting information to learn, apply, and use.

5. **Opportunities for advancement.** The health care field provides many opportunities for upward mobility if you are willing to continue learning and adding to your skills. Many jobs offer opportunities for on-the-job learning that enable you to increase your value to your patients and employer, as well as your eligibility for promotion. In addition, many occupational specialties in health care present the opportunity for career laddering. **Career ladders** comprise jobs within one occupational area that require different levels of

knowledge and skills. The higher-level positions almost always require further education and additional **certifications** or **licenses**. (You will learn more about these approvals in Chapter 2. Career laddering is discussed in more detail in Chapter 17.)

Prescription for Success: 1-7
My Philosophy of Work

1. What meaning does work have for me?
2. What needs do I want to be filled by work?
3. Why did I choose a career in health care?
4. What do I hope to accomplish?
5. What do I hope to contribute?

Q & A with a Health Care Professional

Charlie McKnee

Charlie McKnee provides direct care to older adults in a long-term care facility. Charlie answers questions about beginning a career in health professions and his own experiences.

Q What would you say to someone who is starting a career in health care?

A First, I would say, "Congratulations, you've chosen a very honorable profession." As such, you're an honored and increasingly valuable person. People who take care of others for a living tend to be very giving. I think health care providers need to understand themselves and their own needs—and then take care of themselves, too. If they sacrifice themselves completely for the sake of others, this leads to burnout and their own health problems.

Q What can health care professionals do to take care of themselves?

A First, they need to understand their own importance and give themselves the respect they deserve. Realistically, patients aren't always able to show their appreciation because of their own problems. So health care professionals really have to recognize their own value—give themselves a pat on the back for work well done. They should also review their own strengths and limitations. They need to take care of their mental as well as their physical health. My personal belief is that mental health comes before physical health, so I'm really big on this one.

Q It sounds like you have a holistic view of health, right?

A Absolutely. I really believe that as health care providers we should be aware of the emotional, spiritual, and social needs of our patients and residents. We leave too much out of the equation if we just focus on the physical. We need to see the multiple aspects of health if we are to truly experience love, concern, and purpose in our work.

Q Your specialty is working with older adults. Why do you find this work satisfying?

A I believe that older people have been stigmatized. Society says, "They're old, they have problems, they need our help." At the same time, many people kind of give up on them. They assume they are in decline and work from a disease model—that is, just taking care of any acute problems. I prefer to work from a wellness model. That means helping the people I work with to set goals and think about improving and being able to do more. Just sitting in a wheelchair—that shouldn't be how a person lives out their later years. I believe that older adults have many strengths. I like to do what I can to help them reach their potential. And to see what I—and we—as a society, can learn from them.

Work Preferences

It is also a good idea to begin thinking about the kinds of tasks you like to do and the working conditions you prefer. A wide variety of work settings exists for health care professionals. Being clear about your own preferences will help you choose and prepare for the most appropriate types of positions in your career area.

Prescription for Success: 1-8 What Do I Want?

Think about the characteristics you would like to find in your place of employment.

1. Type of facility
   Examples: large, small, urban (in the city), rural, inpatient (such as a hospital), outpatient (such as a clinic), home care
2. Type of population served
   Examples: economic status, age range, gender, ethnic groups
3. Work schedule
   Examples: steady employment with one employer; per diem (daily, contracted to different facilities); flexible, changing hours; fixed hours; frequent overtime; days only; evenings and weekends
4. Specialty
   Examples: emergency care, orthopedics (bones and muscles), hand therapy
5. Type of supervision
   Examples: closely monitored, work more independently
6. Work pace
   Examples: fast, moderate (There is no slow-paced work in health care!)
7. Amount of interaction with others (All health care professionals are part of a team, although some work more independently than others.)
8. Range of duties performed
   Examples: wide variety of tasks, concentrate on a few, somewhere in between

---

Greg worked in roofing and construction from the time he graduated from high school. He got a job with a company owned by a buddy's father and worked his way up from doing clean-up to full-time work as a roofer. He liked the physical nature of the work, being outside most of the day and having a beer with his fellow workers at the end of the day.

One fall day as his work team was trying to finish a job before the rainy weather got any worse, Greg slipped from a steep incline and fell onto a cement patio. He broke his leg and fractured two vertebrae in his back. He recovered the use of his leg, although he was in pain a good deal of the time. His roofing and construction days were over.

Being unable to work posed a huge problem for Greg. He and his wife, Kathy, had two children to support and Kathy's job was only part-time and did not provide any benefits. On the advice of a friend who worked at a local clinic, Greg looked into a career in health care. Although the idea of working inside all day wasn't appealing to him, it seemed as though there were many job openings in health care and the work was steady.

He and Kathy talked it over and she encouraged him. "You know," she said, "my friend Louise has been working for Dr. Lewis for years as a medical assistant and really likes the work." Greg had some doubts. "Don't you think there might be lifting and other heavy work helping patients? My back might not take that kind of work."

"Well," said Kathy, "I did talk with Louise about that and she said that there are *administrative* medical assistants. They work in the office greeting patients, doing billing and other kinds of paperwork."

"Gosh," said Greg. "I've never done that kind of work. I don't know if I'd be any good at it."

Kathy reassured him. "Honey, I know you can do whatever you set your mind to."

Greg had his doubts, but he enrolled in a medical office administration program at the local college. Kathy's friend Louise gave him some help with his studies and he managed to complete the program with passing grades. The family's finances were approaching the point of desperation and he knew he had to finish his program and look for employment.

Greg worked hard at finding a job. He pursued every lead and presented himself well at interviews. It wasn't surprising, then, that he had a job just a few weeks after graduation, greeting patients and doing front-office work for a local doctor. His outgoing personality made him popular with patients, but he found the appointment scheduling, data inputting on the computer, and other paperwork tedious and not to his liking. Sitting all day in a small area made him feel closed in and uncomfortable. He stayed with the job and did his best because he didn't want to let his family down. But he was never happy with his work and knew inwardly that someday he would have to find something else.

Questions for Thought and Reflection

1. What do you think of Greg's reasons for studying medical assisting?
2. What effect did Kathy and Louise have on Greg's decision?
3. What could he have done to learn more about the job?
4. Do you think he should have explored other career options?
5. Is there anything Greg can do now to improve his situation?

Alignment with Employers

Although it is important to try to meet your personal needs when seeking employment, you must also have realistic expectations. An essential activity in career planning is to compare your work preferences with the needs of potential employers to see how well they match. Students sometimes have unrealistic expectations of the positions they hope to fill immediately after graduation. Recent graduates are qualified for *entry-level* positions. You can avoid frustration and disappointment if you understand the workplace and adjust your expectations.

Formal training is only the beginning of your journey in developing competence as a health care professional. Your skills will continue to grow and be refined as you accumulate hands-on practice and everyday experience in the field. When starting a new career, it may be wise—even necessary—to trade your "perfect job" requirements for opportunities that lead to long-term career success. Consider looking for a first job in which you can do the following:

1. Gain self-confidence
2. Work with a variety of people
3. Acquire additional knowledge
4. Increase your skill base
5. Explore specialties within your field of interest
6. Network with other professionals
7. Demonstrate your abilities

Your first employer is giving you the gift of his or her confidence in your abilities. You will be entrusted with serious responsibilities that may include patient welfare, the accuracy and confidentiality of important records, and other matters that influence the reputation and success of the facility. You will have the chance to prove your value by learning as much as possible, finding ways to help your employer and co-workers, and contributing to the overall success of the organization. Entry-level jobs, performed well, can be the first important step leading to positions that meet all your hopes for a fulfilling career.

Alignment with Your Profession

Health care professions vary in the type of work performed. You need to be aware of the daily tasks and working conditions of the occupation you have chosen. For example, respiratory therapy and radiology require the technical aptitude to work with complex equipment. Occupational therapy requires the ability to apply oral communication skills to teach patients and their families. Health information technology and insurance coding require accuracy and attention to detail when creating, filling out, and organizing medical records and forms.

You may need to consider tradeoffs to obtain a balance that offers maximum career satisfaction. For example, a recent nursing graduate who wants the excitement of a hospital emergency room and the convenience of a 9:00 AM to 5:00 PM weekday schedule may be faced with a conflict. To avoid a mismatch between your expectations and the real world, learn as much as possible about the specific requirements of your future profession so you can rethink your requirements, if necessary.

Adjusting your short-term expectations doesn't mean giving up your long-term goals. In fact, purposeful planning now can help you arrive at where you want to be in the future. If you discover that the specific type of job you want requires previous work experience, you can set short-term goals to serve as stepping stones to acquire that experience. Find out now what skills are emphasized in your target position and look for opportunities to learn as many of them as possible during your studies, **externship**, and first job. For example, Rosa wants to work as a back-office medical assistant with a plastic surgeon, helping the physician with outpatient procedures. Her research shows there are only a few plastic surgeons in her area and they prefer to hire assistants with previous work experience. Rosa decides to look for a job with a general practitioner or pediatrician who does minor surgery in the office. Her short-term goals are to gain experience with **sterile techniques**, **standard precautions**, surgical assisting, and patient care. While in school, she asks her instructor to recommend books and articles about plastic surgery and allow her to spend extra practice time in the lab so she can reach a high level of competence with sterile techniques, surgical instruments, wound care, and related topics. (Goals are discussed in more detail in Chapter 3.)

Employees who are willing to meet the expectations of their employers are often rewarded with additional (and interesting) responsibilities and promotions. Some employers even create new positions so they can use the talents of their employees. For new health care professionals who are well prepared and contribute enthusiastically to the success of their employers, entry-level jobs can serve as launch pads for future career success. You, too, may benefit by having new and interesting responsibilities added to your job description, receiving a promotion, or having a job created that brings you satisfaction. Serving the needs of others can provide you with opportunities to meet your own needs.

Prescription for Success: 1-9 Conduct an Informational Interview

Conducting **informational interviews** gives you opportunities to learn more about the specific needs of employers in your career area, the skill requirements, and the everyday duties performed by professionals. Supervisors, as well as working professionals, are excellent sources of information. The purpose of this type of interview is *not* to seek employment; it is to seek information. You may already know someone you would like to interview. If not, ask your instructor or the career services department at your school for suggestions. If you are a student member of a health care professional organization, this can be a good source of leads.

Once you have a contact, call and make an appointment. Explain that you are a student and want to learn more about your career area. Be considerate of the person's time, and if he or she is very busy, ask if you can schedule 15 or 20 minutes. Arrive a few minutes early and dress professionally. (Professional dress is discussed in Chapter 2.) Afterward, be sure to send a thank-you note to the person you interviewed.

Take along a list of prepared questions and a small notebook and pen. Here are some suggestions of questions for a supervisor:

1. What skills are most important to be successful as a _____?
2. What personal characteristics do you look for in a candidate seeking work as a _____?
3. What type of work is performed by a _____ in your facility?
4. What type of orientation or on-the-job training is given to new employees?
5. What is your best advice for someone who is interested in becoming a _____?
6. What learning and opportunities for promotion are available for professionals who work in this field?

Examples of questions to ask a working professional include the following:

1. What are the typical duties of a _____?
2. What percentage of the day is usually spent on each duty?
3. Describe a typical day. (Is there a typical day? If not, describe a typical week.)
4. How many patients do you see in a day? How many tests do you perform? How many reports do you transcribe?
5. How much independent decision-making is required?
6. What is most challenging about your work?
7. What is most satisfying about your work?

To keep a record of what you hear, take brief notes during the interview or summarize the information as soon as possible afterward.

What did you learn?

What else do you need to find out?

Describe anything you learned in the interview that surprised you.

On the basis of what you learned in the interview, describe anything you plan to work on while you are in school.

Prescription for Success: 1-10 Job Shadowing

Job shadowing means spending time with a professional as he or she works and performs typical duties. Many health care facilities offer programs to which you can apply. Typical requirements include: a sincere interest in a health care career, a recent tuberculosis test, signing a confidentiality agreement, filling out a health-screening questionnaire, receiving the required immunizations, and maintaining a professional appearance. Some facilities only allow students to participate if job shadowing is required by their school. Others welcome anyone who is interested.

Health care facilities may manage their own job shadowing programs, sometimes through a student placement coordinator's office. The Internet contains information about many programs. Enter the search terms "health care job shadowing" along with your geographic area. For example, "health care job shadowing St. Louis."

If you participate in a job shadowing program, take notes of what you observe and learn. Use the opportunity to ask questions like those in Prescription for Success 1-10. For future reference, keep records of the facility information (address, phone number, etc.), the department, the dates you attended, who you accompanied, his or her contact information, and a summary of what you learned.

Prescription for Success: 1-11 Paint an Occupational Portrait

Use what you learned from your research—informational interview, job shadowing, the National Healthcare Foundation Standards, the *Occupational Outlook Handbook* (see "To Learn More" in this chapter), and/or your professional organization—to write a summary report about your future career. Include the following:
1. Major responsibilities
2. Typical duties performed
3. Skills and personal characteristics required
4. Job outlook and salary information
5. Sources of continuing education
6. Opportunities for promotion
7. What you find most interesting about the career

Prescription for Success: 1-12 Are My Expectations Realistic?

Review the information you have gathered about your chosen occupation. Compare this information with your preferences and what you know about your personal qualities.
1. Do your preferences and personal qualities fit the occupation you have chosen?
2. How may you have to adjust your expectations?
3. What can you start doing now to ensure you are fully prepared for the requirements of your chosen occupation?

Summary of Key Ideas

- Your career as a health care professional starts now.
- Study skills are also job skills.
- As a student, you have both rights and responsibilities.
- An effective health care professional needs more than good technical skills.
- Preparing for a new career is like creating and marketing a new product.

Internet Activities

For active links to the websites needed to complete these activities, visit http://evolve. elsevier.com/Haroun/career/.

1. The Occupational Outlook Handbook (OOH), developed by the U.S. Department of Labor, is available online. Choose a health care occupation to review and list 10 facts you learn from the OOH profile.
2. Many of the general skills and characteristics employers seek when hiring new employees are described in an article featured by Quintessential Careers. Read the article, then choose the five skills and characteristics you believe to be most important for succeeding in a health care career. Include your reasons for selecting each.
3. The National Healthcare Foundation Standards and Accountability Criteria are available from the National Consortium on Health Science Education. Read the 11 standards and the criteria listed under each one.
   a. Choose three accountability criteria under "Foundation Standard 2: Communications," and explain the importance of each in delivering high-quality health care.
   b. Review the accountability criteria under "Foundation Standard 4: Employability Skills" and explain how you can use this information now to begin preparing for your career.
   c. Go to "Foundation Standard 8: Teamwork." Explain why, in your opinion, an entire standard is devoted to teamwork.
4. Do a Web search using the key words "marketing yourself." Explore some of the websites listed to read about the importance of self-marketing in planning and conducting a job search. Based on what you learn, write a short paper describing what you can do, as you begin your education, to make yourself more marketable.
5. Do a Web search using the key words "informational interview." Read about conducting an effective interview. List five techniques and 10 questions you can use to set up and conduct your interviews.

To Learn More

About.com: Health Careers

http://healthcareers.about.com
Website containing links to articles about choosing and succeeding in a health care career.

American Hospital Association: The Patient Care Partnership

http://www.aha.org/advocacy-issues/communicatingpts/pt-care-partnership.shtml

Brochure informs patients about what they should expect during their hospital stay with regard to their rights and responsibilities.

Covey SR: The 7 habits of highly effective people, New York, 2004, Free Press

Popular book lists and discusses seven principles that help individuals live effective lives. You may find it helpful to learn about the seven habits, which are as follows:

- Habit 1: Be Proactive: Principles of Personal Choice
- Habit 2: Begin with the End in Mind: Principles of Personal Vision
- Habit 3: Put First Things First: Principles of Integrity and Execution
- Habit 4: Think Win/Win: Principles of Mutual Benefit
- Habit 5: Seek First to Understand, Then to Be Understood: Principles of Mutual Understanding
- Habit 6: Synergize: Principles of Creative Cooperation
- Habit 7: Sharpen the Saw: Principles of Balanced Self-Renewal

Explore Health Careers

http://www.explorehealthcareers.org

Noncommercial website containing general information about working in health care, as well as articles about specific careers.

Family Educational Rights and Privacy Act

http://www2.ed.gov/policy/gen/guid/fpco/ferpa/index.html

Description of the Federal law that protects the privacy of a student's educational records.

Health Care Career Professional Organizations

All health careers have organizations that set standards and provide support and information for both students and working professionals. Many organizations are listed, along with contact information, in Appendix A.

My College Success Story

www.mycollegesuccessstory.com

Dozens of stories from students about how they succeeded in college, including tips on personal organization, studying, and overcoming obstacles. There is also a section containing academic success tools.

National Consortium on Health Science Education

www.healthscienceconsortium.org

Information about health careers, as well as the Foundation's standards developed for the health care student. Reviewing these standards will give you an idea of what employers expect of their employees.

U.S. Department of Labor: Occupational Outlook Handbook

www.bls.gov/ooh

A source of detailed information about hundreds of careers, including typical job descriptions, educational requirements, and average salaries. It is updated every 2 years.

What Work Requires of Schools: A SCANS Report for America 2000

http://wdr.doleta.gov/SCANS/whatwork/whatwork.pdf

Report containing the competencies sought by employers, along with workplace scenarios demonstrating how the competencies are applied.

References

1. National Consortium for Health Science Education. "National Healthcare Foundation Standards and Accountability Criteria." Healthscienceconsortium.org/docs/foundation_standards_ac_jan2011.pdf (Accessed 3/3/14).
2. Anderson R, Barbara A, Feldman S: "What patients want: a content analysis of key qualities that influence patient satisfaction." www.drscore.com/press/papers/whatpatientswant.pdf (Accessed 8/15/14).
3. Binghang M, Stryker S: *Career choices and changes*, Washington, UT, 2005, Academic Innovations.

CHAPTER 2

Your Resume Starts Now

OBJECTIVES

1. Begin to create a product—your professional self—that you can offer with confidence to prospective employers.
2. Develop a professional appearance that is appropriate for the health care field.
3. Use the contents of your future resume as a planning tool for managing your personal and professional development.
4. Start collecting items you can put in your professional portfolio.
5. Begin self-promotion techniques such as professional networking and identifying references.

KEY TERMS AND CONCEPTS

Affirmation A positive statement, said out loud declaring something to be true.

Civic Organizations Groups that are devoted to improving the community.

Hygiene Practices that contribute to cleanliness, good health, and the prevention of disease.

Networking Meeting new people for the purpose of personal and professional development.

Optional Not required.

Portfolio An organized collection of items that provides evidence of your job-related skills and capabilities.

Proactive Taking positive action before it is necessary or required.

Reference A person, such as a former supervisor, who agrees to vouch for your professional skills and capabilities.

Resume A written document that summarizes your qualifications, professional skills, and capabilities.

Self-Fulfilling Prophecy A prediction made by a person that influences his or her actions, resulting in the prediction coming true.

Syllabi Handouts prepared by instructors to let students know what they will learn, what the instructor expects from them, and how the students will be evaluated. Some instructors consider the syllabus to be a form of contract between themselves and their students.

Transferable Skills Skills, such as organizing and tracking supplies, which can be applied to different types of occupations.

Visualization A technique in which you create detailed pictures in your mind of something you want to have or become.

Production: The Second "P" of Marketing

"You have to take life as it happens, but you should try to make it happen the way you want to take it."

—Old German Proverb

In Chapter 1, you read about the first step in the marketing process, Planning. The second of the "5 Ps of Marketing" is Production: using the information gathered from market research to design and put together a product that meets the needs of the customer. Your market research was finding out what patients and employers want and need from health care professionals.

Human beings have the unique ability to create their own lives. They can generate ideas, form mental images, and plan ways to achieve what they imagine. You have already generated the idea of becoming a health care professional and have completed the first step toward achieving that goal by enrolling in school. Whether you graduate and find satisfactory employment will depend, to a great extent, on your belief in your ability to succeed and your willingness to take the necessary actions to achieve your goals.

Henry Ford, who not only created fame and riches for himself, but changed the history of transportation, is quoted as saying, "Whether you think you can, or you think you can't, you're right." The tendency for people to get what they expect is known as a **self-fulfilling prophecy**. Our beliefs about ourselves, about what we can achieve, are more important than any other factor. Many prominent Americans, such as Abraham Lincoln and Thomas Edison, experienced many failures before finally achieving great success. Lincoln experienced business failures and lost elections before becoming one of our most famous presidents. And Edison conducted thousands of experiments before perfecting the electric light bulb: an invention that dramatically changed the world.

You can apply the principle of expecting success as you begin your career journey. All achievements begin as ideas, and what you picture mentally can become your reality. Positive images of yourself succeeding as a student act as powerful motivators. In addition to visual suggestions, your self-talk influences your success, or lack of it. We are continually holding conversations with ourselves that either encourage us ("I know I can pass this test.") or put us down ("I'll never be able to get this report finished."). By taking control of the pictures and words in your mind, you can apply their power to help you create the life you want.

A related and very powerful concept you can apply to your life is to behave as if you already are what you hope to become. You can increase your chances of becoming a successful health care professional if you start approaching life as if you already were that professional. Practice behaviors now that you know

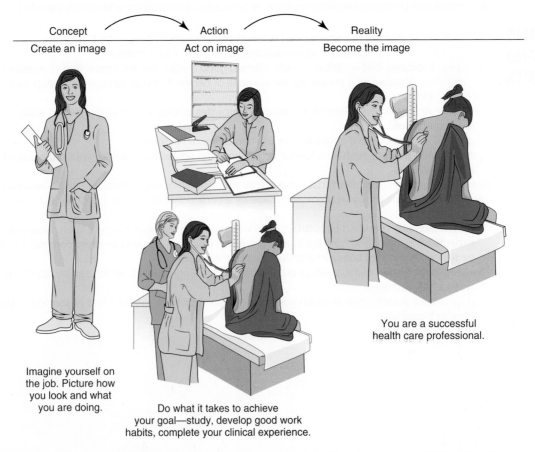

Concept	Action	Reality
Create an image	Act on image	Become the image

Imagine yourself on the job. Picture how you look and what you are doing.

Do what it takes to achieve your goal—study, develop good work habits, complete your clinical experience.

You are a successful health care professional.

FIGURE 2-1 Self-fulfilling prophecy. *Spend some time each week as you progress through your program imagining yourself in your occupation. Be specific and visualize yourself performing the tasks you are learning in your classes.*

will be expected on the job. For example, because accuracy and efficiency are important characteristics for the health care professional, complete all class assignments as if the well-being of others depended on your accuracy. Working effectively with others as part of a team will be required in your work, so start using every opportunity to develop your teamwork skills. Cooperate with your classmates and instructors. Figure 2-1 illustrates how

creating a mental picture of yourself as a health care professional can encourage behaviors that lead you to achieve your career goals. Be **proactive** and look for opportunities to increase your personal and professional growth. Turn mistakes into lessons and learn from them. Approach personal difficulties as opportunities to learn and grow. By the time you graduate, you will have become the health care professional you aspire to be.

Prescription for Success: 2-1 Using Visualization

Visualization is a popular technique for harnessing the creative power of the imagination. If your goal is to become a medical assistant, for example, create a detailed mental picture of yourself working as a professional in a doctor's office or clinic. See yourself performing the tasks of your chosen occupation. Try the technique for yourself by following these steps:

1. Find a quiet, private place where you won't be disturbed.
2. Close your eyes.
3. Imagine yourself as a member of the occupation of your choice.
   A. Create the details. Attempt to make the image as real as possible.

1. What are you wearing?
2. Who are your co-workers?
3. What is the setting? A hospital? A physician's office? A business office?
4. What are you doing? Interacting with a patient? Performing a procedure? Working on a computer?
   B. Create positive thoughts and feelings for yourself in the scene: "I am competent." "I work well with patients and co-workers." "I like what I am doing."
4. Try to keep your imaginary scene going for a few minutes. Make it as specific as possible and keep filling in the details. The idea is to have a clear, firm image of yourself successfully carrying out the duties of your chosen profession.

Prescription for Success: 2-2 Affirmations (Positive Self-Talk)

Filling your self-talk with positive statements is another technique for creating the future you want. These statements are called **affirmations** and like visualizations, they are based on the principle that we become what we create in our minds. Here are a few examples:

- I, Rosa Maria, am a highly skilled dental assistant.
- I, Kenisha, perform my radiology duties with confidence.
- I, Jaime, conduct accurate laboratory tests.
- I, Andrea, am a competent, caring nurse.

- I, Pham, help patients with my therapeutic skills.
- I, Bill, am an efficient health information technician.
  Note that each affirmation:
- Is stated in the present tense
- Includes your name
- Is positive
  Try writing a few affirmations on cards to carry with you or post them where you will see them every day. The important thing is to repeat them daily over a period of time.

Case Study 2-1

Something to Offer

Amber's mother was at it again. She returned from work to find Amber in the kitchen working to put together the family's dinner as she was expected to do every evening. Amber didn't mind doing the cooking; after all, her mother had to work to support the family after her father died in a car accident. But it was hard to take the constant criticism. This time it was how she cooked the potatoes.

"For crying out loud, Amber," shouted her mother. "How many times do I have to tell you not to overcook the vegetables?! No one wants to eat a pile of mush."

Amber's lip trembled. "I'm sorry Mom. I thought you'd be home sooner and we'd have eaten by now."

"Do you ever listen?" asked her mother. "I told you I had a meeting this afternoon and would most likely be late getting home."

Amber mumbled another apology and went about finishing the preparations for a meal she knew she wouldn't enjoy eating. Later that night, alone in her room, she thought about what had happened that day and almost every day. She couldn't seem to do anything right. And

Continued

Something to Offer

now her mother was insisting that she "do something worthwhile with her life" like other young people instead of hanging around the house. Although Amber was pretty sure she would fail at whatever she tried, she decided to talk with her Aunt Jessie, a medical biller and coder at Good Health, a large clinic in town.

Amber sometimes spent time with Jessie, her father's older sister. Jessie was more patient than Amber's mother and recognized that her niece's lack of self-confidence was likely to hold her back in life.

"You know, Amber, why don't you spend some time with me over the next few days?" asked Jessie. "We could talk about some career options. There's a good job shadow program at Good Health that you might want to apply for. You can take a look at what's out there."

Lacking self-confidence and believing herself to be incompetent, Amber couldn't see herself working with doctors or patients. But she agreed to fill out the application for the program and when accepted, spent time at her aunt's workplace. Observing the work of those who work directly with patients, such as nurses, medical assistants, and therapists, reinforced Amber's belief that this wouldn't be the work for her. But she did think that maybe working mostly on her own in an office like her aunt might work for her. She could see that coding required accuracy and attention to detail and worried about being too dumb and making mistakes. But with her aunt's encouragement, she visited a local college that had a coding training program.

Amber decided to enroll in the program. She was very nervous about attending college but decided to try her best. She was so worn down by her mother's constant put-downs that she was desperate to find a way to provide for herself and live on her own. Although Amber's mother resented the time her daughter spent studying, Aunt Jessie helped Amber understand her homework assignments and provided moral support to help her succeed.

The instructors at Amber's school recognized her potential, but realized that she lacked self-confidence. Ms. Ross, the terminology and insurance instructor, invited her to her office one day.

"I don't think you realize what you have to offer an employer," she told Amber. "You're doing well in my classes; your homework is always accurate and completed on time. And you've done well on your quizzes."

"Well," Amber explained, "I don't want to let my aunt down. She's been so helpful to me."

"It sounds as if she's been a good mentor. I'd like to go one step further and help you realize what you have to offer a future employer."

Ms. Ross went on to recommend that Amber start listing the qualities and skills that would make her a valued employee. She suggested that Amber begin by noting her good attendance, her ability to complete work on time, and her respectful attitude in class. Then she gave her some ideas about skills she could list: knowledge of medical terminology and insurance requirements so far.

"I want you to keep this list up as you go through your program," advised Ms. Ross. "Think about what employers are looking for and what you are learning in your classes."

Questions for Thought and Reflection

1. Do you think Amber made a good decision to study medical billing and coding? Why or why not?
2. In what ways has Aunt Jessie helped Amber?
3. What do you think of Ms. Ross's advice?
4. What else might Amber do to improve her self-image?
5. Do you think Amber will finish school and graduate? Why or why not?
6. If Amber graduates, do you think she will succeed in finding a job? Why or why not?
7. If Amber becomes employed, do you think she will succeed on the job? Why or why not?

Packaging: The Third "P" of Marketing

Even an excellent product may not sell if it is poorly packaged. Companies know this and invest a lot of time and money to make their products visually appealing to customers. Appearance can make the difference between a product selling or collecting dust on the shelf. Most of us package ourselves to impress others or to fit into a specific social group. Americans spend billions of dollars annually on clothing, cosmetics, accessories, and hair care in an effort to create what we believe to be a pleasing appearance.

Appearance is especially important in the health care field because many patients form their opinions about the competence of health care professionals based on their appearance. Your effectiveness in meeting patient needs can be influenced by your appearance because patient satisfaction increases when health care professionals "look as if they know what they are doing."

So what are the desired characteristics of a health care professional's appearance? The first is to be fairly conservative in dress and grooming. It is best to avoid fashion trends such as brightly colored hair, tattoos, and body piercing. At the same time, it is true that employers are becoming more accepting of these trends. The problem is that some patients may interpret them as signs of rebellion, immaturity, and a lack of common sense. Others are offended or even frightened by this type of appearance.

Even clothing that is not extreme may be inappropriate for work. Dressing for work is different from dressing casually for recreation or for social functions. For example, low-cut tops that reveal cleavage may be in style and generally accepted but they are not appropriate in the health care workplace.

What is perfect for a party may be totally out of place for a job interview or for the job itself.

A second consideration is to strive for an appearance that radiates good health. An important responsibility of the health care professional is to promote good health, and this is partly achieved by example. If you smoke or are overweight, putting you at risk for serious health problems, this would be a good time to adopt new healthy living habits. In addition to being harmful to health, smoke clings to hair and clothing, resulting in unpleasant odors that may offend others. Other conditions such as teeth that need dental work, badly bitten fingernails, and dandruff indicate a lack of self-care, and this is inappropriate in a profession that encourages the practice of good personal health habits. The way you present yourself reflects your approach to life and your opinion of yourself. Failure to care for yourself can project a lack of self-confidence and can undermine a patient's faith in your effectiveness. Chapter 3 discusses self-care issues such as managing stress, eating properly, and getting adequate physical exercise.

Third, the issues of cleanliness and **hygiene** are vitally important for professionals whose work requires them to touch others. Patients literally put themselves in the hands of health care professionals and must feel assured that they will benefit from, and not be harmed by, any procedures performed. It is natural to want the professional to look clean and neat and be free of unpleasant odors. For example, although the hands of a dental assistant may be clean and gloved, dirty uniforms or shoes (or even shoelaces!) give an unfavorable impression to the patient, who may wonder whether proper attention was given to sterilizing the equipment and cleaning the work area.

Finally, professionals must consider the safety and comfort of both patients and themselves. Perfumes and scented personal products cannot be tolerated by many patients. Long fingernails, flowing hair, and large dangling earrings may be attractive and appropriate for a social event, but in a health care setting they can scratch patients, contaminate samples, get caught in equipment, or be grabbed by young patients. Safety on the job cannot be compromised to accommodate fashion trends. Some clothing customs are determined by one's culture, such as head coverings and flowing skirts. These customs may also have to be modified to ensure the safety of both yourself and the patient. (See Figure 2-2 for an example of a professional appearance.)

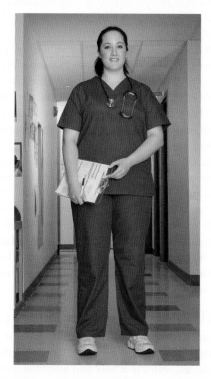

FIGURE 2-2 Appearance counts! *Name 5 aspects of this young woman's appearance that demonstrate professionalism. Do you think patients would believe her to be competent based on her appearance? Why or why not?* (From Bonewit-West K, Hunt S, Applegate E: *Today's medical assistant: Clinical & administrative procedures,* ed 2, St Louis, 2013, Saunders.)

Trouble Ahead? 2-1

Crystal is one of Amber's classmates in the medical billing and coding program. Like Amber, she prefers working alone. Unlike Amber, Crystal believes in herself to the extreme. She thinks that "doing her own thing" is her right and frequently believes that her way is better than the one recommended by others, including her instructors.

When Ms. Ross, the instructor who took an interest in Amber, talks to the class about the importance of a professional appearance when working in health care, Crystal rolls her eyes. Later, she tells her mom, "I don't understand what all the fuss is about. Who's going to see me working at a computer all day?"

Her mom is somewhat of a free spirit and agrees with her daughter. "I know, dear, it's interesting how others seem to know best, isn't it? What's wrong with expressing ourselves as individuals?"

Crystal thinks it over. She understands that learning to bill and code accurately is important; that makes sense to her. But having to cover up her tattoos, remove some of her piercings, and dress more conservatively doesn't make sense and she's not sure she's willing to make these changes.

Questions for Thought and Reflection

1. Why are billing and coding instructors concerned about the appearance of their students?
2. What is your opinion of Crystal's attitude?
3. Do you think Crystal will be successful as a medical biller and coder? Why or why not?

Presentation: The Fourth "P" of Marketing

Your **resume**, a written outline of your qualifications for work, is an important tool for presenting yourself and what you have to offer to prospective employers. The main purpose of a resume is to convince an employer to give you an interview, and in Chapter 13 you will learn how to write and organize an effective resume. The focus of the rest of this chapter is on learning about the content of the resume and how you can use it as a guideline to create your professional self. Starting to plan your resume now will help you do the following:

1. Recognize what you already have to offer an employer
2. Build self-confidence
3. Motivate yourself to learn both the technical and nontechnical skills that contribute to employment success
4. Identify anything you might want to improve about yourself
5. Know ahead of time what kinds of experiences will enhance your employability
6. Get started gathering information and collecting examples to demonstrate your value and skills

Your Resume as a Guide to Success

"Begin with the end in mind."

—Stephen Covey

Thinking about your resume at the beginning instead of waiting until the end of your educational program turns your resume into a checklist of "To Dos" for creating a product, your professional self, which you'll be able to offer with confidence to prospective customers: health care employers. The various components of a resume, listed in Box 2-1, are explained in this chapter, along with suggestions on how to make them work for you while you are still in school.

Each resume component lines up with a Resume Building Block included in this chapter. These Resume Building Blocks, all interspersed through this chapter, are intended to be used to

BOX 2-1   Resume Building Blocks

1. Introduction
2. Education
3. Professional Skills and Knowledge
4. Work History
5. Licenses and Certifications
6. Honors and Awards
7. Special Skills
8. Volunteer Activities
9. Professional and Civic Organizations
10. Languages Spoken

build your resume throughout your education program. Complete the "To Do Now" section as you proceed through your classes. Some ask you to start collecting information; others give you ideas about activities to increase your employability; still others give you a chance to set goals to best take advantage of your education. The second section, entitled "Writing Your Resume," is to use later when you are putting together a resume for your job search. You will do this in Chapter 13, "Finalizing Your Employment Presentation Materials."

Building Block 1: Introduction

The introduction, or first section of your resume, can be written as a career objective, professional or career profile, or as a summary of your qualifications. Until recently, most resumes began with an objective: a brief description of the job the applicant was seeking. For example: "Occupational therapy assistant in a pediatric facility." A typical objective might also include a short statement of what the applicant can offer the employer: "Position in an orthopedic office where I can apply my excellent human-relations skills working with patients and fellow professionals."

Many career experts are now advising job applicants to omit the career objective from their resumes because it comes across as being more about what *you* want rather than about what you can offer the employer. They suggest that instead you provide a career profile or list of your qualifications for the target job. Use Resume Building Block # 1: Introduction to begin defining the kind of job you want and to begin listing your qualifications. Keep the list up-to-date as you progress through your training and acquire new skills.

Building Block 2: Education

The education section contains a list of all your education and training, with emphasis on health care training.

Start your list with the school you attended most recently. Include your grade point average and class standing (not all schools rank their students by grades) if they are above average. Use Resume Building Block #2: Education as a motivator to do your best academically.

Building Block 3: Professional Skills and Knowledge

Professional skills and knowledge refer to the technical skills and knowledge that contribute to successful job performance.

Resume Building Block #1 Introduction

Complete the "To Do Now" section as you proceed through your classes. Complete the "Writing Your Resume" section as you read Chapter 13, "Finalizing Your Employment Presentation Materials."

To Do Now

1. Career Objective: Start to think about the kind of job you want. You may change your objective for your first job several times while you are in school as you learn new subjects and get ideas from your lab and externship experiences. Even if you decide not to include an objective on your resume, creating one can provide motivation and help you focus on your future. List at least two sentences that describe your objective, as you see it now, for your first job in health care.
2. Personal Profile: Begin a list of the qualifications that apply to your occupational area.

Writing Your Resume

1. Write your career objective.
   OR
2. Write your career profile.

Resume Building Block #2 Education

Complete the "To Do Now" section as you proceed through your classes. Complete the "Writing Your Resume" section as you read Chapter 13, "Finalizing Your Employment Presentation Materials."

Your education is more than a list of schools you've attended. Take steps to get all you can out of your training program.

To Do Now

1. List five things you can do to get the most from your education.
2. Write three academic goals.

Writing Your Resume

1. List the schools, workshops, and other training you have attended, starting with the most recent.

The way you organize this section when you actually write your resume depends on your educational program and the number and variety of skills acquired. You can list them individually if there are not too many (such as "Take vital signs") or as clusters of related skills (such as "Perform clinical duties").

Listing individual skills or clusters of skills is a good idea if your previous work experience is limited and you want to emphasize the recent acquisition of health care skills as your primary qualification. Even if you decide not to include a skills list on your resume, starting a list now will keep you aware of what you know and have to offer an employer. Employers report that many recent graduates do not realize just how much they really know, and therefore they fail to sell themselves at job interviews.

Find out if your school provides lists of program and course objectives and/or the competencies you will master. Some

Resume Building Block #3 Professional Skills and Knowledge

Complete the "To Do Now" section as you proceed through your classes. Complete the "Writing Your Resume" section as you read Chapter 13, "Finalizing Your Employment Presentation Materials."

To Do Now

1. Track the skills you are learning by keeping an inventory for each of your subjects. Here are some examples of the kinds of skills to include:
   • Setting up dental trays for common procedures
   • Accurately completing medical insurance claim forms
   • Creating presentations using PowerPoint
   • Teaching a patient to use different ambulatory devices

Writing Your Resume

1. You can organize your professional skills and knowledge into clusters or write a list of individual skills.

instructors give their students checklists to monitor the completion of assignments and demonstration of competencies. Other sources of information include handouts from your instructor, such as **syllabi** and course outlines; the objectives listed in your textbooks; and lab skill sheets. Develop your own inventory of what you have learned using Resume Building Block #3: Professional Skills and Knowledge to begin a personal inventory of your skills. An additional benefit of tracking your progress is the sense of accomplishment you gain as you see the results of your hard work. You will be amazed by how much you are learning!

Building Block 4: Work History

The work history is a list of your previous jobs, including the name and location of the employer, your job title and duties, and the dates of employment.

You can benefit from this section of your resume even if you have no previous experience in health care. There are three ways to do this. The first is to review the duties and responsibilities you had in each of your past jobs. Which ones can be applied to health care work? Skills that are common to many jobs are called **transferable skills**. Take another look at the general skills listed in the SCANS report (see Box 1-2 in Chapter 1). Do you see any that you have used? Here are a few examples of general and more technical skills common to many jobs:

• Working well with people from a variety of backgrounds
• Creating efficient schedules that reduce employee overtime
• Purchasing supplies in appropriate quantities and at competitive prices
• Resolving customer complaints satisfactorily
• Performing word processing duties
• Managing accounts receivable
• Providing customer service
• Providing appropriate care for infants and toddlers

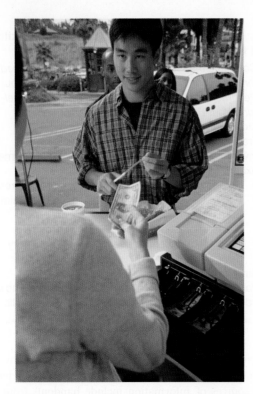

FIGURE 2-3 Many health care students have held jobs in which they developed transferrable skills. For example, a good cashier in a fast food restaurant provides quality customer service, arrives at work on time, works efficiently, and follows good hygiene standards when handling food. *List five skills from jobs you have had that apply to your future health care occupation.* (Copyright Steve Mason/Photodisc/Thinkstock)

Identifying transferable skills is especially important when you are entering a new field in which you have little or no experience. There is actually a type of resume that emphasizes skills and abilities rather than specific job titles held. It is called a "functional resume," and the format is described in Chapter 13. At this time, start compiling a list of possible transferable skills such as the ones illustrated by the cashier in Figure 2-3.

The second way to maximize the value of the work history section of your resume is to state what you achieved in each job. In a phrase or two, describe how you contributed to the success of your employer. When possible, state these achievements in measurable terms. If you can't express them with numbers, use active verbs that tell what you did. Here are some examples:

- Increased sales by 20%
- Designed a more efficient way to track supplies
- Worked on a committee to write an effective employee procedure manual that is still in use
- Trained five employees to use office equipment correctly

If you had jobs that didn't provide many opportunities for measureable accomplishments such as those listed above, think about what you *learned* from each job. For example, personal organization so that you always arrived at work on time; handling the responsibility of accepting cash from customers; and following the directions of your supervisor.

A third way to add value to this section is to include your externship experience. Although you must clearly indicate that this was a part of your training and not paid employment, it still serves as evidence of your ability to apply what you learned in school to practical situations. For many new graduates, this is their only real-world experience in health care. Some students make the mistake of viewing their externship experience as simply an add-on to their program; just one more thing to get through. They fail to recognize the impact their performance can have on their career. Remember that clinical supervisors represent future employers. (In some cases they *are* future employers because some students are hired by their externship sites.) Their opinion of you can help launch your self-marketing efforts successfully or cause them to fizzle, so commit to doing your best during your externship experience. The inclusion of a successful externship experience on your resume increases your chances of getting the job you want.

Use Resume Building Block #4: Work History to start compiling your work history.

Note: Do *not* be concerned if your work experience is limited or you can't think of any achievements. You may have finished high school recently or perhaps you spent several years working as a homemaker. Employers understand that everyone starts with a first job and you are receiving training to qualify you for work. And homemakers, as well as parents and others who care for family members, gain experiences that are valuable to employers. Examples include caring for others, practicing time management, and handling family finances.

Building Block 5: Licenses and Certifications

Some professions require you to be licensed or have specific types of approval before you are allowed to work. Nursing is one example. Others include physical or occupational therapy and dental hygiene. The kind of approvals needed vary by state and profession. Most licenses and certifications require certain types of training and/or passing a standardized exam. It is important for you to clearly understand any professional requirements necessary or highly recommended for your profession. Some professions, such as medical assisting, have certifications and registrations that are not required but that increase your chances of being hired.

Learn as much as you can now about the requirements for the occupation you have chosen. It is not advisable to wait until the end of your studies to start thinking about preparing for the required exams. Ask your instructors about review classes, books, and computerized material. Check with your professional organization. (See the contact list in Appendix). Become familiar with the topics on the exams, and plan your studies accordingly. Knowing the format of the questions (multiple choice, true-false, etc.) is also helpful. Increase your chances for success by preparing over time, the proven way to do well in exams. (Taking exams is covered in detail in Chapter 8.) Use Resume Building Block #5: Licenses and Certifications to start gathering information about certifications for your occupation.

Building Block 6: Honors and Awards

The section on honors and awards is an **optional** resume section. Your school may offer recognition for student achievements and special contributions. Community and professional organizations to which you belong may also give awards. Acknowledgments received for volunteer work can also be included in this section.

Investigate what you might be eligible for and use these rewards as incentives for excellent performance. Keep this in perspective, however. Awards should serve as motivators, not indicators of your value. They are nice to have but certainly not essential for getting a good job.

Use Resume Building Block #6: Honors and Awards to find out about the availability of awards for which you may qualify and the necessary requirements.

Building Block 7: Special Skills

Special skills are those that don't fit into other sections but do add to your value as a prospective employee. Examples

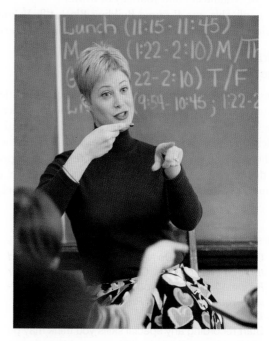

FIGURE 2-4 Many skills, such as sign language, enhance the value of the health care professional. *What skills do you already have that you can use in your future work?* (© Stockbyte/Stockbyte/Thinkstock)

include a proficiency in desktop publishing or the ability to use American Sign Language as illustrated by the teacher in Figure 2-4.

Research the needs of employers in your geographic area. Do you already have special skills that meet these needs? Would it substantially increase your chances for employment if you were to acquire skills outside the scope of your program; for example, becoming more proficient on the computer? If (and only if!) time permits, you may decide to attend workshops in addition to your regular program courses, do extra reading, or take a course on the Internet. Use Resume Building Block #7: Special Skills to record any skills that might supplement your qualifications.

Building Block 8: Volunteer Activities

Volunteer activities can be included on your resume if they relate to your targeted occupation or demonstrate any desired qualities such as being responsible and having concern for others. If you are already involved in these types of activities, think about what you are learning or practicing that can help you on the job. If you aren't, consider becoming involved if you have a sincere interest and adequate time available. Adult students face many responsibilities outside class, and the additional activities mentioned in this chapter should be taken as suggestions, not must-dos. Mastering your program content should be your first priority.

Box 2-2 contains examples of locations and programs that typically need volunteers. To find opportunities in your area, check the local newspaper or search the Internet by entering the term "volunteer" and your city or town.

If applicable, use Resume Building Block #8: Volunteer Activities to investigate opportunities and record your service.

Building Block 9: Professional and Civic Organizations

Professional organizations provide excellent opportunities to network, learn more about your field, and practice leadership skills. (See Appendix for a list of professional organizations.) Participation in **civic organizations**, groups that work for the good of the community, promotes personal growth and demonstrates your willingness to get involved in your community. Consider joining and participating actively in a professional or civic organization while you are in school. Find out whether your school or community has a local chapter. Use Resume Building Block #9: Professional and Civic Organizations to record your participation.

Building Block 10: Languages Spoken

In our multicultural society, the ability to communicate in a language other than English is commonly included on the resume. Find out whether many patients speak a language other than English in the area where you plan to work. Consider acquiring at least some conversational ability or a few phrases to use to reassure patients. Appendix contains a list of useful Spanish phrases for the medical professional. If your school offers these languages as elective courses, they would be good choices. Patient benefit greatly, during the stress of illness or injury, when health care professionals know at least a few phrases of their native language. Even speaking just a few basic phrases can increase your value to employers. Also consider learning about the customs,

---

Resume Building Block #7 **Special Skills**

Complete the "To Do Now" section as you proceed through your classes. Complete the "Writing Your Resume" section as you read Chapter 13, "Finalizing Your Employment Presentation Materials."

To Do Now
1. Start recording any special skills you think may be applicable to a job in health care.
2. How did you or how can you acquire each of the skills you listed?
3. How does each skill apply to health care?

Writing Your Resume
1. Describe your special skills.

Resume Building Block #8 **Volunteer Activities**

Complete the "To Do Now" section as you proceed through your classes. Complete the "Writing Your Resume" section as you read Chapter 13, "Finalizing Your Employment Presentation Materials."

To Do Now
1. List any volunteer activities you could use on your resume. Do you have time while you are in school for new or additional activities that are directly related to your career goals?
2. What skills have you acquired from your volunteer work?
3. What personal qualities have you demonstrated while volunteering?

Writing Your Resume
1. Describe your volunteer work and community service.

Resume Building Block #9 **Professional and Civic Organizations**

Complete the "To Do Now" section as you proceed through your classes. Complete the "Writing Your Resume" section as you read Chapter 13, "Finalizing Your Employment Presentation Materials."

To Do Now
1. List any professional and/or civic activities you could include on your resume. Are there any organizations you can join to gain experience and enrich your educational program?
2. What skills have you acquired or expect to acquire from these activities?

Writing Your Resume
1. Describe the professional and civic organizations you have joined.

BOX 2-2   Examples of Places and Programs that Need Volunteers

- Homes of seniors and the disabled
- Homeless shelters
- Assisted living and senior centers
- Hospices
- Hospitals
- Meals on Wheels
- Volunteers in Medicine
- Adaptive sport programs

especially the ones related to health practices, of ethnic groups in your community. (Cultural differences are discussed in Chapter 10.) Use Resume Building Block #10: Languages Spoken if you have or plan to acquire knowledge of another language.

Portfolios

A **portfolio** is an organized collection of items that document your capabilities and qualifications for work. A portfolio can give you a competitive edge at job interviews.

Starting to plan your portfolio now can cast your class assignments in a new light. More than work you hand in to your instructor, they can serve as demonstrations of your abilities to an employer. Strive to perform consistently at your highest level, producing work that will represent you well.

As you complete each course, save assignments that might be suitable for your portfolio. Store them in a folder or large envelope so they stay in good condition. In addition to written assignments, there are nontraditional ways to showcase your abilities. The items you collect need not be limited to evidence of your technical skills. For example, it is appropriate to include documentation of other activities, such as organizing an event for charity. No standard list of items to put in your portfolio exists, although your school may have prepared a list for students. In any case, only accurate and neat work should be included. How to finalize the contents and assemble your portfolio for presentation is covered in Chapter 13. See Box 2-3 and Figure 2-5 for examples of portfolio contents.

Promotion: The Fifth "P" of Marketing

Think about how companies use promotional campaigns to give new products maximum exposure. They advertise (sometimes endlessly, it seems!) on television, in magazines and newspapers, and on the Internet to spread the word to as many consumers as possible about how the product will fulfill their needs. You will undertake a similar campaign when you conduct your job search. As with your resume and portfolio, you can begin to prepare now. Networking, references, and the job interview are the three main ways to promote yourself during the job search.

Resume Building Block #10 Languages Spoken

Complete the "To Do Now" section as you proceed through your classes. Complete the "Writing Your Resume" section as you read Chapter 13, "Finalizing Your Employment Presentation Materials."

To Do Now
1. List the languages you speak other than English.
2. List the languages spoken by the patients in your geographic area.
3. Name any opportunities there may be to learn another language (even a few phrases are useful in the health care setting).

Writing Your Resume
1. What languages do you speak?

BOX 2-3　Examples of What to Include in Your Portfolio

1. Assignments
   - Accurately filled out insurance form
   - Accounting forms
   - Perfectly typed or word processed letter
   - Lab reports
   - Sample medical history form, filled out
   - Charting entries
   - Research report
2. Certificates of completion or achievement
   - Proof of having completed courses, seminars, and workshops
   - Proof of skill mastery, such as cardiopulmonary resuscitation (CPR), first aid, or the Burdick electrocardiographic (ECG) procedure, or documentation of the number of successful performances of an important procedure, such as venipunctures, injections, and x-ray studies
   - Documentation of word processing or data entry speed
   - Recognition of special achievements, such as honor or merit roll or perfect attendance
3. Grade records or transcripts
   - Consider including these if your grades are above average. If they started out as average or even below average and then improved as you advanced through your program, you could use them to demonstrate your persistence and progress.
4. Employer reviews or evaluations
   - You can include these from your previous employment if they demonstrate the attitudes or skills applicable to work in health care. A positive review from your externship supervisor can be very valuable because it is recent and relates directly to health care.
5. Recognition of your contributions
   - Thank-you letters you received
   - Proof of participation in activities such as walk-a-thons to raise money for worthy causes
6. Attendance record
   - An excellent addition if you have very good attendance
7. Honors and awards
8. Licenses or certifications (copies)
9. Photographs
   - Use these to document activities in which you played a major role, such as organizing a fundraising activity or planning and coordinating a school picnic.
10. Letters of recommendation

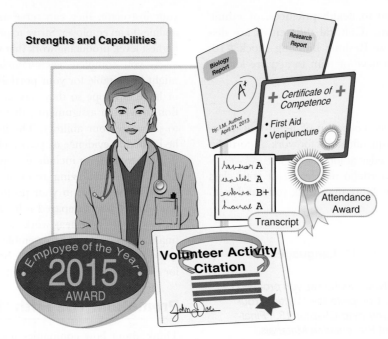

Strengths and Capabilities

Biology Report

A⁺

by: I.M. Author
April 21, 2013

Research Report

Certificate of Competence
• First Aid
• Venipuncture

A
A
B+
A

Transcript

Attendance Award

Employee of the Year
2015
AWARD

Volunteer Activity Citation

FIGURE 2-5 A professional portfolio supports your qualifications. *Start now to collect evidence of your qualifications for a job in health care.*

Q&A with a Career Services Professional

Melva Duran

Melva is the former director of Career Services at Kaplan College in San Diego. Melva shares insight on how new graduates can get a first job in the health field and the salary they should expect.

Q You usually work with students as they graduate and begin their job search. Do you have any recommendations for students as they begin their training for a job in health care?

A I think it's important for them to consider what they need to earn in terms of dollars and what they can reasonably expect when they are beginning a new career. Ideally, they will have researched starting pay for the career they've chosen to train for before they actually start school. Even if they haven't, it's important for students to understand that it might take time to work up to either a higher position or pay raises as they gain experience.

Q Do you suggest that students develop a budget?

A Absolutely. They should track their expenses to see what they need for the basics. If they are changing careers, they may earn less for a while. Knowing what they are spending helps them see where they can cut back until they are earning more.

Q Do you have examples of students who have done this?

A Well, I once had a student who was changing from a career in a financial institution to a career in medical billing. She had earned over $60,000 and was hoping to earn that much in the health field. I had to tell her that she would be starting out at about half that much but that with hard work and promotions, she could earn well in the billing field. We discussed how she could set short-term goals and plan to live on less until she got established.

Q Are there ways that graduates can increase the amount they earn in first-time jobs?

A Wages do vary from one part of a city to another and for the type of care offered or insurance accepted. As you know, reimbursement from a private insurance, Medicare, and so on varies and influences what employers can pay. Websites such as salary.com can give graduates a general idea of salaries but they are not always accurate for a specific geographic area or working conditions. It is best for students to do their own direct research on employers rather than depending on the information they find on the Internet.

When the job market is good, a qualified graduate may want to research a variety of employers. Sometimes traveling extra distance to a job is worth it if the pay and benefits are higher than with employers who are closer to home. Work schedules, such as a night shift, which are a little less convenient, may offer higher pay. This is why students should think about what they need so they can consider all the pros and cons of jobs that are available when they are ready to begin working.

Write down all your regular expenses for a three-month period for the following items. Include items that you are not paying now but can expect to pay in the future, such as student loan payments.

Mortgage or rent
Utilities
- Gas and/or electricity
- Television
- Telephone
- Internet access
- Garbage
- Water and sewer

Food
Child care
School expenses for children
Student loan payments (future)
Payments
- Car
- Credit card(s)
- Other

Transportation
- Fares
- Gas
- Car repairs
- Car registration and license

Nonfood grocery items
- Cleaning supplies
- Paper goods

Personal
- Grooming
- Haircuts
- Clothing
- Gifts
- Entertainment
- Vacation
- Savings

Add the three monthly totals and divide by three to calculate your average regular monthly expenses. This number will be total A.

Now list the expenses for items that occur less frequently.

Insurance
- Homeowner or renter
- Car
- Health
- Life
- Other

(*Note:* Health and disability insurance may be offered as employment benefits. This is discussed in Chapter 15.)

Property taxes
Income taxes

Divide the total by 12 to get the average monthly amount needed for these annual expenses. This number will be total B.

Add A and B totals to see how much you need to cover your expenses.

Networking

Networking, as we are using the word here, refers to meeting and establishing relationships with people who work in health care. It is an effective way to learn more about your chosen career. At the same time, it gets the word out about you and your employment goals. Many career experts report that networking is the best source of leads for job seekers. Examples of networking opportunities include attending professional meetings and career fairs; going on class field trips to health care facilities; and listening to guest speakers who come to your school.

There are many ways to begin networking. At a professional meeting, introduce yourself to other members; after hearing a guest speaker in class, ask questions; at a career fair, ask a local employer for advice about what to emphasize in your studies. Be sure to follow up with a phone call or thank-you note (traditionally mailed or e-mailed) to anyone who sends you information or makes a special effort to help you.

Another benefit of networking is building your self-confidence as you introduce yourself to people. You can improve your speaking proficiency and increase your ability to express yourself effectively. These are valuable skills you will use when attending job interviews. Start now to create a web of connections to help you develop professionally and assist you in your future job search and career.

To increase the effectiveness of your networking, consider making or purchasing personal business cards to give to people you meet. It adds a professional touch and ensures that they have the information they need to contact you. Companies such as Vistaprint.com enable you to create your own cards at a very reasonable cost.

Personal Reflection

1. What opportunities can I take advantage of now for professional networking?

Megan was eager to start her studies to become a surgical technologist. She had excelled in science, especially biology, in high school and had considered applying to the state university to study pre-med. However, her parents had struggled financially since the economic depression of 2009 when her father lost his managerial job. Megan realized that the cost of years of medical training would be prohibitive, even with scholarships, so she decided to train for a career that would allow her to begin work within two years.

Megan investigated the training programs in her city and decided to enroll in a certificate program that she could complete within a year. In one of her first classes, the instructor, Dr. McArthur, took some time to discuss career strategies and encourage the students to begin planning for their future. Dr. Mac, as the students call him, pointed out that although the health care industry was growing, students couldn't automatically assume they would find a job easily when they graduated.

"The demand for surgical technologists is growing," he explained, "but I would still urge you to get out there and network and get to know people who are working in the field." He then described the school's surgical technology club in which students could share ideas. He also gave the name of a local hospital that had a job shadow program for students.

Megan had never been very sociable, a "bookworm" her family called her, and found it hard to get excited about getting involved with clubs and programs that involved interaction with others. She only had a couple of close friends. As she told Andrea, one of them, "I like my classes, but I avoided all that social stuff in high school and I'm really not interested in getting started now!"

"I know you mostly like to keep to yourself," said Andrea. "Sometimes it's like pulling teeth to get you out of the house! Anyway, what kind of 'social stuff' are you talking about?"

"Oh, the school has some kind of a club for surgical technology students. Why would I spend time with them outside of class? I have enough to do with studying."

Andrea considered what Megan said. "You know, it wouldn't hurt to go to a meeting and see what it's about. If your instructor recommended it, maybe it has some value."

Megan responded, "I don't know. I'll think about it. But there's even more; he wants us to consider applying to St. Francis Hospital to job shadow and meet the professionals there. Can you see me doing something like that? I already dread having to face job interviews after I graduate but going and asking if I can hang out in the hospital when I don't even have any training? I just don't know."

Questions for Thought and Reflection

1. Why did Dr. Mac encourage the students to start thinking about their future job search and career while they were still in school?
2. What would you recommend to Megan if you were her friend?
3. Do you think Megan will have a difficult time becoming employed? Why or why not?

References

References are people who will confirm your qualifications, skills, abilities, and personal qualities. In other words, they endorse you as a product. Professional references are not the same as personal or character references. To be effective, professional references must be credible (believable) and have personal knowledge of your value to a prospective employer. Your best references have knowledge of both you and the health care field. Examples include your instructors, externship supervisors, and other professionals who know the quality of your work. Previous supervisors, even in jobs outside of health care, can also be good references.

Recall the discussion in this chapter about becoming a health care professional by conducting yourself as if you already were one. Start now to project a professional image to everyone you meet, including your instructors and other staff members at your school. Become the person others will be happy to recommend. When competition for jobs is intense, good references may be your key to landing the job you want.

Prescription for Success: 2-4 Planning Ahead

1. Who do you already know who would be a good professional reference?
2. What can you start doing now to ensure you have access to at least four positive recommendations when you begin your job search?

Job Interview

Job interviews provide the best opportunities to promote yourself to prospective employers. Interviewers often ask for examples of how you solved a problem or handled a given situation. Start thinking now about your past experiences and begin to collect examples from your work as a student, especially from your externship experience, that will demonstrate your capabilities. It is not too early to start preparing so you can approach your future interviews as opportunities to shine, be at ease and confident that you are presenting yourself positively like the applicant in Figure 2-6. Job interviews are discussed in detail in Chapter 14.

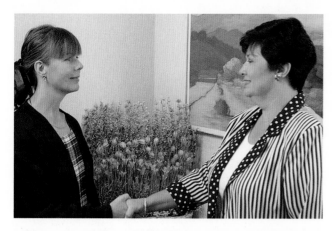

FIGURE 2-6 Put your best foot forward! *How is the job candidate on the left demonstrating self-confidence as she meets the employer for an interview? What can you start doing now to ensure you attend future interviews with confidence?* (From Bird D, Robinson D: *Modern dental assisting,* ed 11, St Louis, 2015, Saunders.)

Summary of Key Ideas

- Your attitude and expectations influence your future.
- A professional appearance has a positive influence on patients.
- The components of your resume can serve as a guide for career preparation and self-motivation.
- It is not too early to start networking and preparing for your job search.

Positive Self-Talk for This Chapter

- I have many qualities that will be of value to my future employers.
- I have a plan for preparing to become a successful health care professional.
- I am on my way to a great future.

Internal Activities

ⓔ For active links to the websites needed to complete these activities, visit http://evolve.elsevier.com/haroun/career/.

1. Use the search term "affirmations" and explore the websites listed. Then choose five affirmations to use for at least a week. Do you think using affirmations is helping you?

2. Use the search term "career networking" to find sites with information about this important job-search tool. Name five reasons to use networking. Include the names and addresses of the sites where you find the information.

3. Search "professional portfolio." Why is using a professional portfolio recommended in today's job search? Include the names and addresses of the sites where you find the information.

To Learn More

Covey S.R.: The 7 Habits of Highly Effective People, New York, 1990, Fireside

This book remains popular today in helping individuals apply a principle-centered approach to solve their personal and professional problems. Covey emphasized promoting personal success through fairness, integrity, honesty, and dignity. A summary of the habits is available at: www.stephencovey.com/7habits/7habits-habit1.php

Erupting Mind

www.eruptingmind.com
This website contains dozens of reader-friendly articles that offer self-improvement advice. The topics covered include self-esteem, success skills, and using mind power with affirmations and visualization.

Gawain S.: Creative visualization: use the power of your imagination to create what you want in your life, Novato, Calif, 2002, New World Library

This book, originally published in 1977, remains a classic in the use of visualization and affirmation to attain personal success. Creative visualization has been used in the fields of health, education, business, sports, and the arts. The author explains how to use mental imagery and affirmations to produce positive changes in one's life.

Key Career Networking Resources for Job Seekers

www.quintcareers.com/networking_resources.html
This website contains links to many articles and additional websites about career networking.

O*Net Online

www.onetonline.org
This website contains summary reports for hundreds of occupations that include tasks, the tools used, the required knowledge, skills, abilities, work activities, credentials, and more. Check out your occupational area to learn more.

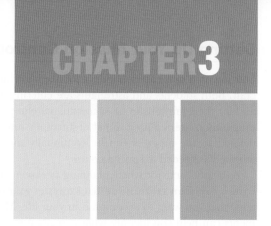

CHAPTER 3

Developing Your Personal Skills

OBJECTIVES

1. Create a personal mission statement.
2. Set achievable goals to help guide your life.
3. Recognize the advantages of maintaining a positive attitude.
4. Develop time-management and organizational strategies to improve your personal efficiency.
5. Incorporate stress-reducing habits into your life.
6. Practice healthy eating habits.
7. Engage in regular physical activity.
8. Identify and use personalized learning strategies.
9. Improve your ability to retain information.
10. Understand the benefits of having a mentor.

KEY TERMS AND CONCEPTS

Burnout Physical and emotional exhaustion, often caused by overwork and feeling that one's efforts are not appreciated.

Cholesterol Oily substance essential for body functions; at higher-than-normal levels, it is a major risk factor for heart disease and stroke.

Diet The kinds of foods a person usually eats (not to be confused with a plan to lose weight).

Efficiency Getting the most done with the least effort and waste of time.

Insomnia The inability to sleep well. It can be caused by worry, anxiety, or physical disorders.

Learning Styles Different ways of taking in, processing, and retaining information.

Linear Organized in a structured manner.

Mentor A knowledgeable advisor or coach.

Mission Statement A statement of your fundamental beliefs that serves as the foundation for your actions.

Peers People with whom you have something in common, such as other students and co-workers.

Prioritize Put in order of importance.

Procrastinate Put off doing something that needs to be done.

Refined Grains Grains that have been milled to remove the bran (outer layer) and germ (part of the seed). These two components contain healthy fiber and nutrients that are lost during the milling process. Examples of refined grain products include white bread, white flour, and white rice.

Relevant Meaningful or important.

Saturated Fats A type of fat that is solid at room temperature and tends to increase cholesterol levels in the blood. Examples of sources include butter, meat fat, and coconut oil.

Stress Physical and emotional reactions to life's events.

Trans Fat (also called: trans-fatty acid; partially hydrogenated oil) Fats created when hydrogen is added to liquid vegetable oils to make them solid.

Values Beliefs about what is important in life.

Setting Up Your Mission Control

Starting on a new career path is a lot like launching a spacecraft. Both students and astronauts are entering new worlds, and for their missions to be successful, careful planning and preparation are required. Final destinations must be clearly defined so the progress can be continually monitored and adjusted as needed to stay on course.

A helpful activity when planning a career launch is to write a **mission statement** that expresses your basic beliefs and what you want to accomplish in your life. Mission statements can help you identify what is really important to you and keep you on track to accomplish your goals. Individual mission statements are based on personal values. **Values** are our beliefs about what is important in life. They are the result of the teachings of our family, school, religion, and friends as well as our experiences in life. Values provide a foundation for making important life decisions, such as what we hope to contribute to the world, how we perform our work, and what we believe our obligations are to others and to ourselves.

Mission statements should be written out but there is no set format. You may want to write yours as a list, a series of paragraphs, or even a letter addressed to yourself. If you prefer, you can create a poster or collage, with each picture illustrating a value. Box 3-1 contains a sample mission statement written by Sarah, a student of medical assisting.

Mission statements can serve as powerful motivators. For example, if you are committed to the well-being of your future patients, this value, rather than simply the need to pass a test, should guide your studying. Suppose you have an anatomy test tomorrow morning. It is 10:00 PM and you have just finished a day filled with classes, work, and family responsibilities. Studying the skeleton becomes more meaningful when placed in the context of your dedication to helping future patients. You are not simply memorizing a collection of bones. You are learning about the source of Mrs. Jones's painful arthritis, and the more you know and understand about the bones and joints, the more you will be able to help her. Figure 3-1 illustrates the importance of focusing on what is really important to you—your major goals in life.

Keep in mind throughout your program that your future patients will be directly affected both by what and how you are studying now, so you should be guided by your highest values. Here's another example: suppose that your mission statement includes the statement, "Provide high-quality care to all patients." You have an important exam for which you feel unprepared, and you are offered an opportunity to cheat. Cheating may take care of what you believe to be your most urgent need—getting a passing grade. But the consequences of this action—not learning the material and compromising your integrity—do not align with your stated goal of competently serving the needs of future patients.

Prescription for Success: 3-1 Create Your Own Mission Statement

Develop a mission statement for your life as a student and future health care professional. Use the following questions as a guide for what to include. You may write out your mission statement or express it in another way, such as with drawings, pictures taken from other sources, your own photographs, or any other medium that works for you.

1. What do you most admire in other people?
2. How do you want to be remembered by people who matter to you?
3. Who do you most respect? Why?
4. If you could accomplish only three things in life, what would they be?
5. What makes you happiest? Why?
6. Which activities give you the greatest sense of purpose and satisfaction?

Exercise adapted from Covey S, Merrill AR, Merrill RR: *First things first,* New York, 1995, Simon and Schuster.

BOX 3-1 Sarah's Mission Statement

My decisions and actions will be based on my dedication to:

- Maintaining my health and that of my family
- Balancing my work and family life so that neither is neglected
- Doing my best to master the professional skills of a medical assistant
- Serving the needs of all patients with whom I work
- Continuing to learn about my profession
- Being loyal to my family, friends, and employer
- Keeping a positive attitude
- Seeking to understand rather than to judge others

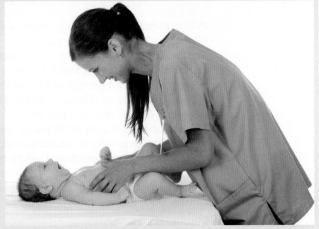

(Copyright Zdenka Darula/iStock/Thinkstock.)

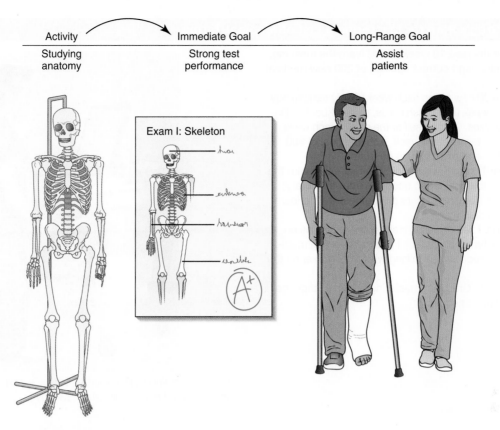

Activity	Immediate Goal	Long-Range Goal
Studying anatomy	Strong test performance	Assist patients

Exam I: Skeleton

A+

FIGURE 3-1 Keep your values and purpose in mind. What you do now as a student will influence the success of your future career. *Can you name three things you can do now to help you reach an intermediate goal? A long-term goal?*

Goals—Signposts on the Path to Success

"Success is steady progress toward one's personal goals."

—Jim Rohn

Goals are based on your mission statement and serve as signposts, giving your life direction and measuring your progress on the road to success. Use them to motivate yourself and mark your accomplishments. Effective goals have the following characteristics:

- They are based on your values and mission statement: The goals help you achieve what you believe to be important in life.
- They are reasonable: You may have to work hard but you can accomplish them.
- They are measurable: You'll know when you have achieved them.
- They are clearly stated and written: Writing down goals greatly increases your chance of reaching them.

Here are two examples of well-stated goals for a health care student:

1. Over the next 10 weeks, I will learn the definition, pronunciation, and spelling of 150 medical terms.

2. Within the next month, I will attend one professional meeting and talk with at least two people I have not met before.

Making Goals Work for You

"Discipline is the bridge between goals and accomplishments."

—Jim Rohn

Many people fail to achieve what they want in life because they fail to set clear goals for themselves. The first step, then, to is to spend some time deciding what it is you want to accomplish. The next step is to put together an action plan in which you outline what you need to do to reach each goal. Include reasonable deadlines for completing these actions. This is also the time to identify and locate any resources you may need to carry out your action plan. Examples of resources include people, materials, classes, equipment, and money. Greg, a nursing student, is studying medical terminology. He knows that he will need a good knowledge of terminology in his career. Box 3-2 contains his plan to learn 300 medical terms.

Incorporate working toward goals into your daily life. What can you do each day—even if it is something small—to move closer to achieving them? Long-term goals can be put aside in the scramble to meet everyday obligations, so it's a good idea to periodically review your goals and track your progress.

- *Goal:* Over the next 10 weeks, I will learn the meaning, pronunciation, and correct spelling of 300 new medical terms.
- *Plan:* Learn 30 new terms each week. Study terminology 4 hours per week using flash cards, the workbook, CDs, and self-quizzes. Quiz myself at the end of each week.
- *Deadline:* 30 terms each week. Achieve goal of 300 words at the end of 10 weeks on (date).
- *Resources:* Text and workbook; CD that came with the textbook; additional tapes and CDs from the library; suggestions from instructors on the best way to learn; the medical dictionary.
- *Visualization:* I see myself in class receiving 100% on the medical terminology test. I see myself using medical terms correctly when talking with a co-worker on the job.
- *Affirmation:* "I, Greg, am mastering medical language easily and on schedule."

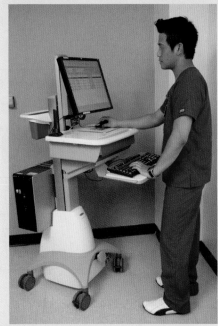

(From Sorrentino S, Remmert L: *Mosby's textbook for nursing assistants*, ed 8, St Louis, 2012, Mosby.)

Long-Term Goals

"When it is obvious that goals cannot be reached, don't adjust the goals, adjust the action steps."

—Confucius

Create and write out your major, long-term goals first; then prepare short-term supporting goals. Link them together in a progressive series so each one supports the next (see Figure 3-1). Let's look at an example: Jaime's long-term career goal is to become successfully employed as an x-ray technician in a large city hospital. Here is his plan:

- Long-term goal: Employment as an x-ray technician
- Short-term goals: Graduate from an approved x-ray training program
  - Take a study skills course
  - Earn at least a B in all courses
  - Maintain perfect attendance for all classes
  - Complete all homework assignments on time
  - Receive a rating of at least "above average" on clinical experience
  - Pass the state licensing exam on the first try

As we discussed in Chapter 1, you may have to set short-term employment goals as a means of achieving your long-term ideal job goal. In Jaime's case, he discovers that the large urban hospital where he wants to work hires only technicians who have had at least 1 year of experience. Furthermore, they prefer technicians who are able to perform specialized x-rays not taught in most x-ray technology programs. So Jaime adjusts his goals as follows:

- Long-term goal: Employment in x-ray department at Grand Memorial Hospital
- Short-term goals: Receive a rating of "Excellent" on clinical experience
  - Improve communication skills
  - Work for at least one year in a facility that performs a variety of x-ray studies
  - Complete three specialized x-ray courses
  - Network with local professionals
  - Become active in the x-ray professional organization's local chapter

Jaime knows his clinical experience will provide valuable opportunities to demonstrate his hands-on competence as a technician. This will serve him well when he applies for his first job after graduation and will also supplement his work experience when he applies at Grand Memorial. His action steps to achieve his short-term goals include arranging reliable transportation (his old car is no longer dependable) so he can always arrive at his clinical site on time. By planning ahead, setting goals, and identifying appropriate action steps, Jaime has greatly increased his chances of achieving what he really wants.

Success Tips for Achieving Your Goals

- Visualize yourself achieving your goals.
- Use affirmations.
- Work on goals even when you don't feel like it. (Especially then!)
- Don't give up!

Planning Ahead

Rosa Gonzalez, introduced in Chapter 1, is the first child in her family to go to college. Her parents have worked hard to support their family and encouraged their children to take advantage of all educational opportunities. However, money is scarce and Rosa has a part-time job to help pay for school expenses. It is not easy working and going to school, but she believes that it is through a good education that she will be able to get ahead in life. She wants to not only train for a career in health care, but also to serve as an example for her younger brothers and sisters.

Rosa is studying medical assisting. She wants to do well so her parents will be proud of her. Her career goal is to work as a back-office assistant with a plastic surgeon, helping the physician with outpatient procedures. Her interest in plastic surgery began when she saw the miraculous work performed on a young cousin who was disfigured after being burned in a fire.

Early in her program Rosa did some research and found that there were only a few plastic surgeons in her town and they all preferred to hire assistants with previous work experience. Rosa decides not to let this information discourage her and creates a plan of short- and long-term goals to help her achieve her career dream.

While in school, Rosa asks her instructor to recommend books and articles about plastic surgery and allow her to spend extra practice time in the lab so she can reach a high level of competence with sterile techniques, surgical instruments, wound care, and related skills. At the same time, Rosa works hard in her classes, asking for help when necessary and completing all homework assignments.

On graduating, Rosa decides to look for a job with a general practitioner or pediatrician who does minor surgery in the office. Her entry-level job goals are to gain experience with sterile techniques, standard precautions, surgical assisting, and patient care. She knows that this experience will help her reach her goal of working with a plastic surgeon some day.

Questions for Thought and Reflection

1. Why do you think Rosa wants to serve as an example for her siblings?
2. What would have happened if Rosa had not researched her career goal before she completed her medical assisting program?
3. How do Rosa's short-term goals serve as stepping stones for reaching her long-term goal?
4. Do you think Rosa will achieve her goal of working with a plastic surgeon? Why or why not?

Prescription for Success: 3-2 **Name That Goal**

1. Write down a goal and then determine the following information to achieve your goal:
   - Deadline
   - Action step 1
     - Deadline for the action step
     - Resources I will need
   - Action step 2
     - Deadline for the action step
     - Resources I will need
2. Explain how your goal relates to your mission statement and supports your values.
3. Think of a visualization to help you achieve your goal. Briefly describe it.
4. Write two affirmations to help you achieve your goal.

On the Job

Using Goals on the Job In addition to promoting your own growth and progress, the ability to set appropriate goals and take action to achieve them increases your effectiveness as a health care professional. Patients often benefit from goal setting, for example, when they are recovering from an illness or injury, arranging to pay a large medical bill, or attempting to follow a weight-loss plan. By developing your own goal-setting skills, you can share this knowledge and help patients plan the steps necessary to achieve their goals.

In some professional areas, such as physical and occupational therapy, goal setting is an integral part of the rehabilitation plan. Working with clients to set goals that are both realistic and challenging is an important part of therapy. You can use the same principles for both personal and patient/client-focused goal setting.

It's All in the Attitude

"Man is not disturbed by the things that happened, but by the perception of things that happened."

—Confucius

Your attitude, the way you mentally look at things, can be your strongest ally or your worst enemy. It is more powerful than physical strength, more important than natural talents, and has helped people overcome seemingly impossible difficulties. Many survivors of concentration and prison camps, for example, attribute their survival to having a positive attitude. The best thing about attitude is that it does not depend on other people or circumstances. It is yours alone, one of the few things in life over which you have complete control.

We hear about positive and negative attitudes to describe how people interpret things. Is the weather partly sunny or partly cloudy? Is a difficult class an opportunity to grow intellectually or a nightmare? Dr. Philip Hwang, a popular professor at the University of San Diego, tells his students he prefers to interpret a popular offensive gesture as "half a peace sign." He chooses his reaction, and this is the key to the power of attitude: we all can choose how we react to any situation.

"Well," you may say, "that doesn't make sense. If someone insults me or I'm having a bad day, it's natural to get angry or feel frustrated." It does seem natural because we are in the habit of responding negatively to situations that are annoying or upsetting. But how does this benefit you? For example, if you develop a negative attitude about a class ("I'll never learn how the endocrine system works," or "She really can't expect us to perform 20 perfect venipunctures after 2 weeks!"), you are working against yourself. Your attitude, whether positive or negative, will not change the circumstances. A negative attitude, however, can make it more difficult for you to understand the endocrine system or master venipunctures. A negative attitude is distracting, drains your energy, and interferes with your ability to concentrate. Choosing to approach life with a positive attitude releases you from the control of the circumstances and frees you to focus fully on the actions that are in line with your mission and goals. Table 3-1 contains a list of suggestions for developing a positive approach to life.

Prescription for Success: 3-3 It's All How You Look at It

Scenario 1 Your medical terminology class is more difficult than you expected. You must memorize long lists of words and parts of words and take quizzes twice a week. To make matters worse, the instructor is quite strict and does not seem very sympathetic. For each of the following options, decide whether it reflects a positive or negative attitude. Then describe the probable outcome of each attitude.
- Be angry with the instructor and his "ridiculous" expectations.
- Focus on the fact that learning terminology relates to your goals of becoming a health care professional.
- Complain to your classmates about the unfairness of the situation.
- Organize a study group with your classmates.
- Meet with the instructor privately and ask for study suggestions.
- Look for ways to apply your learning style (discussed later in this chapter) to learning the terms.

- Skip class whenever possible because it doesn't really do any good to attend.
- Think up and say affirmations stating you are mastering the vocabulary.
- Don't waste your time studying because you won't remember the words anyway.
- Think about how you will use medical terminology on the job.

Scenario 2 You are working as a physical therapist assistant for a home health agency. Overall, you like your job and enjoy helping patients in their homes to regain their mobility and strength after surgery and injuries. However, one of your clients is a teenager who is recovering from a cycling accident. You find her very difficult to work with. She is rude and seems to resent your efforts to help her. List six ways of handling this situation, and label each as being either a positive (effective) or negative (ineffective) reaction.

TABLE 3-1
Focusing on the Positive

Suggestion	Ask Yourself
Do an inventory of the good things in your life	What do I have to be thankful for? Good health? Friends? Family? Decent living conditions? Opportunity to attend school? Ability to succeed in school and start a new career?
Keep things in perspective	How important will this problem or situation be to me in 1 month? In 1 year?
Fix your sights on your mission and goals	Should I distract my focus and waste energy on negativity? How will a positive attitude be better in helping me get what I want and need?
Distinguish between what you can and cannot change, and concentrate your efforts on what you can change	What action can I take? Which negative people and situations can I avoid? What changes can I make to improve the situation?
Find sources of help and inspiration	Who can give me support? Who can give me advice? Do I have problems, such as depression or substance abuse that could be helped with professional assistance?
Visualize the satisfaction you can receive by overcoming a difficult situation	How will this contribute to my personal growth? What can I learn from this?
Challenge your negative beliefs	Is this belief based on facts or on false perceptions and old ideas?

Tripped Up by Your Thoughts

"The only thing we have to fear is fear itself."

—Franklin D. Roosevelt

In Chapter 2, you read about how what we expect is often what happens—we get or become what we think! In fact, negative expectations can be just as powerful as positive ones, sometimes even more powerful. This is because our mental images, whether positive or negative, help create our reality. It is important to understand that doubts and worries can actually bring about the outcome you fear. For example, Melinda thinks her supervisor dislikes her, so she avoids him and reacts defensively whenever he makes suggestions about her work. As a result of Melinda's behavior, the chances are good that the supervisor will have a problem with her. Tripped up by her thoughts, Melinda ends up creating what she expects and fears. Graciela, pictured in Figure 3-2, uses a different approach with her supervisor.

The fact is, your attitude greatly influences your performance in school and your ability to secure and succeed in the job you want. Expect the best for yourself and you are more likely to get it.

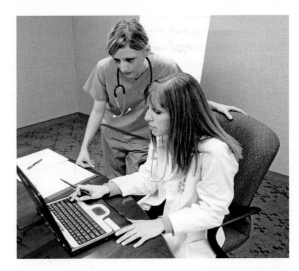

FIGURE 3-2 When Graciela makes a mistake inputting data, as sometimes happens with employees who are new on the job, she seeks help from her supervisor. Instead of fearing that her supervisor will dislike her—or even discipline her for the mistake—she approaches the situation as an opportunity to learn. *How does Graciela's attitude differ from that of Melinda? Who do you think is the most successful employee?* (From Yoder-Wise PS: *Leading and managing in nursing,* ed 6, St Louis, 2015, Mosby.)

On the Job

Attitude on the Job Employers know that health care professionals with a positive attitude contribute to the success of their facility because their attitude can promote the well-being of patients and improve the spirit of teamwork among the staff. Patients seek health care in times of need, and they bring with them an assortment of fears and doubts. They want hope and encouragement along with solutions to their health problems. Your cheerfulness, energy, and enthusiasm can assist in their recovery and increase their satisfaction with the care they are receiving. Your goodwill is an important part of the example you set as a role model. In short, your positive attitude can make a difference in the lives of those you serve. Happiness is contagious and is one thing we want to both give to others and catch from them!

Make Time Work for You

"Plan your work and work your plan."

Your success in life depends, to a large degree, on how you manage your time. Learning to use it to your advantage requires planning and self-discipline but the payoffs are well worth the effort. One fact of life is true for everyone: there will never be enough time for everything you want to do. There are ways, however, to use your time more effectively. Two key strategies are prioritizing and practicing efficiency. **Prioritizing** means deciding what is most important and taking care of those tasks first. Your goals should determine your priorities. What do you most want to accomplish? Are you spending enough time and energy on the activities that will help you achieve your goals? For example, if your goal is to graduate from a medical lab

technician program with honors, are you spending the necessary time attending class, studying, and developing the work habits required of a lab technician? Or are phone conversations, Internet surfing, television viewing taking up a lot of your time?

Efficiency means planning and making the best use of time—getting the most done with the least effort. Examples of inefficiency include running to the grocery store to pick up a forgotten item, spending time looking for misplaced homework, and stopping for gas when you're already late for class rather than filling up the tank the day before. It's easy to feel very busy and yet be inefficient. Pay attention to how you spend your time. A short break from studying to "rest your eyes" can stretch into an evening of lost hours in front of the television set.

Keeping a calendar is an important part of good time management. Many types of calendars and planners are available. Especially popular today are those available on phones. They allow you to store lots of information, including your schedule, telephone numbers, and other reference information. The important thing is to select the best kind for you—one you will use. It should be convenient to carry with you and should have room to list several items for each date.

Collect all the sources of important school and class dates: schedules, catalogs, and class syllabi. Mark important items on your calendar, including dates of quizzes and tests; due dates for assignments, projects, and library books; school holidays (for both you and your children); and deadlines for handing in the required paperwork, such as financial aid and professional exam applications, and for paying fees. Add important personal dates: birthdays of family members and friends, deadlines for bills and taxes, doctors' appointments, and back-to-school nights for your children. If you work, note the dates you need to remember, such as the company potluck party, your performance review, and project deadlines.

Success Tips for Managing Your Time

- Consider your priorities and goals when you plan your schedule and decide how to spend your time.
- Write out a weekly schedule. Take a few minutes every week to plan ahead. This allows you to coordinate your activities with family members, plan ahead for important days (to avoid trying to find just the right birthday present on the way to the party), combine errands to save time, and plan your study time to avoid last-minute cramming.
- Write a to-do list each day. List the activities in their order of importance.
- Schedule study time every day. This is a high priority! Give yourself a chance to succeed. Arrange not to be disturbed, and let friends and family members know that when you are at your desk, the time is yours.
- Schedule around your peak times. We all have individual body rhythms, specific times of the day when we feel most alert and energetic. Some people do their best work late at night. Others accomplish the most between 5:00 AM and 9:00 AM. Class and work schedules cannot always accommodate your needs, but when you have a choice, do the most challenging tasks during your best hours.
- Do the hardest thing first. When you have a number of things to do or subjects to study, try tackling the most difficult one first, when you are freshest. Completing unpleasant tasks gives you a surge of energy by removing a source of worry and distraction from your mind and rewarding you with a sense of accomplishment.
- Be realistic about what you can accomplish and how much time tasks will take to complete. For example, thinking you can complete a research paper in one weekend can be a serious mistake because you may run into difficulties and end up with no time to spare. You will learn more about your work speed as you progress through your program. At the beginning, it is best to plan more time than you think you will need.
- Prevent feeling overwhelmed by breaking work into small segments. (The thought of writing this book was overwhelming until I broke it down into chapters, topics, and pages.) Plan deadlines for each segment, and put them on your calendar.
- Learn to say "no." Your schedule cannot always accommodate the requests of other people. It's difficult, but sometimes necessary, to turn down demands on our time such as an invitation to a party or a request to help at the church rummage sale. An instructor who reviewed this book said the following response works very well: "I'm really sorry but I won't be able to help. I wish you the best in finding someone who can."
- Use down time to your advantage. There are many pockets of time that usually go to waste, such as when waiting for an appointment or using public transportation. Use this time to study flash cards, write lists, review class notes, brainstorm topics for a research paper, review the steps involved in a lab procedure, or summarize the major points of a class lecture. (I did about half the work toward my last college degree while sitting in airports and on airplanes.)

Control of Time, Control of Life

Sam was late again. He had overslept, then couldn't find his car keys. On top of everything else, he discovered that he didn't have clean clothes ready for the day. He dreaded the look—and possible lecture—he would get from his boss, physical therapist Angie Johnson.

The tough part was that Sam loved his job as a physical therapist assistant and didn't want to lose it. He had worked hard, actually struggled at times, to complete his program at Good Therapy Institute, and he didn't want to lose everything now because of his tardiness.

Feeling stressed as he drove to work, he went over in his mind how hard it seemed for him to stay on top of things in his life. He noticed that many of his friends and classmates seemed to have things under control and he wondered why everything seemed so hard for him.

Control of Time, Control of Life

Today felt like the last straw. He was tired of being rushed and worried and decided to see if Angie had any advice. After all, she was well aware of his problem. Maybe if he talked with her, she would realize that he was serious about improving.

There were already patients waiting in the office when he arrived, so he knew Angie would be annoyed with his tardiness again. Fortunately, everyone hurried along and by lunch time the office was on schedule. Sam asked Angie if they could talk in her office. "Sure," she answered. "In fact, we've *got* to have a talk about your work habits."

Once in her office, Angie told Sam that in spite of his being good with patients, it didn't help her when he wasn't there on time to begin the day with the early appointments. "Sam," she said, looking directly at him, "you've got to get yourself organized or you're not going to make it in this office—or in this field, for that matter."

Sam looked down at his hands and said in a soft voice, "I know, Angie, and that's what I wanted to talk to you about. I love this job and I want to be good at it. But I just can't seem to get my act together. I thought maybe you'd have some suggestions."

"Well," she said, "you seem to have a lot of trouble with time management. Tell me, do you write lists and prioritize your tasks so that get the most important things done first?"

"No," said Sam. "I just keep stuff in my head and do what seems right at the time."

Angie asked Sam how he was able to finish his homework and the studying needed to pass his exams at school.

Sam laughed. "I pulled a lot of late nights—even some all-nighters. There always seemed to be other stuff to get done, so a lot of times I didn't sit down to study till maybe 10 or so at night."

Angie thought for a few moments and said, "We may have identified part of the problem—and it has to do with prioritizing. When you say you had "other stuff to get done," I want you to think about it—was it more important than studying? Keep in mind that you had a big investment in school—and that you did want to work in physical therapy. Do you like your job here?"

Sam sat up in his chair. "Absolutely. I really like working here."

"I thought so," said Angie, "and you *are* good at it. But you've got to get control of your time, arrive at work promptly, and"—she smiled—"make time to do your laundry. We'll start by talking about prioritizing. I'm also going to recommend a couple of books on time management that I think will help you."

Sam was so appreciative that he had found someone to help him—his boss, no less. He promised himself that he would do his best to learn about and practice time management and personal organization. He had so much to gain.

Questions for Thought and Reflection

1. What made Sam finally seek help for his tardiness and disorganization?
2. Why do you think Angie was willing to help him?
3. How would learning to prioritize improve Sam's life?
4. Do you think Sam will be successful with time management? Why or why not?

Prescription for Success: 3-5 **Beat the Clock**

1. Based on your goals, which activities should receive the most of your time and attention while you are in school?
2. Using your planner or calendar, set up a personal schedule. Include all the important dates for the next month.
3. Plan a more detailed schedule for next week. Write in the major tasks you want to accomplish each day.
4. Identify your peak times, and describe how you can best use them.

On the Job

Time Management on the Job A growing concern in the United States today is providing health care in a cost-effective manner. As a consequence, efficient scheduling and good use of time are increasingly important for health care facilities. A major expense for any employer is paying employees, which translates to paying for the time they are on the job. Using your time efficiently at work will contribute to the overall financial success of the organization.

A specific application of time management on the job is patient scheduling. In a clinic or doctor's office, scheduling may be performed by the receptionist or administrative medical assistant. The first part of this important responsibility is to properly schedule appointments for smooth patient flow. The second part is working throughout the day to coordinate office activities and ensure that, with the exception of emergencies, everyone is kept on schedule. Waiting to see the doctor is reportedly the most common patient complaint because it gives the impression the office does not value the patient's time. And constantly playing "catch up" is stressful for the staff. Good time management creates a better work environment and increases the quality of customer service.

Defeating the Procrastination Demon

To **procrastinate** is to put off doing what needs to be done. Procrastinating can cause late assignments, failed tests, poor recommendations, and increased stress. Yet many of us fall victim to this self-defeating habit. Although it's natural to delay what you perceive to be difficult, tedious, or overwhelming, there are steps you can take to break the habit.

The first step is to identify the reason for your procrastination. What is holding you back? Are you afraid of failing? Do you believe you lack the ability to do what needs to be done? Does the task seem so unpleasant you cannot motivate yourself to start it? Is the project so large you feel overwhelmed and are the victim of "overload paralysis"? Once you have identified the reason, examine it carefully. Is it true you don't have the ability? Can the job be broken down into manageable portions?

The next step is to set a time to start, even if you simply work on planning what you are going to do. Accomplishing a small amount can inspire you to keep going. Look for ways to break large projects into manageable pieces and plan deadlines for each. Develop a controlled sense of urgency (not panic!) to encourage yourself to meet self-imposed deadlines.

If you find yourself stuck, identify sources of help, such as your instructor, your supervisor, or a friend. Perhaps you need additional materials or more information to get started. Try using affirmations such as, "I am capable of understanding how the nervous system functions." "My presentation to the class will be interesting and well organized." Visualize yourself completing the work. Experience the feeling of satisfaction. Finally, focus on your future. Think about how completing the work on time will help you achieve your goals to graduate and get a good job.

Prescription for Success: 3-6 Defeating the Demon

Note: Students who never procrastinate may skip this exercise.
1. What have you been putting off doing?
2. Why do you think you have been procrastinating on this task?
3. Which of the techniques listed in this chapter do you think would help you most?
4. Develop a plan to get started, including the date you will begin.

Personal Organization: Getting It All Together

"A vital key to success is learning to work smarter, not harder."

The purpose of personal organization, like time management, is to make life easier. Organizational techniques build consistency and predictability into your daily routines, saving you time and energy. Surprise-filled adventures are great for vacation trips but efficiency is a better way to ensure academic and career success. Hunting for your keys every morning and arriving late for class is a waste of your time and a sign of inconsideration for your instructor and classmates. On the job, a lack of organization can reduce patient satisfaction. No one wants to wait while the massage therapist scurries about to gather clean sheets or the relaxation music CD she wanted to play.

Organization, however, should never be an end in itself. It doesn't mean keeping a perfectly tidy house, with clothes arranged according to color and season. It does mean surveying your needs and developing ways to avoid unnecessary rushing, repetition, and waste.

Success Tips for Getting Organized

- **Write lists.** Most people today, especially students, have too many things on their minds to remember grocery lists, all the day's errands, who they promised to call, which lab supplies to take to class, and so on. Scraps of paper are easy to lose. Commercial organizers and planners, both paper and electronic, give you a place to record phone numbers, the addresses of stores, recommendations from friends, ideas you think of throughout the day, and so on.
- **Carry a big bag.** A typical student's day may include classes, work, shopping, and errands such as picking up a prescription. Start each day—either in the morning or the night before—by checking your calendar and to-do list to see what you need to take with you. If you go directly to class from work, pack your books, binder, uniform, and other necessary supplies. Take along a healthy snack to avoid having to raid the vending machines. Always carry your planner or calendar and/or phone.
- **Stock up.** Running out of milk, shampoo, or diapers can lead to a frustrating waste of time and energy. Even worse is discovering at 11:30 PM, while finishing a major assignment due in the morning, that your printer cartridge is empty and you don't have another. (Cartridges seem to be well aware of deadlines and choose to dry up accordingly!) Keep important backup supplies on hand. A handy way to monitor these is to keep a shopping list on the refrigerator and instruct everyone in the household to list items as they run low.
- **Give things a home.** Keeping what you need where you can find it saves search time. It also prevents redoing lost assignments or paying late fees on misplaced bills. If your study area is a dual-use area such as the kitchen table, try keeping your books and supplies in one place on a shelf or in a box or basket where everything can stay together. This way you can set up an "instant desk" when it is time to study. Organize your class notes and handouts by subject in a binder. Color-coded files work well for keeping ongoing projects and notes from previous classes in order.
- **Keep things in repair.** Life is easier if you can depend on the car and other necessities. If money is tight, focus on keeping the essentials in working order and look for ways to economize elsewhere.
- **Cluster errands.** Modern life requires trips to the grocery store, the mall, the children's school, the post office—you name it, we go there! Save time and money by doing as much as possible on each trip. Look for shopping centers that have many services to avoid running all over town.

- **Take advantage of technology.** Take advantage of your computer, tablet, and/or phone to shop, pay bills, and perform other tasks.
- **Handle it once.** If you find that mail, bills, announcements, and other paperwork accumulate in ever-growing piles, try processing each item as it comes in. Sort the mail quickly each day and do something with each piece: discard the junk, pay the bills (or file them together for payment once or twice a month), read messages and announcements, and place magazines in a basket to be looked at when you have time. Handle other papers that come into the house—permission slips for the kids, announcements from work—the same way.
- **Get it over with.** Certain disagreeable items, like parking tickets and dental work, come into everyone's life. It's easy to spend time worrying about them. A good strategy is to get them over with as quickly as possible: pay the ticket or make an appointment with the dentist. Procrastinating and worrying can drain your energy and interfere with your concentration.
- **Plan backups.** Prearrange ways to handle emergencies: a ride to school if the car breaks down, childcare to cover for a sick babysitter, a study buddy who will lend you notes if you miss a class. Backups are like insurance policies—you hope you won't need them but if you do, they're good to have.

If getting organized seems like a waste of time, too much work, or just "not your style," consider the alternative: losing even more time and energy in unproductive ways that result in frustration and inconvenience. You can start now to help yourself get it together at the same time you develop organizational skills that are valuable in all health care occupations.

On the Job

Organization on the Job A typical job description for a medical assistant includes many organizational duties that correspond closely with the success tips listed in this section:
1. Sort and handle the mail daily. (Handle it once.)
2. Monitor warranties on equipment, and call for maintenance and repair. (Keep things in repair.)
3. Check inventory and order administrative, laboratory, and clinical supplies. (Stock up.)
4. Organize and store supplies and equipment. (Give things a home.)
5. Complete all tasks as directed by the physician. (Write lists.)

Taking Care of Your Health

Achieving and maintaining good health will pay tremendous rewards for you as a student and future employee. Working in health care can be stressful and physically demanding. Therefore, managing stress, keeping physically fit, and having good eating habits can help you to thrive rather than simply survive.

What Is this Thing Called Stress?

We hear a lot about stress these days. One friend says, "I'm so stressed over this exam." Another exclaims, "I just can't take any more of this stress." **Stress** refers to our physical and emotional reactions to life's events. These reactions can either help us or hurt us, depending on the circumstances. "Good stress" motivates us when we are called on to perform outside our usual comfort or physical ability zone. For example, if you witness a car accident and stop to help the victims, your body will likely experience certain reactions: your heart rate speeds up, your blood pressure rises, and the blood vessels in your muscles and the pupils of your eyes dilate. These changes increase your energy, strength, and mental alertness so you can best deal with the situation.

You can draw on these natural reactions to help you in important, although less dramatic, situations such as taking a professional licensing exam, giving a speech in class, or planning your wedding. This is making good use of stress to maximize your performance. The excitement experienced when you pass the exam and start a new career or get married and begin a new life with the person you love is also a form of good stress.

Pressure and unresolved worries experienced over long periods of time can create "bad stress." When the physical responses to stress are repeated over and over, with no resolution or action taken, they can actually decrease your ability to cope with life's ups and downs. In a sense, your body wears itself out as it continually prepares you to handle situations that are never resolved. Signs of long-term stress include **insomnia,** headaches, digestive problems, muscular tension, fatigue, frequent illness, irritability, depression, poor concentration, excessive eating and drinking, and the use of illegal substances. It's easy to see that these don't work in your favor and are likely to increase your stress level. It's possible to get caught in a vicious cycle of ever-increasing stress that leads to feelings of hopelessness. Your mental images become dictated by worry and fear and as previously discussed, may bring about the very thing that you fear.

Sources of Stress

The first step in dealing with long-term stress is to identify its source. The following list contains some of the common sources of stress (stressors) for students:
- Financial difficulties
- Family problems: an unsupportive partner, abuse, children's behavior, overdemanding parents
- Poor organizational skills
- The inability to manage time; having too much to do
- A lack of self-confidence and poor self-esteem
- Feeling unsure about study skills and your ability to learn
- Loneliness
- Health problems, pregnancy
- Believing that instructors are unfair or don't like them

- Poor relationships with **peers**
- Believing the assignments and tests are too difficult or not **relevant**
- Difficulty in following school rules and requirements

The second step in handling stress is to examine the source to see whether it's based on fact or fiction. For example, if you worry about failing your courses because you are not "smart enough," this may be based on a false belief about yourself. It is very likely you are intellectually competent. But believing you aren't can create stress that discourages you from even trying. After all, what's the point of making a significant effort if you're going to fail anyway? (The self-fulfilling prophecy at work!) A better approach is to seek guidance from your instructor or student services. You may simply need to work harder on some subjects.

Finally, look for a practical solution. What are your options? Can you distance yourself from the stressor (for example, a negative friend who constantly asks why you are returning to school at your age)? Can you get help to resolve the problem (free financial counseling for budget and credit problems, tutoring in a difficult subject)? Can you empower yourself (math refresher course, improved time management)? The important thing is to face the stressor and look for ways to take control. Convert bad stress into good stress by using it as a signal that you may have issues that could prevent you from achieving your goals and attaining the success you want and deserve.

Success Tips for Handling Stress

The very nature of being a student and working in health care brings a certain amount of ongoing stress that cannot be avoided entirely. Many of the practices that promote good health are excellent for relieving stress: exercise, adequate sleep, eating properly, and avoiding excess caffeine. Here are some other things you can try:

- **Practice mentally.** If your stress is caused by an upcoming event such as a job interview, you can anticipate and practice the event in your mind. Athletes use this technique to prepare for the big game. They "see" themselves performing the perfect tennis serve or making the free throw. Use your stress to motivate you to prepare in advance.
- **Use time-management and personal organization strategies.** Try the techniques suggested in this chapter to help you take control of your life. Work on eliminating the conditions that have you feeling as if you're racing downhill with no brakes.
- **Seek the support of others.** People do better when they have the support of others. Many studies have demonstrated that having a network of supportive relationships contributes to psychological well-being. High levels of social support even contribute to good physical health and longevity. So, spend some time with trusted friends, family members, classmates, or school personnel.
- **Perform relaxation exercises.** Meditation, yoga, deep breathing, and muscle relaxation, described in Box 3-3, can relieve physical discomfort and promote emotional well-being. See also Figure 3-3.

BOX 3-3 Relaxation Exercise

Eliminating muscular tension helps relieve anxiety and fatigue. Try this simple exercise to help you release this tension and prevent headaches and other pain.
1. Sit comfortably in a place where you won't be disturbed. Choose a chair that supports your back and allows you to place your feet flat on the floor.
2. Close your eyes.
3. Begin at your toes and tense each group of muscles. Hold for a few seconds and then release. Work from the bottom of the body to the top, tensing and relaxing each area. Pay special attention to the shoulders and jaw muscles, common areas of tension.
4. As you proceed, focus on the feelings of tension and then let go.
5. When you finish, sit quietly and say to yourself, "I am relaxed."

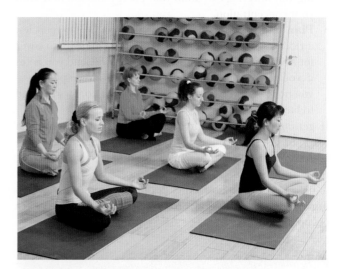

FIGURE 3-3 Yoga is a positive way to manage stress. It has been shown to have numerous health benefits, such as increasing strength and flexibility, lowering blood pressure, and promoting better sleep. *Which of the suggestions for relieving stress do you think might work best for you?* (Copyright Alexander Novikov/iStock/Thinkstock.)

- **Engage in physical exercise.** Even a short walk can be a very effective stress reducer. Find something you enjoy doing and make a little time for it on a regular basis.
- **Adjust your attitude.** Focus on your goals, acknowledge all your progress, and concentrate on the benefits you will receive.
- **Keep your sense of humor.** Look at the humorous side of life and its events. Laugh therapy has been found to strengthen the immune system and positively affect health.
- **Use school and community resources.** Refer to the list of resources you prepared in Prescription for Success 1-2. Helpful information may be available from student services, your religious organization, or the local community center.

- **Make use of this book.** Chapters 3 through 10 contain many suggestions for developing effective study and life skills. Try them out and use the ones that work best for you.

On the Job

Stress on the Job Good stress can serve the health care professional by providing extra energy and increased mental alertness to handle emergency situations properly, provide competent patient care, and maintain a busy schedule. Your success in assisting a fallen patient, performing first aid, and getting through a hectic day of processing medical bills are examples of using good stress. "Bad stress," however, can have negative results, so it is important to incorporate stress-reduction techniques into your daily work life. The tragic results of an excessive buildup of stress among health care workers include **burnout,** addiction to painkillers, and alcoholism.

Learning to handle stress will benefit not only you, but your future patients as well. Illness and injury are major stressors, and an important part of patient education is helping patients deal with both physical and emotional stress. At the same time, stress can be the cause of illness. Research has shown that the majority of visits to the doctor are for stress-related conditions. If the health care staff is showing signs of stress, this can trickle down to patients, and this is certainly the last thing they need.

Personal Reflection

1. Do you believe you may be experiencing long-term stress?
2. If yes, what are the signs?
3. Can you identify the cause or causes?
4. List at least three strategies you will try for dealing with stress.

Healthy Eating

Eating a balanced **diet** and avoiding becoming overweight can be challenging in a world of fast food, vending machines, and busy schedules. We are fortunate to have abundant supplies of food in our country, but as of 2012, this has resulted in a population in which 69% are either overweight or obese.[1] This has led, in turn, to an increase in the conditions and diseases brought about by this extra weight (Box 3-4).

The U.S. Department of Agriculture has designed a graphic called *ChooseMyPlate* to illustrate the recommended portions of the various food groups. Half of the plate is allocated to fruits and vegetables, a little more than a quarter to grains, and a little less than a quarter to proteins (Figure 3-4). Much more detail is contained in *The Dietary Guidelines for Americans, 2010*. This report emphasizes three major goals for Americans to:
1. Balance calories with physical activity to manage weight.
2. Consume more of certain foods and nutrients, such as fruits, vegetables, whole grains, fat-free and low-fat dairy products, and seafood.

BOX 3-4 Health Problems Associated with Overweight and Obesity

- Type 2 diabetes (becoming an epidemic)
- Heart disease
- High blood pressure
- Nonalcoholic fatty liver disease (excess fat and inflammation in the liver of people who drink little or no alcohol)
- Osteoarthritis (pain, swelling, and stiffness in one or more joints)
- Some types of cancer: breast, colon, endometrial (related to the uterine lining), and kidney
- Stroke

National Institute of Diabetes and Digestive and Kidney Diseases. Overweight and obesity statistics. Available at: http://win.niddk.nih.gov/statistics/index.htm.

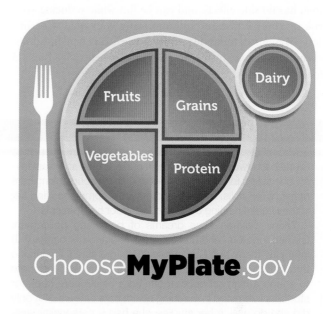

FIGURE 3-4 ChooseMyPlate was designed to be an easy guide to healthy eating. It illustrates the need for variety in our diet and shows how we should eat more from some food groups—vegetables and grains—than others—proteins, fruits, and dairy. *How do your eating habits coincide with the ChooseMyPlate suggestions?* (From U.S. Department of Agriculture: ChooseMyPlate, 2011, http://www.choosemyplate.gov.)

3. Consume fewer foods with sodium (salt), **saturated fats, trans fats, cholesterol,** added sugars, and **refined grains.**[2]

To help consumers determine the contents of the food they eat, the Food and Drug Administration developed the nutrition facts label that appears on most food products. It contains information about calories, fat, the sodium content, and more, for each serving. Pay special attention to the number of servings noted on the label. Some cans and packages appear to contain one serving but in fact, may contain several. Make a habit of checking these labels when you shop for food and snacks.

Create a good diary in which you record everything you eat for one week. The diary can be on paper, your computer, your phone, or any other electronic device. It should be something you can carry with you. At the end of the week, answer the following questions.

1. How did your diet compare with the Choose MyPlate and other government guidelines for nutrition?
2. If your diet needs improvement, what are some easy ways you can eat more healthily?

BOX 3-5 Benefits of Physical Activity

- Increases energy levels
- Promotes feelings of well-being
- Reduces anxiety and depression
- Manages stress
- Decreases risk of heart disease and stroke
- Reduces high blood pressure
- Helps prevent type 2 diabetes
- Prevents back pain
- Prevents being overweight and obesity
- Promotes bone formation to lower risk of osteoporosis[3]

Physical Activity

Physical activity has been called the "magic pill": it can be free, has no side effects, and can be fun while reducing your risk of chronic diseases and improving your quality of life. Just 30 minutes a day five times a week can benefit adults; even more activity further increases the benefits. See Box 3-5 for examples of the benefits of physical activity.

Finding the time for physical activity can seem overwhelming to a busy student. But consider that exercise can increase your level of concentration and feeling of well-being, therefore making up for the time you spend on it. Find something that's easy—perhaps walking—and that you enjoy. If it becomes drudgery, the chances are you won't keep up any type of exercise program.

Trouble Ahead? 3-1

Carrie had always wanted to be a nurse. When she was seven, she asked for a toy nurse's kit and spent hours taking care of her "sick" dolls. Carrie's mother would sometimes find her in the kitchen heating up canned soup for her "patients."

Many children have dreams of becoming policemen, firemen, doctors, and nurses. Most find another career that interests them but Carrie remained interested in nursing throughout elementary and high school. She was fortunate to attend a high school that offered a health care track for students interested in pursuing health care careers. Not only did she do well in her studies, she had a personality well-suited to nursing. She was patient with her younger brothers and sisters who were a boisterous bunch and could be a handful to take care of. She had empathy for others and was especially good at helping with an autistic brother who presented challenges for the family. And she was good at communicating—her siblings often came to her with their problems, knowing she would listen to what they had to say.

Having working parents and several brothers and sisters meant that Carrie had quite a few responsibilities. After school, she looked after her siblings, did some of the housework, and got dinner started in the evening. Later every evening and on weekends, she studied and did her homework. Not having much time to socialize or take part in school activities, she missed out on a lot of the fun of being a teenager. She began to take comfort in food, especially sweet things like cookies, donuts, and ice cream. These became a substitute for what she felt she was missing. By the time Carrie graduated from high school, she was 55 pounds over a healthy weight.

Carrie did well enough to earn a scholarship to pursue her nursing education and because she was living at home, was able to afford to complete her degree. The work was challenging, and sometimes she was bothered by self-doubts. She worried about her progress. Each approaching test in her classes made her nervous. And living at home, with continued responsibilities, left her no time to make friends at college, join study groups, or take part in social activities. Once again, she found herself turning to food. She continued to gain weight and worse, began to smoke as a way to calm herself. She never intended to become a smoker. She knew about the negative effects on health—she certainly had learned enough about that in her health care studies. What she thought would be an occasional time-out with a cigarette became a regular habit. When she was up to a pack a day, she became alarmed and tried to quit. But the withdrawal seemed overwhelming and she decided that now was not the time to give it up. Maybe after she graduated.

Once Carrie graduated and passed the nursing license exam, she began her job search. Because she had good communication skills and her commitment to nursing was evident when she interviewed at the local hospital, she was hired. Her first assignment was in the oncology ward. Carrie was surprised at how physically demanding the work was. When she did her clinical rotations during her training, she was busy but there were down times when her group met with their instructor. But now she was on her feet almost all day long. And some of that time it seemed like she was running from one task to another. In addition, she was moving and lifting patients and equipment, responding to calls from patients and doctors—it seemed to go on nonstop. By the end of each day, all Carrie could think about was getting off her feet and having a good meal—followed by a cigarette. By the end of the first three weeks, she began to wonder if after all these years and all her struggles, she had chosen the wrong career.

Questions for Thought and Reflection

1. Do you think Carrie chose the wrong career? Why or why not?

2. What might she have done as a teenager to prevent the problems she is having now?
3. What effect might Carrie's habits have on her patients?
4. What advice would you give her now that she has become a nurse?

Personal Reflection

1. How would I rate my level of health and fitness?
2. Do I need to improve my eating habits?
3. Do I need to get more physical exercise?
4. What can I start doing now to take action?

Learning for Life

Learning means much more than just getting by in school and remembering information long enough to pass tests. It means storing information mentally and mastering hands-on skills that you can retrieve and use when you need them on the job. Furthermore, it means being able to apply what you have learned to solve problems and make informed decisions. For example, if you are learning about the circulatory system, you are not simply memorizing the parts of the heart and the path of blood through the body. You are acquiring information to help real patients who have heart problems. If you are studying a form of therapy, your study of the muscular system will have practical applications. Your purpose for learning is far more important than simply studying to earn a grade. Your future patients and clients will depend on your knowledge, and they deserve your best efforts to learn now.

How Do You Learn Best?

We know that people tend to learn in different ways. For many years now, the idea of **learning styles** has been popular. By identifying your own preferred learning styles, you can be more successful in your studies. The three styles most commonly discussed are grouped by the senses used when acquiring and processing new information: auditory (listening), visual (seeing), and kinesthetic (hands-on). Table 3-2 contains a description of each of these styles. (Note: In recent years, researchers have begun to question whether there is evidence supporting the existence of different learning styles. In fact, it is now recommended that students engage as many senses as possible when learning new material.)

There are other learning preferences, in addition to the styles related to our senses. Table 3-3 describes six other approaches to learning. None of us learns in just one way. And it is important to understand that there is not a "best way" to learn. Just as we have different personalities, we have different combinations of learning styles. The purpose of discovering your preferred learning style is to help you study more efficiently and effectively. Table 3-4 gives examples of the many study techniques possible for learning the names and locations of the major bones.

TABLE 3-2
Three Major Learning Styles

Learning Style	How Student Learns Best	Examples of Effective Learning Activities
Auditory	Through *hearing.* Remembers information from lectures and discussions better than material read in a textbook. Prefers music over art and listening over reading. Understands written material better when it is read aloud. May spell better out loud than when writing. Misses visual cues. Prefers doing oral rather than written reports.	Lectures, CDs, tapes, music, rhymes, speaking
Visual	Through *seeing.* Remembers information presented in written or graphic form better than in lectures and discussions. Often needs people to repeat what they have said. Takes notes when oral instructions are given. Prefers art to music and reading to listening. Understands better when the speaker's face is seen. Prefers doing written rather than oral reports.	Reading, pictures, diagrams, charts, graphs, maps, videos, films, chalkboard, overhead projections
Kinesthetic (hands-on)	Through *doing.* Remembers information acquired through activities. Reads better when moving lips and saying words silently or moving finger along the page. Enjoys moving around while studying. Likes to touch things, point, use fingers when counting or calculating. Prefers doing a demonstration rather than an oral or written report.	Lab activities, skills practice, experiments, games, movement, building models

TABLE 3-3

More Approaches to Learning

Specifics Versus the Big Picture	
Specific to General (Big Picture)	**General (Big Picture) to Specific**
Some students want to learn facts before forming generalizations (the big picture). They prefer to memorize dates, study individual events, and know the details first. When learning about the circulatory system, for example, they would rather study the various parts of the system before learning how they all work together to circulate the blood.	Other students want to see and understand the big picture that they then use as a framework for learning the details. When learning about cells, for example, they want to know the purpose and function of the cell before learning the individual components.
Linear Versus Global	
Linear	**Global**
Linear thinkers learn best when material is organized in a logical sequence. They like to do things in order, building on material previously learned.	Global thinkers like to work with all the facts, regardless of the order. They are interested in forming relationships within the material.
Individual Versus Interactive	
Individual	**Interactive**
Individual-type learners prefer to work on learning tasks alone. They like to figure out all the aspects of assignments and projects on their own.	Interactive-type learners like to work with another student or in groups. They want to share their ideas and hear the ideas of others (Figure 3-5).

TABLE 3-4

Developing Learning Strategies That Work for You

Learning Style	Examples of Learning Strategies for Learning the Names of the Bones
Auditory	Say the names of the bones out loud. Listen to a CD of the names and locations of each bone. Make your own CD of the names and locations. Create a song, rhyme, rap, or jingle. Silly is good because it helps you remember. ("There are fourteen phalanges in my little handies.") Clap or tap out a rhythm as you repeat the words. Make flash cards and say the words and/or definitions out loud. Create sound-alike association. Remember, silly is okay. ("The cranium holds the brain-ium.")
Visual	Look at photos or drawings of the bones as you study their names. Label a drawing of the skeleton. Color the bones on a drawing. Create mental pictures of associations (a crane lifting a huge cranium). Put up a labeled drawing of the skeleton where you will see it often—the bathroom mirror, your bedroom wall, near your study desk. Make flash cards with a picture of the bone on one side and its name on the reverse.
Kinesthetic	Point to or touch each bone as you learn its name. Use drawings, a model (inexpensive anatomical models are sold in toy stores), or your own body. Make two flash cards for each bone: one with the name of the bone, the other with the location. Mix the cards, then study by sorting and matching each set. Stand, move, or walk around as you study. Associate movements with the bones as you learn. For example, lift and bend your arm when studying the humerus, ulna, and radius. Write the name of each bone several times.
Specific to General	Start by learning the name and location of each individual bone.
General to Specific	Start by looking at the whole skeleton. Look at the relationships and connections between bones. Consider how the bones contribute to body function.
Linear	Study the bones in a structured order, such as by area (arms and legs) or from top to bottom (shoulder to hand).
Global	Study from a labeled diagram that includes the entire skeleton or all the bones of a given area.
Individual	Use the suggested learning techniques by yourself. Set goals for how many bones you'll learn each day. Create a reward system for yourself.
Interactive	Form a study group with classmates. Ask a friend or family member to quiz you. Organize a group or class competition (Figure 3-5).

The three checklists below represent three learning styles. As you read through each list, give yourself one point for every statement with which you agree or that best describes you. Total your score for each checklist. The checklist with the highest number of points is likely to be your strongest or preferred learning style.

Auditory Checklist
- I follow oral instructions better than written ones.
- I enjoy listening to music more than looking at art.
- I would rather listen to a lecture than read the material in a textbook.
- I prefer to listen to the news on the radio rather than read the newspaper.
- I spell better out loud than when writing words out.
- When I read, I sometimes confuse words that look like other words.
- I remember things the instructor says better than what I read.
- I don't copy well from the board.
- I enjoy jokes told orally more than cartoons.
- I like games with action and noise more than quiet board games.
- I understand material better when I read it aloud.
- Sometimes I make errors in math because I don't see the sign or I read the numbers or directions incorrectly.
- I am often the last one to notice something new that requires observation—for example, if a room is painted or a wall display is changed.
- Reading a map is difficult for me.
- I like to use my finger as a pointer when I read. Sometimes when reading I get lost or skip lines.
- I often sing, hum, or whistle to myself.
- I frequently tell jokes, tell stories, or make verbal analogies to demonstrate a point.
- Matching tests are difficult for me, even when I know the answers.
- I often talk to myself when I'm alone.
- I sometimes need to have diagrams, graphs, or printed directions explained orally.
- *Score (total of all checked items)*

Visual Checklist
- I often have to ask people to repeat what they have just said.
- The best way for me to remember something is to picture it in my head.
- I typically prefer information to be presented visually on the board, on PowerPoint slides, etc.
- I often find myself "tuned out" in class when the instructor is talking.
- Sometimes I know what I want to say, but I just can't think of the exact word.
- I am good at drawing graphs, charts, and other visual displays.
- I take notes during lectures so I can look at them later to review what was said.
- I can usually follow written instructions.
- I can understand maps and use them to find my way.

- I have difficulty understanding instructors or speakers when their backs are turned and I can't see their faces.
- Other people sometimes accuse me of not listening to them.
- I'd rather show someone how to do something than explain it in words.
- I prefer board games to games that require listening.
- I have trouble remembering things that are announced unless I see them written down or write them down myself.
- Sometimes I confuse words when I am speaking, especially words that sound similar.
- When trying to recall the order of letters in the alphabet, I have to go over most of it from the beginning. For example, recalling whether "j" comes before or after "g."
- I would choose art over music activities.
- I do better when the instructor demonstrates how to do something instead of just explaining it in words.
- I often forget things I've been told, such as phone messages, unless I write them down.
- I often draw pictures or doodle on the edges of my notes, on scrap paper, etc.
- *Score (total of all checked items)*

Kinesthetic Checklist
- I read better when I say the words quietly to myself.
- I often draw pictures or designs when taking notes in class to help me concentrate and remember the lecture.
- When I shop, I frequently touch the items displayed for sale; when I walk through a room, I tend to touch the furniture.
- I often count on my fingers.
- I like to smoke, eat, drink, or chew gum while I study.
- I am comfortable being touched by others. I often hug others or touch them when I'm speaking to them.
- I learn best by doing an activity, rather than reading or hearing about it.
- I enjoy hobbies that involve making things.
- I like to be able to move around as I learn. For example, moving about in the classroom helps me concentrate on the lesson.
- I would rather do a demonstration than give an oral or written report.
- I fidget a lot, such as tapping my pen or jiggling my leg.
- I usually prefer to stand while working.
- I use my hands more than the average person to communicate what I'm trying to say.
- I'm pretty coordinated and good at sports.
- I'm always on the move.
- I tend to talk and eat faster than most people.
- I would rather participate in an activity, such as a ball game, than watch it.
- It's hard for me to sit still for long periods of time.
- I work well with my hands to make or repair things.
- I enjoy labs more than lecture classes.
- *Score (total of all checked items)*

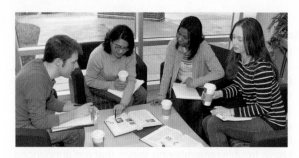

FIGURE 3-5 Starting or joining a study group has a number of advantages. It helps prevent procrastination in preparing for tests, provides different perspectives, decreases test anxiety, and enhances communication and teamwork skills. *Do you think a study group would help you?* (From Yoder-Wise PS: *Leading and managing in nursing,* ed 6, St Louis, 2015, Mosby.)

Developing Effective Study Habits

Current research on the brain and how we learn has revealed some interesting findings about good study habits. For example, one experiment showed that students who studied the same material in two very different rooms did much better when tested on the material than students who studied in only one location. This seems to challenge the idea that we should develop the habit of always studying in one place. (The scientific explanation: the different environments force the brain to make multiple associations with the same material, thus making more connections in the brain.)[4]

Other studies have shown that it is better to study a variety of related topics during a study period rather than the same topic intensely for the entire time. For example, reviewing one type of insurance claim form over and over may not be as effective as reviewing various types of claim forms. Comparing and contrasting the information appears to reinforce learning. It follows that learning to think in this way will help you make decisions on the job when you are confronted with a variety of situations and circumstances.[5]

As in the case of finding your best "learning styles," experiment with different study techniques to see which work best for you. For example, one person may find music distracting, while another finds it difficult to work in silence. Or you may discover that music helps when you are writing, but is not helpful when you are reading a textbook. Apply your own experiences and what you know about yourself and how you have learned most successfully in the past.

Trouble Ahead? 3-2

Robert joined the military when he was 18, just out of high school. His uncle had been in the Marine Corps and Robert enjoyed hearing his stories about Vietnam. In spite of the disagreements in the U.S. about that war, his uncle had been proud of his contribution. Robert was attracted by the reported exclusivity of the Marines: "The Few. The Proud. The Marines."

Robert participated in sports in high school to develop his fitness and kept his grades above average in the hope of qualifying for the Corps.

After graduation, he contacted a recruiter, went through the application process, and was thrilled to be told to report to the San Diego Recruit Depot. Robert liked the challenge of boot camp—basic training. He toughened up physically, learned to follow orders, and developed self-discipline.

While serving two deployments in Afghanistan, Robert faced many traumatic situations. He became accustomed to the adrenaline rush of battle and the constant need to remain vigilant. He saw some pretty brutal action and lost a few friends while overseas. In spite of the challenges, Robert remained on active duty for eight years.

After his discharge, he returned to his parents' farm in North Dakota and spent a few months making the transition to civilian life and thinking about what he wanted to do next. Part of his Marine training was in first aid in which he learned to treat injuries like fractures and flesh wounds. Part of his gear included a first aid kit. Although helping the wounded in the field could be gruesome, he liked the feeling of knowing he could help. He decided that a career as a paramedic would be a good fit for him and enrolled in a local community college.

Robert thought that after what he'd been through in the last eight years, attending school would be easy. But a few weeks after he started his classes, he ran into some challenges. He had little in common with most of his classmates. He missed the comradery he had experienced in the Marines. The daily routine seemed boring after living in a battle zone. The complaints and problems of his fellow students seemed trivial. And the type of learning required was different. In the Marines, he was used to getting hands-on, in-the-moment training. Now he was faced with reading and writing assignments, quizzes, and final exams. These seemed like a waste of time and sitting in class listening to lectures was frustrating. He found himself getting lost when studying and did poorly on his tests.

On the advice of his mother, an elementary school teacher, he visited the learning center at his college. There he talked with a counselor who suggested he take a learning styles inventory, take a reading test, and answer a number of questions about his study habits. He spent a few minutes on the inventory, but thought to himself how ridiculous all this seemed. After all, he had successfully completed eight years in the military. These questions seemed silly. He left the learning center and decided he just needed to use more self-discipline when he studied.

Questions for Thought and Reflection

1. What do you think about Robert's attitude?
2. How might he better approach his new role as a student?
3. Do you think he will complete his paramedic classes and graduate? Why or why not?

Learning on the Job The ability to provide good patient education is an increasingly important skill for today's health care professionals. Shorter hospital stays have resulted in patients and their families being responsible for care that was once provided by nursing staff. Patients must be taught about home care and the signs of complications.

Many of the major health problems affecting patients today are influenced by lifestyle factors, such as weight, exercise, smoking, and stress. In fact, the three leading causes of death in the United States, cancer, heart disease, and lower respiratory disease, are strongly influenced by personal habits. Teaching patients about self-care and healthy habits is easier and more effective when you understand that people learn in different ways. Health care professionals may need to provide information in a variety of ways, including oral explanations, pictures and written materials, and hands-on demonstrations of procedures.

Prescription for Success: 3-9 Make Your Learning Styles Work for You

Apply what you know about learning styles to create five strategies you believe would help you learn the name and purpose of 25 vitamins (or any other material for a class you are taking).

Down Memory Lane

Memorizing is not the same as learning but it is an important component of the learning process. Although you may be able to rely on your short-term memory to complete assignments and pass tests, it is the material stored in the long-term memory that will serve you throughout your studies, when taking your professional exam, and afterwards on the job. There are many ways to improve your memory and better retain the material you study.

Start by making sure you understand the new material. Experiments have shown it is much more difficult to remember nonsense syllables or lists of unrelated numbers than material that has meaning. In other words, it is very difficult to remember what you don't understand in the first place.

Repeat, repeat, repeat. The proven best way to retain new material is repetition over an extended period of time. In fact, the length of time information is remembered is often in direct proportion to the length of time taken to learn it. Review new material as soon as possible after you first encounter it and continue to review it on a regular basis, at least weekly.

Use a variety of learning strategies. For example, if you are learning numerical formulas you can: listen to or say them over and over; post the formulas on the bathroom mirror; write each new formula 10 times. Use your imagination.

Studying does not necessarily mean working quietly at a desk. Create rhymes or funny images. Make up movements associated with each item you have to remember. One learning method, called "pegging," has you place imaginary pegs on walls around the house. On each one, "hang" a fact or idea you must remember. As you walk through the house each day, review the material on each peg.

Look for ways to relate new information to your own experience by connecting it to something you already know. And try to use new information in your daily life—or picture in your mind how you would use it in your future job.

Success Tips for Improving Retention

- **Relax.** Your ability to store and remember things does not work well when your body is tense and your mind is distracted with worry. Try doing a relaxation exercise before starting a study session.
- **Remove distractions.** Studying for mastery requires concentration. Find a place where interruptions are limited and where you can use your chosen techniques.
- **Break up your study sessions.** Most people can't concentrate fully for very long periods of time. The great thing about reviewing over time, rather than at the last minute, is that you can take time for short breaks.
- **Overlearn.** Continue to review and repeat material you already know. This helps to firmly lock it into your long-term memory.
- **Quiz yourself.** Make up your own quizzes. Review one day and take the quiz several days later to evaluate your retention. It has been shown that testing yourself is one of the most powerful learning tools available to students.

Prescription for Success: 3-10 Memory Test

Choose something you want or need to memorize, such as the facts for an upcoming quiz. Use the memory techniques to help you learn and remember the material.
1. Which techniques did you choose?
2. How did they work for you?
3. Which ones seemed to work best?

The Perils of Cramming

Cramming is a well-known student activity consisting of frantic last-minute efforts, sometimes fortified with coffee and junk food, to finish assignments and prepare for tests. The major problem with cramming is that it serves only the immediate goal of meeting a school deadline. True learning rarely occurs. The conditions required for learning, such as the opportunity for repetition over time, are absent. Most of what is crammed is forgotten within a few days—or hours! Work in health care demands a higher level of competence than you are likely to achieve as a result of cramming. Do your future patients deserve your best efforts to learn, or are the bits you may remember after a night of cramming good enough? This is an important consideration for students who claim that cramming works well for them because they can study only at the last minute when the deadline is close. This is true only if passing the test is their only goal.

Another problem with cramming is it leaves you with few options. If you are writing a paper the night before it is due and you discover that the information you have is inadequate (and the Internet is not available), you have no time to consult other sources. If you are studying for a test and realize there are several points you don't understand, it's too late to ask the instructor to explain them.

Finally, cramming adds more stress to an already busy life in which you may be balancing various responsibilities. If it costs you a night's sleep, it can deplete your energy and interfere with your ability to concentrate. You end up creating a nonproductive cycle consisting of a continual game of catch-up and the danger of creating ongoing stress.

The reality is that things happen, you get behind, and you run out of time. Almost every student occasionally finds it necessary to cram. Here are some tips to make the best of a bad situation[5]:

1. Don't beat yourself up and waste energy feeling guilty. You'll only distract your attention from what you have to do. Just make a mental note to change your study habits to avoid the need for cramming in the future.
2. Do a very quick visualization in which you see yourself accomplishing what you need to do in the time you have available.
3. Minimize all distractions. For example, see if you can find someone to watch the children.
4. Focus on the most important material. What is most likely to be emphasized on the test? What are the main requirements of the assignment?
5. Use the learning and memory techniques described in this section. Draw on your learning style to help you learn the necessary material.
6. Try to stay calm. Physical tension distracts from mental effort. Breathe deeply, stretch, and do a quick relaxation exercise.

Mentors Make a Difference

"People seldom improve when they have no other model but themselves to copy."

—Oliver Goldsmith

A **mentor** is an advisor you choose for yourself, someone who has the experience and background to give you sound advice about your studies and career. This is a person you respect—and who is respected by his or her colleagues—and whom you see as a positive role model. Your chances of succeeding are greatly increased when someone you respect cares about your progress. This has been proved in both school and business settings. Where can you find such a person? It could be an instructor, school staff member,

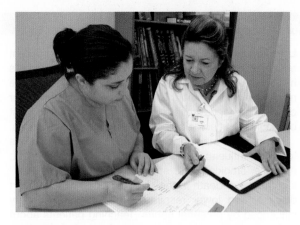

FIGURE 3-6 Working with a mentor increases your chances of both academic and career success. *Is there someone you can contact now about becoming your mentor? In what ways might this person help you succeed in school? On the job?* (From Yoder-Wise PS: *Leading and managing in nursing,* ed 6, St Louis, 2015, Mosby.)

administrator, or someone who works in health care. You might find a graduate of your school who is working successfully. Once you have graduated, you might choose a mentor who is currently working in your career field. It is important to choose someone with whom you feel comfortable (Figure 3-6).

Once you have identified a person you would like to have as your mentor, ask for an appointment. Let him or her know you want to talk about mentoring. At the meeting, explain that you are pursuing a career in health care and that you would like him/her to serve as your mentor and give you guidance. Ask how much time he or she has to meet with you. If the first person you approach does not have the time or is not interested, don't be discouraged. Continue your search—it will be worth the effort! (You may want to have more than one mentor—perhaps one at school and another who is working in the field.)

Mentors who work in health care can give you information about the current state of your targeted occupation, suggest what you should emphasize in your studies, and introduce you to other health care professionals. Other ways they can help you include:

• Giving you direct, constructive feedback about your performance
• Sharing the knowledge they have gained during their career
• Helping you resolve problems, such as a conflict with your supervisor
• Letting you know about employment opportunities
• Advising you about whether to accept a job
• Helping you understand and deal with organizational culture and politics

You should meet or talk with your mentor periodically to ask questions and stay motivated. Be clear about what you want in the relationship; perhaps set some goals together to keep you on track. Finally, be sure to show your appreciation for their time and advice.

Personal Reflection

1. What would you look for in choosing a mentor?
2. Who do you know who might be a good mentor?
3. What can you do to find a mentor who works in health care?

Summary of Key Ideas

- Let your goals be your guides.
- Never underestimate the power of attitude.
- If managed well, time can work for you.
- Work smarter, not harder.
- Good health can help you succeed.
- You can use stress to work for you instead of against you.
- Learning how to learn will increase your ability to learn.
- A mentor can help you succeed.

Positive Self-Talk for This Chapter

- I have worthy goals and am on track to achieve them.
- I manage my time efficiently.
- I am well organized and in control of my life.
- I practice good health habits.
- I use effective study strategies.

Internet Activities

ⓔ For active links to the websites needed to complete these activities, visit http://evolve.elsevier.com/Haroun/career/.

1. Use the search terms "setting goals," "achieving goals," and "achieving personal goals" to locate information about using goals successfully. Assume the role of a "success coach" and use what you learn to write a short article for students.
2. Using the search term "effective time management," find five facts or suggestions on time management not covered in this chapter.
3. Search for information about the benefits of having a positive attitude. Use the information you find to write a short report on how a positive attitude can contribute to school and career success.
4. MedlinePlus, a public health information website sponsored by the National Library of Medicine, has many links to scientific and health organizations. Choose an article on stress, weight control, or physical activity and write a report about its effects on health. Explain how this information can benefit both you and your future patients.
5. Search for information about learning and memory using search terms such as "learning strategies," "learning techniques," and "improving memory." Find and describe three techniques you would like to try.

Building Your Resume

1. Review the Resume Building Block #1 form at the end of Chapter 2. Think about how your goals relate to your career objective.
2. Review the Resume Building Block #2 form in Chapter 2. How can identifying your learning styles help you get more from your education?
3. Do you have good time-management and/or personal organization skills you can apply to a health care job?

To Learn More

Chapman E: *Life is an attitude!*, Menlo Park, Calif, 1992, Crisp Publications

Elwood Chapman has been an "attitude guru" since the 1950s. This is a great little book on how to control your outlook on life by beating negativity, eliminating doubts, and setting positive goals. Although full of helpful hints, it is short and easy to read.

Covey S, Merrill AR, Merrill RR: *First things first,* New York, 1995, Simon and Schuster

Also available on a CD.

This classic book connects mission statements and goals with time management. Rather than describing ways to get more done, it explains how to do what you decide is the most important. Covey teaches a method of categorizing tasks to help you focus on what is really important, not just on what is urgent. As he puts it, "Doing more things faster is no substitute for doing the right things." He suggests that you focus on a few key priorities and then identify small goals for each week.

Hansen K: The value of a mentor: Students and job-seekers... how to find yourself a mentor

http://www.quintcareers.com/mentor_value.html
This article includes tips on finding and benefiting from a mentor as you pursue your career goals.

Lakein A: *How to get control of your time and your life,* New York, 1989, Penguin Group (USA)

Although first published 43 years ago, this book is still a classic. Many consider it to be the authoritative source on which all other time-management books are based. Lakein explains the importance of prioritizing tasks and learning to work smarter, not harder.

Mind Tools

http://www.mindtools.com
This website contains hundreds of helpful articles about important life and career skills, including time management, memory improvement, and stress management.

U.S. Department of Agriculture

http://www.ChooseMyPlate.gov
This government agency website has information on current recommended eating guidelines, as well as tips on eating healthy food on a budget, meal planning, sample menus, and lots more helpful information.

References

1. Fast Stats, Obesity and Overweight. Centers for Disease Control and Prevention. http://www.cdc.gov/nchs/fastats/obesity-overweight.htm
2. Office of Disease Prevention and Health Promotion: Dietary guidelines for Americans. 2010. Available at http://www.health.gov/dietaryguidelines/2010.asp.
3. Health benefits of physical activity. Available at: http://www.medicinenet.com/script/main/art.asp?articlekey=10074.
4. Carey B: Forget what you know about good study habits. Available at: http://www.nytimes.com/2010/09/07/health/views/07mind.html?pagewanted=1&_r=1.
5. Ellis D: *Becoming a master student*, ed 12, Boston, 2009, Houghton Mifflin.

CHAPTER 4

Strategies for Adult Students

OBJECTIVES

1. Describe the portrait of an adult student, confront and manage fears you may have about returning to school, and recognize how your experiences as an adult can help you succeed as a student.
2. Develop advanced time-management skills.
3. Learn positive ways of working with your children to help with your decision to return to school.
4. Create relationships with family and friends to support your role as a student and recognize the importance of balancing work and school schedules.
5. Review and strengthen your academic skills.

KEY TERMS AND CONCEPTS

Academic Abilities Specific abilities and skills related to studying and learning, such as reading, writing, and calculating.

Adult Student A student who is over 25, who has been out of high school for at least 5 years, and who may have dependents and be employed. (Also called a *mature* or *nontraditional student*.)

Irrational Without cause; unreasonable.

Learning Center A dedicated section of a school that offers help with academics and study skills.

Study Group A group of students who meet together on a regular basis to study, discuss, and support one another's learning.

Study Skills Skills used for learning and mastering material.

Support Group A group organized to help its members with specific types of problems.

Tutor A person who helps others learn specific subjects or skills in a one-on-one or small-group setting.

Portrait of the Adult Student

Just what is an **adult student?** There are a variety of definitions, depending on the source. Generally, adult students have one or more of the following characteristics:

- Have been out of high school for at least 5 years
- Are over the age of 25
- Work either full- or part-time
- Have children or other dependents

Come Join the Crowd

"Through education, you hope to give a new direction to life."
—Linda Simon

If you've been out of school for a number of years, you may be quite nervous about the idea of returning to school. Something you should know is that returning to school after a few—or even many—years is becoming much more common these days. In fact, the crowd of older students is getting larger. Some sources report that up to 50% of all college students are over the age of 25. The world is changing rapidly, and education is becoming increasingly important for securing good jobs and moving up in careers. This is especially true for health care careers.

Continuing your education will ultimately add to the quality of your life—and to the lives of those around you. But you may be experiencing a number of fears and wondering if you have made the right decision. It is not unusual for adults to have concerns about their ability to succeed as students. Table 4-1 lists common fears, along with suggestions for overcoming each one.

One proven way to deal with fears is to share and discuss them with other people who are in the same situation. You may discover that you are not the only one feeling the way you do and that your fears are not **irrational.** Talking

TABLE 4-1
Common Fears of Adult Students

Fear	Suggestions for Overcoming
My brain is rusty and I won't be able to learn quickly.	Think of it this way: you may not have been in school but if you have been working and/or raising a family, your brain has had plenty of workouts! You have simply been using it in different ways, but they all involve thinking and learning.
I won't be able to compete with younger students.	You actually have certain advantages over younger students. These are described in the next section of this chapter.
My **academic abilities** are not that great. I didn't do well in math/science/English, etc.	This book can help you review basic skills and overcome special fears such as math anxiety. See Chapters 7, 8, and 9. Take advantage of any resources available at your school, such as the **learning center** and **tutors.**
I don't have a computer or Internet access.	Computers have become quite affordable. If purchasing one is not an option, check with your school and the public library. Most have computers that students and the public can use.
I don't know how to use computers like the kids do.	Technology does have a way of moving on, and it's not uncommon to feel left behind. (The manual for the last car I bought was 506 pages long!) If possible, take a computer class. Your school may have them. If not, they are often available free of charge or for a small fee at public libraries, adult schools, and community centers. There are also many good books and websites for beginners.
I might not be able to do it all—work, study, and raise a family.	This is a problem faced by many students. See the suggestions in this chapter as well as the sections in Chapter 3 on time management and personal organization.
My family will feel neglected.	There are actions you can take to help prevent your family from feeling this way. This chapter contains many specific ideas.
I worry that people in my life may try to sabotage my efforts.	People who truly care about you will support your efforts to improve your life. It may be that they feel threatened or left out. This chapter contains some suggestions you can try to gain their support.
The thought of taking tests worries me.	Taking tests is a skill discussed in detail in Chapter 8.
Instructors might not like older students.	Actually, many instructors believe that older students are more motivated and committed.

Adapted from Siebert A, Karr MK: *The adult learner's guide to survival and success,* ed 6, Portland, 2008, Practical Psychology Press.

with someone else, however, should not simply be an "ain't it awful, this is tough" gab session. Rather, use it as an opportunity to help each other focus on the positive, exchange ideas for managing difficulties, and share resources. Examples of such resources include the following:

- Trading childcare
- Car pooling
- Teaching each other, such as computer skills
- Sharing class notes when one of you is absent

According to Al Siebert, an expert in helping adult learners, "Creating a personal **support group** and issue-specific learning teams is the most effective thing you can do to help assure your success in college."[1] This makes sense because research has shown that social support—relationships with other people—has powerful positive effects. For example, people with good social support have been shown to have reduced stress, improved resistance to disease, and improved recovery from illness.

Once you have graduated, consider maintaining your support group as you navigate the job search and for the first few months on the job. You will likely encounter new challenges, and sharing these experiences can help smooth the road during these times.

Another suggestion for overcoming fears is to grit your teeth and face them head on. Ask yourself if the fear is based on reality. Then think about ways you can deal with it: ask for help; take advantage of school and community resources; use the suggestions in this book. Do your best to get through what needs to be done and then reflect on your success. Over time, with each new triumph, your fears will decrease.

Advantages of Being an Adult Student

It is quite possible that you have a number of advantages over more traditional students—those who are entering college directly from high school or who have been out of school for only a couple of years. Perhaps you left school to get married and raise a family, join the military, or go to work. If so, you have almost certainly accumulated a wealth of experience that will help you as a student. In fact, it is likely that as an older adult you have acquired many skills you can apply at school. Examples of these are listed in Table 4-2. Many educators believe that lessons learned from life are the most valuable.

Certain life experiences are especially helpful for health care students. If you are a parent, for example, you have undoubtedly taken your children to the doctor. You understand how important it is to have faith in those who are caring for your loved ones. You yourself may have had health problems. These experiences can motivate you to do your best in school to become a truly qualified health care professional.

Okay, now you're feeling more confident about being a mature student. At the same time, adult students who find themselves with instructors and classmates younger than themselves should take care not to assume a know-it-all attitude. Adults who are used to being in charge at home—and perhaps even on the job—can find it difficult to become a

student and follow the directions of others. You may believe that you have more practical experience than the instructor and many of the other students. Recognize the need to learn from individuals who, although younger, have health care experience and knowledge. On the other hand, don't hesitate to share your experiences when these are appropriate for the topics being presented in class. Offer your comments courteously, and take care not to dominate the discussion.

Prescription for Success: 4-1 What Are the Benefits?

1. List all the ways that attending school and pursuing a career in health care will help your family.
2. Share the list with them and ask them to add ideas of their own.

Meeting New Challenges

"Believe in yourself and take things one day at a time."

—Al Siebert

The greatest challenge faced by most adult students is the matter of time—having enough of it! Adults have multiple responsibilities that may include running a household, caring for children, and holding down a job. They may even include helping elderly parents and holding volunteer positions in the community. Balancing these demands can be stressful, even

TABLE 4-2
Skills Acquired Through Life Experience

Skill	Application in School
Meeting deadlines	Turning in assignments on time
Handling several activities at the same time	Coordinating studying, caring for children, and completing household tasks
Interacting and working with others	Developing working relationships with instructors; getting along with other students
Solving problems	Determining the best ways to learn; balancing adult responsibilities so you can study; completing assignments that require solving problems
Adapting to new situations	Adjusting to being in school; adapting to the role of student
Having patience and knowing that situations will improve over time	Staying with your studies even if the going gets tough

overwhelming. At times your responsibilities may seem like acceptable excuses for being late for class, or even absent. You may feel that your instructors are not caring or understanding if they don't accept your excuses. But you must remember that the goal of health care education is to prepare you for a career. You will have important responsibilities in this career, and your employer and your patients will count on you to know what you are doing. Being prepared to serve requires attending your classes regularly. If instructors were to let students slide through school because they have good excuses and good intentions, the instructors would be doing a disservice to their students and to their future employers and, most importantly, the future patients of these students.

Personal Reflection

1. Which of the life skills listed in Table 4-2 do you believe will most help you in your role as a student?
2. Can you think of others that you can apply to help you succeed in school?

Time Management—Advanced Techniques

This section is called "Advanced Techniques" because good time management is especially important for adult students. The fact is, there are only 24 hours in a day. When you combine typical adult responsibilities with attending class and studying, no day will seem long enough to take care of everything you believe needs to be done. Adding the role of student to your other responsibilities may require some major adjustments and new strategies.

As discussed in Chapter 3 in the section on time management, prioritizing is the key to the effective use of time. Remember that prioritizing means determining which tasks are the most important and then making sure that they are completed. Start by determining which activities are critical to your success as a student and focus on these. If you are a parent and/or a spouse, maintaining these relationships will also be high on your list of priorities. For example, when time is short, spending an hour with a child may be more important than dusting and vacuuming the house or performing volunteer activities. The fact is, you may have to temporarily put off some of your customary activities. Attending school—and putting in the necessary time to study—is a big commitment and will almost certainly require some sacrifices. You may have less time for social and volunteer activities and household chores. See which of these can be put off, without endangering your health or that of your family, until after you graduate.

In addition to the ideas presented in Chapter 3, adult students may benefit from the following suggestions:

- Let family members and friends know your schedule. Consider putting up a large calendar where everyone can see it. Mark the dates when assignments are due and you have tests so everyone knows when you will be especially busy. Include events that are important to others as well, such as a child's music recital.

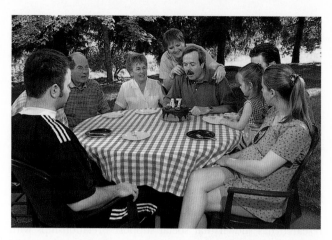

FIGURE 4-1 Although school and your studies must be high priorities, your family is an essential part of your life. *What can you do to include them in your plans and achievements? What activities can you plan now to ensure they do not feel left out as you pursue your studies?* (From de Wit S, O'Neill P: *Fundamental concepts and skills for nursing*, ed 4, St Louis, 2014, Saunders.)

- Work with your family to delegate tasks. Organize a family meeting to discuss your need for study time and assign age-appropriate chores. Have follow-up meetings to evaluate how things are going and make any needed adjustments to schedules and tasks.
- Schedule fun time with your family. Plan activities together that everyone enjoys. Aim for days that follow a major exam or project due date (Figure 4-1).
- Treat your studies as you would a job. After all, you wouldn't just leave your job to visit a friend or stay on the phone for an hour catching up on the latest news.
- Plan to study each day, even if some days it is for a short period only. Don't wait until you have long periods of uninterrupted time—this luxury may happen rarely, if at all! (I have learned that 20 minutes here and there eventually results in a completed book.)
- Add 15 minutes to each day, either by getting up earlier or staying up later. This will add 91 hours a year to your waking—and hopefully productive—hours.[2]

Prescription for Success: 4-2 Breaking It Up

1. Handling your various roles won't seem so overwhelming if you break what you need to do into bite-sized pieces. Choose a project or task you are currently working to achieve. Break it into a series of steps (at least five separate ones).

Managing with Children in the House

Being a parent presents special challenges for adult students, especially if you are a single parent. In spite of comments throughout this book about dedicating yourself to your

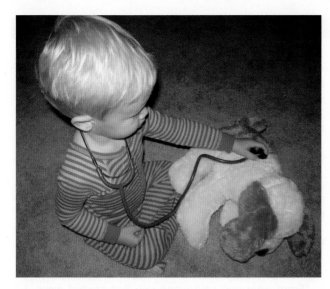

FIGURE 4-2 Make an effort to involve your children in your education. *How can you teach your children about what you are learning? In what activities can they be involved?* (From Gerdin J: *Health careers today,* ed 5, St Louis, 2012, Mosby.)

studies, the truth is that your children are your top priority. If they are young, finding appropriate childcare is critical. Even with a good provider, you should develop a backup plan to cover emergencies. For example, preschools can close during severe weather, individual caretakers can become ill, or your child can get sick and be required to stay at home.

Your children's school and the adults who care for them should be able to reach you in an emergency. Make sure they have your school's phone number. If your instructors require you to turn off cell phones during class (not an unreasonable request), ask the administration about their policy for taking emergency calls and notifying students in class.

Handling childcare issues now is excellent preparation for later when you are employed. Although employers understand true emergencies, they cannot tolerate employees who regularly miss work because of child-related issues. Employers must make patient care and achieving work goals their highest priorities.

Your children may be upset by any changes in your schedule, absences from home, and limitations in the time you have to spend with them. It can help if they know where you are spending your time and what you are doing. Ask your school for permission to show your children the classrooms, labs, and other areas. Explain how you are learning new things to help others and to help them have a better future. Show them a picture of a health care professional, and tell them about your future job. Make it a habit to tell them about your day in school, something interesting that happened, and what you learned (Figure 4-2).

Make time for each child for activities you enjoy doing together, talk about their concerns, and let them know how much they mean to you. Focus on them during this time so they feel included and loved. My neighbors have a busy family with two working parents and four school-age children. They eat dinner together whenever possible and during the meal each person is allotted 2 minutes (they set a timer) to give a presentation about their day. The message is that each person, regardless of their age, has something of value to contribute.

When your children help around the house, show appreciation. Even if the beds aren't made perfectly or dinner isn't as nutritious as you would like, let them know that you are grateful for their efforts. Al Siebert offers the following ideas[1]:

• Say "thank you."
• Buy or fix their favorite food.
• Give hugs and kisses.
• Give treats or little gifts.
• Leave nice notes for them; send cards.
• Share something interesting from your day.
• Speak highly of them to others.
• Let them feel that your success is their success.

Finding quiet time to study can be challenging when children are present. Here are a few suggestions:

• If your children are old enough, work on homework together.
• Have young children "help" you by drawing, coloring pictures, filling in sticker books, or performing other "desk work."
• Try turning your study time into a positive experience for the kids by saving their favorite videos, toys, and other activities for the times when you are busy.
• Set up a special place for children to play quietly while you study. Childproof a room in the house where older children can play while you study.
• Set a timer for quiet periods. If children know there is an end to the quiet time, they may be more willing to oblige.
• Let children help you study, such as by showing you flashcards or asking you questions.

Working with your children in these ways can be a win-win situation. Not only will you accomplish more, but you will serve as a positive role model for your children. They will see your behavior as a disciplined, goal-oriented person who enjoys learning and self-improvement.

Explore combining resources with other students. For example, see about organizing a study group with classmates who have children. Contribute to a babysitting fund, and hire someone to watch all the children while you study together. Or you could exchange childcare with one other student, trading off watching the children for an afternoon. For older children, investigate activities such as day camps, sports teams, and craft classes. Organizations such as churches and community centers offer these at reasonable prices. There may also be opportunities for single parents who are continuing their education.

Finally, if it becomes necessary, try studying before and after classes in the school library. You may accomplish more there in shorter periods of time than if you are at home with constant interruptions.

Working with Your Children

Chuck Graham teaches the Introduction to Health Care course at Sano College. Many of his students are older adults. Many work part- or even full-time, some have families and most are feeling a little overwhelmed with everything they have to do.

Several of Mr. Graham's students have had difficulty keeping up with the class work. They frequently turn in their assignments late and do poorly on weekly quizzes. He knows they are serious about training for a career in health care, so he decides to talk to the students individually about their lack of progress.

Rachel Schneider is one of the students he is most worried about and he asks her to meet with him after class.

"I guess I know why you wanted to talk with me," says Rachel. "I'm not doing well. Are you kicking me out of school?"

"Not at all," Mr. Graham reassures her. "But I am concerned about how you're doing in my class. Are you finding the work too difficult?"

"Not the work I'm able to get done," Rachel answers.

"Can you tell me what you mean by that—'the work you're able to get done'?" asks Mr. Graham.

"Well, I just don't have much time to study and do the homework. It's my kids—I have three and they take up a lot of my time. They're pretty demanding."

"How do they feel about your being in school?" Mr. Graham asks.

"Oh, they think I'm crazy! At least that's what they tell me. My son told me the other day he thought I was too old to be in school—that school is for kids!"

"What did you tell them when you were thinking about going back to school?" he asks.

"Well, honestly, not much. I had a lot of discussions with my husband because he works two jobs and we knew it would be hard covering everything at home. But I figured the kids would go along with whatever I needed. They've always been pretty good about things."

Mr. Graham explains, "Rachel, this is a really different situation for them. You worked in the past—in retail, right?"

Rachel nods. "When you got home from work, I'm guessing you devoted time to them."

"Yes," responds Rachel. "We did a lot of things together. I spent time helping them with homework, things like that."

"And now you just don't have that kind of time with them, do you?" asks Mr. Graham.

"Actually, that's just the thing. I feel guilty not sharing with them like I did before I went back to school. So I wait for them to go to bed before I start studying—but by then I'm usually just too tired…"

"And that's why your assignments aren't getting done," finishes Mr. Graham.

Rachel looks down. "That's it. I just feel like I need to be a good mom to my kids."

"From what you said when you first started class, I know you believe that training for a career will benefit your children in the future. As I recall, there were other students in the class who also have families and other responsibilities—and were hoping to better provide for them."

Rachel looks up. "Oh, I know some of the others are really busy. We've talked some about problems with our kids."

Mr. Graham has an idea. "How about I check with the class and see who would like to get together to talk about family issues? Maybe you all could share some ideas. Last year one of the classes organized a family gathering— kind of a picnic—here at the school on a Saturday. The kids were invited and we showed them what their moms and dads were learning—even let them peek through the microscopes and listen to their hearts through the stethoscope. It seemed to go over pretty well."

Questions for Thought and Reflection

1. Why was it a mistake for Rachel not to discuss her decision to attend school with her children?
2. What do you think of Mr. Graham's advice?
3. If you were in the group of student-parents, what suggestions would you offer?

Mary Jo grew up in a small town and married her high school boyfriend, Bruce, when she was 19. She and Bruce wanted children and decided they both preferred Mary Jo to be a stay-at-home mom until the kids were in school. After having their first child, they moved to a large city where Bruce would have more job opportunities. After 15 years at home, Mary Jo decided to explore her career options. She had always been interested in health care and liked working with her hands. She knew she would need some kind of education for any career she chose, but at her age, she didn't want to spend years in school.

After exploring a number of careers, Mary Jo enrolled in the dental assisting program at a local college. At first, she found the classes a bit challenging. "After all," she told Bruce. "I haven't been a student for a long time!" She sought help from her instructors and checked out websites that offered ideas for improving her study skills.

School seemed to be working out until Mary Jo suddenly found herself confronting a series of unexpected problems. Her father, who had lived alone and cared for himself after Mary Jo's mother died three years ago, suffered a debilitating stroke. After being hospitalized for a short time, he was moved to a rehabilitation facility an hour away from Mary Jo's house. Visiting him several times a week took a lot of her time—time she really needed for studying.

Mary Jo asked her sister, Carol, to come from out of town to stay a while and share some of the load. "Mary Jo," said Carol, "I'd love to help out. But I finally got a job myself. You know how long I've been looking. I'm afraid if I ask for a leave now they'll let me go."

When it is time for Mary Jo's father to be released from inpatient rehabilitation, she discusses the situation with Bruce. "Of course he can come live with us," Bruce assures her. "He's family—and a good guy." They prepare the guest room and make some alterations to the house to accommodate her father's wheelchair.

Mary Jo's children were basically good kids, but she had never expected them to do much around the house. She had been the second of eight children and felt that she didn't have much of a childhood, what with all the chores and babysitting. She wanted her kids to have time to focus on school and enjoy themselves in their free time. When she started attending classes herself, Mary Jo believed she could continue to manage the household: shopping, cooking, cleaning, and laundry. She reassured the children, "I'll still be 'mom' and take care of you."

Mary Jo now found herself a member of the "sandwich generation," caring for both her own parent and being a parent to her children. The stress of handling so many responsibilities became overwhelming. While Bruce was supportive of her school and career goals, he found it difficult to help with household chores.

In spite of the difficulties, Mary Jo struggled along and managed to graduate from her dental assisting program. She didn't earn the high grades she had hoped for, nor did she receive a certificate for perfect attendance, but she finished.

When she started her externship with Dr. Gutierrez, a local dentist, the situation reached a crisis point. Her classes had met four hours a day in the afternoon, so she had had time to study and take care of her other responsibilities at home. But now she was expected to be on site for eight hours a day. She found that after pushing so hard for so long to finish school, she was really tired and couldn't seem to get rested. Her father made demands on her time in the mornings, and she was often late getting to the dental office. To make matters worse, her family was complaining about the frequent fast-food dinners, lack of clean clothes, and other things missing from their lives now that Mary Jo was away all day.

Dr. Gonzalez called Mary Jo into his office toward the end of her second week of externship. "I'm sorry, Mary Jo," he started. "You will probably be a good dental assistant, but this just isn't working out. I depend on you to be here, and you have been late six days out of the last eight. And when you're here, you often seem to be just going through the motions."

Mary Jo's eyes filled with tears. "I know and I'm so sorry. I've let you down."

Dr. Gonzalez told her, "Well, it's a matter of my duty to my patients. I've got to be able to count on you, just as I do on my staff. I'm sorry this hasn't worked out."

Questions for Thought and Reflection

1. How did Mary Jo fail to prepare her family for her new role as a student?
2. Where might she find help to care for her father?
3. How can her husband and children be more helpful?
4. How might she persuade them to help?
5. Do you think she will be able to achieve her goal of becoming a dental assistant? Why or why not?

Maintaining Personal Relationships

Most adults have many relationships with others. These may include aging parents, a spouse or significant other, friends, and co-workers. Becoming a student can put a strain on these relationships because you will have less time to devote to them. In addition, your new status as a student may cause others to feel frustrated, jealous, or even threatened.

Include people who are important to you when making your educational plans. Consider throwing a going-back-to-school party. Invite friends and family and tell them about your plans, what you'll be studying, and the great future you anticipate working in health care. Let them know how important this is to you and ask for their support.

When adult students are interviewed, married women report having more difficulties than other students. Their role as "caretaker of family needs" presents obstacles when they assume the role of student.[1] It can be hard for a spouse or significant other to accept your new status as a student. They may worry you will leave them behind or not have time for them, or they may be jealous of your opportunity. Here are some things you can try if you find yourself with an unhappy spouse[1]:

1. Ask your spouse what is really bothering him or her. It will be easier to deal with if you are both clear on the nature of the problem.
2. Focus on the future. Emphasize that attending school is temporary.
3. Discuss how your studies can benefit your relationship.
4. Schedule time together to do something you both enjoy.

Being pulled in many directions can be stressful for everyone, and it is important to make a special effort to include family members in your decisions. If behavior problems develop with members of your family, such as being upset and refusing to talk, allow some time for adjustments. If the reactions of the others are extreme, it may be necessary to seek help such as family counseling. If this is difficult financially, check with your school about free or low-cost services in your community.

When you do spend time with others, try to minimize complaining. That is, don't go on and on about how difficult you are finding a subject, how a certain instructor gives challenging tests, how stressed you feel, and so on. These issues should be addressed with the staff at your school who can help you with these particular problems. If there is already some stress over your attending school, the last thing you need to do is cast a dark cloud over everything when you are home. Describing how tired you are, how difficult your classes are, or how unfair your instructors are will take away from the time you do have to spend with loved ones.

Although personal relationships can cause problems as you begin your studies, strong support systems can increase your chances for success. This is not surprising because studies have shown that social support is associated with good mental health and the ability to handle stress. There is even some evidence that good social support positively influences physical health. For example, the survival rates of individuals who have heart attacks are higher in those who have the greatest emotional support from others.[3,4]

Your personal support system may extend beyond your immediate family and can include anyone who encourages you and supports your goals: your health care provider, spiritual advisor, and members of your place of worship and other groups to which you belong.

There are three basic types of social support, and you can benefit from each:

1. Emotional: provided by people who make you feel loved and cared for and increase your sense of self-worth
2. Instrumental: provided by those who help you with specific tasks such as childcare, household tasks, and transportation
3. Informational: provided by instructors and others who give you the information you need to succeed as a student[5]

Don't hesitate to ask for support: explanations from your instructor, encouragement from your spouse. Show your appreciation and let people know how important their help is to you. And don't forget to give back—even if you are busy, you can offer to provide the same kind of support to others. In fact, giving of yourself is a valuable characteristic of the health care professional.

> ### Prescription for Success: 4-3 **My Support Team**
> 1. List the names of everyone you know who supports your decision to go to school.
> 2. From these names, who can you rely on when you need help?

Combining Work and School

Working takes time, but according to government surveys, many working students believe that employment helps them with their coursework; more than half think it helps them prepare for a career.[6] It may be wise, however, to work as few hours as is financially possible. Working full-time while attending school is doable, but it is difficult for most people.

Try to enlist the support of your employer. Discuss your educational plans and see if there are ways you can tie school assignments to your work. Take care, however, not to use work time inappropriately. If you are seeking a new job, look for a position that permits studying while at work, such as receptionist or security guard. (This would, of course, be with the employer's permission.)

Q&A with a Health Care Professional

Kim Fruge

Kim is a manager and caregiver in a care home for older and disabled adults. She shares her experience going back to school as an adult student with a family and full-time job.

Q When did you return to school to study medical assisting?

A Six years ago. I was married with grown children—they were 20 and 21 at the time—and had worked many years in retail. When I decided to make a change, I was a scan supervisor. That means I was supervising the coding and pricing of items in a large grocery store.

Q Why did you decide to change careers and return to school?

A I never really liked working in retail, but it was something I could do without any education beyond high school. I had always wanted to work in something where I could work directly with people, helping them in some way. I loved raising my kids and we always had their friends around the house. So I checked around and found out I could earn my certificate in medical assisting in a reasonable amount of time.

Q How did your family react when you decided to return to school?

A When I first decided to go back to school, my family thought I was crazy! They didn't think I would do it. But after I started talking about it and what I would achieve, they were 100% behind me. Then, after I started, they thought I would give up. But when they saw how well I was doing and the grades I was getting, they started encouraging me and trying to help me in any way they could. They helped me to study and to research. My son was still living at home. Actually, both my son and daughter helped me with homework and quizzed me. My daughter helped me with math.

When I accomplished something, they were very happy for me and patted me on the back. My son's friends were so nice—they would call me, help me study. Then my children's friends came to my graduation. They were so proud of me and what I had done because I graduated with a 3.8. And that was after 20 years of not being in school!

Q Did you find returning to school difficult?

A Oh, yes. I was still working 40 hours a week at the store, from 4 AM to noon or sometimes 2 PM. I'd go home for a quick nap and then go to class. My classes met Monday through Friday for 5 hours a night, so my schedule was intense. Including my externship, this all lasted about a year.

After not being in school for all those years, trying to learn how to study again was really hard until I found a way to make it easier for myself. I discovered flashcards and that really helped me. I made my own flashcards for whatever we were studying. I learned about these when we used them for medical terminology. Then I started making them for facts and questions in all my subjects. I don't think I could have made it through without those flashcards.

I did get discouraged sometimes—with pharmacology, for example. I had trouble learning to convert ratios so I could calculate medications. Math was always my worst, worst subject. I didn't think I would have to worry about math studying medical assisting but I was wrong about that!

Q What helped you most when you had problems with math?

A Actually, my husband, Jimmy, was great about helping. He could explain things in words so that I understood. Also, my instructors were wonderful. I always stayed after class and got as much help as possible. I always asked lots of questions. I would get help from Jimmy at home and then ask my teachers. Talking with my teachers really helped. I'm a hands-on learner, so once I saw it on paper, I could do it. So, ask for help when you need it!

Q What other advice do you have for adults who are returning to school?

A Set your goals and work to achieve them. Study hard. Do lots of research. Make sure you have the time to spend on school. You have to make this a priority. Always tell yourself what the outcome will be—what you will achieve by doing this. Do lots of research on things you don't understand. I spent lots of my time in the library trying to understand certain things. I did extra practice, too. I did lots more blood draws than were required to make sure I got it.

Q How did you handle time management?

A Very carefully! I stayed on a schedule that worked best for me and my family. I spent all my spare time studying, getting ahead on courses—doing extra homework ahead of time as much as possible because I always liked to be ahead of where we were, always doing extra credit to learn and better understand.

Q How did you handle the pressure of balancing so many activities?

A I took deep breaths and told myself, "I am smart enough to do this." I said that to myself at least once a week. There was a lot of pressure to make sure I got all my classwork done. And at work the pressure was making sure I met all my deadlines. As scan coordinator, I had to be sure the prices were all up to date.

Q How did you balance your job and school?

A The other employees and my boss were really great. I got their support when I started school. For example, when I did my externship from 8 to 5, I worked at the store on the weekends. They were all really good about accommodating me and my scheduling needs.

Overcoming Academic Weaknesses

You may have had difficulties during your previous educational experiences. This is very common for students of all ages who are pursuing career training. You may be a practical person who learns best through hands-on activities. If so, a health care career is a good choice because much of the work is hands-on. At the same time, health care requires background knowledge and theory, so academic skills are needed for reading, writing, and calculating.

If your academic and **study skills** are not what they should be, the first step is to acknowledge this. This is nothing to be embarrassed about. In fact, it is a sign of a strong character to recognize our weaknesses and seek the means to make improvements. It is very important to seek help as soon as you realize you need it. Many health care programs move along quickly. You may have only one month or a few weeks in a class. You cannot wait until just before the final exams to seek help. There are a couple of good reasons for this. First, it may simply be too late to catch up. Second, even if you are able to pass the class, have you really learned what you should? Have you mastered the information and skills you need to perform your future health care duties?

If you believe that your academic skills are not strong, plan to spend a little time each day working on them. For example, spend 15 or 20 minutes working on math skills or spelling.

Over time, you are likely to acquire the skills needed to master your classes.

Here are some ways to improve your study and academic skills:

1. Read the information and try the suggestions presented in this book. They include everything from understanding what you read, to overcoming anxiety about math, to writing a well-organized paper. See Chapters 7, 8, and 9.
2. Investigate the learning resources at your school: learning center, review courses, tutors, writing lab.
3. Look for helpful classes open to the public in your area: computer literacy, basic skills, using the Internet.
4. Organize a **study group** with other students.
5. Don't hesitate to ask your instructors for help. They want successful graduates—in other words, they want their students to succeed!

Many adults have trouble admitting when they don't know something or when they need help. But think of it this way: you are paying for your instructors to help you learn. That is their job and seeking their help is one way to ensure that you are getting what you pay for, just as you would with any other service. One difference with education, of course, is that you must do your part, too, by reading assignments, attending class, and doing the homework.

1. Look over the classes you will be taking and read any available descriptions. List any academic challenges that concern you.
2. What can you do now to improve your skills? Create a plan with resources and timelines.

Achieving academic success is important. At the same time, a common cause of stress among adult students is striving for perfection. You may feel that because you are older, you should do better than younger students. You may believe that others expect more of you. If your previous experiences in school were not all positive, don't stress yourself out thinking you must earn an A in every class. Your goals should focus on learning and preparing yourself for your health care career.

Summary of Key Ideas

- Adult students have different challenges and advantages from traditional students.
- There are effective strategies to handle the challenges faced by adult students.

Positive Self-Talk for This Chapter

- I have many experiences that will help me become a successful student.
- I face up to my fears and concerns and seek help when necessary.
- By attending school, I am making a better life for myself and my family.
- I can master the study skills I need to succeed in school.

Internet Activities

ⓔ For active links to the websites needed to complete these activities, visit http://evolve.elsevier.com/Haroun/career/.

1. Identify a problem you want to work on related to the topics in this chapter. Use search terms, such as "time management," "tips for adult students," or "studying with children" and choose three websites that deal with the topic. Try the suggestions you believe might be helpful and report on the results.

To Learn More

Doolin M: The success manual for adult college students, ed 3, 2006

Available at: http://www.Booklocker.com

Siebert A, Karr MK: The adult student's guide to survival and success, ed 6, Portland, Ore, 2008, Practical Psychology Press

Available at: http://www.adultstudent.com
The Internet companion to the book provides help with study skills and includes success stories and suggestions from other students.

Simon L: New beginnings: a reference guide for adult learners, ed 4, Upper Saddle River, NJ, 2009, Pearson Prentice Hall

References

1. Siebert A, Karr MK: *The adult student's guide to survival and success,* ed 6, Portland, Ore, 2008, Practical Psychology Press.
2. Ellis D: *Becoming a master student,* updated ed 8, Boston, 1998, Houghton Mifflin.
3. Berkman LF, Leo-Summers S, Hoewitz RI: Emotional support and survival after myocardial infarction: a prospective, population-based study on the elderly, *Ann Intern Med* 117:1003–1009, 1992.
4. Williams RB, Barefoot JC, Califf RM, et al.: Prognostic importance of social and economic resources among medically treated patients with angiographically documented coronary artery disease, *JAMA* 267:520–524, 1992.
5. Seeman T: *Social support and social conflict: Section one—social support.* John D and Catherine T MacArthur Research Network on Socioeconomic Status and Health, last revised 2008. Available at: www.macses.ucsf.edu/research/psychosocial/socsupp.php.
6. *Nontraditional undergraduates:* Findings from the condition of education, 2002, National Center for Education Statistics. Available at: http//nces.ed.gov/pubs2002/2002012.pdf.

CHAPTER 5

Strategies for English-as-a-Second-Language Students

OBJECTIVES

1. Identify areas of weakness in your English skills.
2. Use learning strategies to improve your English.
3. Review grammatical points that commonly present problems for English-as-a-second-language students.

KEY TERMS AND CONCEPTS

Consonant All the letters in the alphabet *except A, E, I, O, U,* and sometimes *Y.*

Context The words surrounding an unknown word that may give you clues to its meaning.

Grammar A set of rules for constructing sentences.

Idiom Words that when used together have a different meaning from the dictionary definition of the individual words.

Motivated Having enthusiasm or a purpose for doing something.

Phrasal Verb Verbs that can be combined with prepositions to create phrases that mean something different from what the verb means by itself.

Prepositions Words that show relationships, such as direction, place, time, and cause, between other words in a sentence.

Scan Read quickly to find something specific.

Skim Read quickly to explore or review.

Study Group A group of students who meet together on a regular basis to study, discuss, and support one another's learning.

Syllable The shortest part of a word that can be pronounced as a unit. For example, *contamination* has five syllables: con-tam-i-na-tion.

Vowels The following letters: *A, E, I, O, U,* and sometimes *Y.*

English for the Non-Native Speaker

English may be your second—or even third or fourth—language. This may be because you grew up in a family that spoke another language. Or you may have moved to the United States from another country. In either case, you probably speak English pretty well—perhaps very well. However, you may have concerns such as the following:

- I'm not always sure which verb tense to use. In fact, I could use some help with many parts of grammar.
- English spelling is difficult. How can I remember words that have so many letters that aren't even pronounced?
- I have an accent and am self-conscious about speaking.
- I'm worried about doing writing assignments in school or having to write on the job.

These are natural concerns when English is not your first language, and they, along with other challenges, will be discussed in this chapter. First, let's look at some of the advantages of knowing more than one language. You may have heard the term "global economy," which is evidence of just how interconnected the countries of the world have become. You also know that the people of the United States come from a variety of countries and cultures. Large numbers of people living in the United States do not speak English well. Some do not speak it at all. Knowing at least two languages can be a real advantage in this environment. This is especially true in health care. Think about how frightening it can be for patients who are being treated by someone they can't easily communicate with. If you speak a language that is spoken by many people in your area, this is a valuable and useful skill. You have something extra to offer your future employers.

If you speak a Romance language, such as Spanish, you may be surprised to find that some medical terms you will be learning are similar to everyday words in your language. Table 5-1 contains several examples of terms that speakers of

TABLE 5-1
Medical Words and Everyday Spanish

Medical Term or Word Element	Related Everyday Spanish Word	Nonmedical Term in English
mandible	mandíbula	jaw
costa, costal	costilla	rib
pulmonary	pulmón	related to the lungs
brachi/o	brazo	arm
oste/o	hueso	bone
ot/o	oído	ear
quadr-	cuatro	four
axillary	axila	pertaining to the armpit

Spanish might find easier to learn than students who speak only English.

Personal Reflection

1. What are some reasons you want to improve your English?
2. How would better English help you in school?
3. In your future career?

Prescription for Success: 5-1 My Problems with English

Write a short description of up to five problems you have with English.

Strategies for Improving Your English

"Surround yourself with English; practice it, study it, and you will learn it."

—Kathy Ochoa Flores

To be successful at improving your English, it is important to be committed and **motivated.** This means that you *want* to improve your English communication skills. At the same time, be patient with yourself. Mastering another language is a gradual process, taking time and effort.

A good way to start is to set learning goals for yourself. Think about what you want or need to improve. Write your goals out, along with your plan to achieve them. For example, you might decide to add 50 words to your vocabulary by reading one news article each day for a month. (See Chapter 3 for more about goals.) Setting and achieving goals will keep you on track and seeing what you have accomplished can motivate you to keep learning.

Language teachers agree that to learn or master another language, you need to spend some time—even if it is only 10 to 20 minutes—studying or practicing every day. This is more effective than working on it once a week for several hours. Try using different learning activities each day: reading a short article, practicing your pronunciation, or listening to a talk show on the radio.

Try to make your language study fun. Choose practice materials that interest you. For example, if you have a hobby, a favorite type of music, or a sport you like to watch, find related articles on the Internet. This helps to make learning more enjoyable and effective. Read jokes. (*Reader's Digest* magazine has many sections containing humor; it also contains articles, written in nontechnical language, about a wide variety of topics you might find interesting.) Try playing word games such as Bananagrams, Scrabble, word searches, and crossword puzzles. There are websites with interactive games. One to start with is www.learn-english-today.com that contains dozens of games, quizzes, links to newspapers, grammar explanations, fun activities, and much more. To find more websites, use the search term "word games to learn English."

Kenneth Beare, an English-as-a-second-language expert, suggests doing a short warm-up exercise before you begin an English study session[1]:

1. Think about the subject you are about to study, recalling the vocabulary you will use
2. Sing a song to help your brain focus in a relaxed manner
3. Type a short paragraph in English to activate the part of your brain that learns through physical activity
4. Describe a photo or other image that is related to what you are about to study

Improving Your Speaking

The best way to improve any skill is to practice—a lot. Although this is the best way, it is not always the easiest. For example, you may speak a language other than English with the people with whom you spend most of your time. Perhaps your parents don't speak English. You may be more comfortable with friends who speak your language and understand your cultural background. But if you are serious about improving your English, you need to look for opportunities to use it. Here are some suggestions:

- Make friends with classmates who speak English only. Invite them to have coffee and use the time to practice speaking. This is a good way to learn slang and informal conversational English (Figure 5-1).
- Organize or join a **study group** in which the majority of the members speak English.
- Speak up in class to ask and answer questions. If this is too difficult at first, speak with your instructors outside of class.
- Talk with everyone you can, such as people you do business with: clerks in stores, the librarian, or the receptionist at the doctor's office.

- Speak aloud when you are by yourself: describe what you are doing as you go about your tasks at home; read what you are studying aloud.

It can be scary speaking English with people you don't know, especially if you are self-conscious about your speaking ability. It is especially hard for adults who worry about sounding dumb. But this is the best way to learn. In Chapter 1, we said that students have the right to make mistakes. This is also true for people who want to improve their English—they have the right to make mistakes. In fact, you must give yourself permission to make mistakes. Think about it in this way: if you only repeat what you already know and don't try new things, you won't learn anything new. English instructors believe that their best students are the ones who are willing to take risks. They are not afraid to make mistakes and don't worry about using perfect grammar, vocabulary, or pronunciation. When they make mistakes, they are not discouraged. Instead, they learn from their errors.

Good language students speak with other people (not during class when the instructor is speaking, of course!), ask and answer questions, and interact as much as possible. If your instructors make you work in groups, this is an excellent way to practice. Health care involves working with others and interacting with your classmates is excellent practice for this on-the-job skill. If you sit quietly in class everyday, you will lose many opportunities to learn and practice.

You could also try practicing at home. If you have family members who are interested, teach them new English words and phrases. Teaching others is an excellent way to learn and reinforce what you know.

Improving Your Listening Comprehension

Just as in the case of speaking, the key to improving your understanding of spoken English is to practice listening.

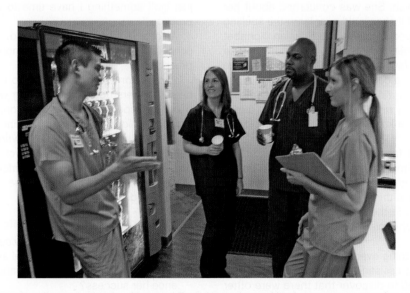

FIGURE 5-1 Become friends with native English speakers with whom you can practice speaking. *Do you have classmates with whom you can study? This week, ask someone if they would be willing to study with you and/or help you practice speaking English.* (From Yoder-Wise PS: *Leading and managing in nursing,* ed 6, St. Louis, 2015, Mosby.)

In class, don't hesitate to ask the instructor if there are words you don't understand. This is especially important if these are vocabulary terms or words you will need on the job.

When listening in any situation, start by listening for the main ideas. Don't try to translate from English to your native language. This distracts your attention from the speaker and can cause confusion as you try to translate and listen at the same time.

In addition to conversing with others and listening to class lectures, listen to radio programs such as news shows and talk programs. The Internet contains a number of websites such as the Voice of America that have audio versions of international news reports. It is available at http://learningenglish. voanews.com. For health and medical related topics, go to www.nlm.nih.gov/medlineplus and click on Videos and Cool Tools. You can watch and listen to dozens of videos.

Case Study 5-1

Gaining Confidence with English

Alyona's family emigrated from Russia to the United States when she was 18. Although English is a required course in Russian schools, much of the emphasis was on grammar and reading. Therefore, no one in the family considers himself or herself to be fluent.

It took some months for the family to become settled and even more time to become a little accustomed to life in a country so different from the one they had left. They became involved in a local Russian Orthodox Church and a community center dedicated to helping immigrants find services, such as a doctor or dentist.

Alyona's parents were well-educated professionals in Russia. Hearing about the high school dropout rate among the children of Russian immigrants, they realized that learning English and helping their children to succeed in school should be high priorities for the family. They spoke with the teachers at the public schools attended by their younger children about helping them mainstream and learn English. Then they located English classes at an adult school for Alyona and themselves.

Alyona enjoyed her English classes, but found that at age 18 it was not easy to master a language as different from Russian as English. She was concerned about her accent and wondered if she would ever learn the spelling of English words, especially since the Russian alphabet is different. But like her parents, she was motivated to succeed and after a few months of class, believed she was ready to look into a career. As a youngster, she was interested in becoming a doctor like her Uncle Leo. But that goal seemed pretty unattainable now that the family had left Russia, so she knew she had to consider other options.

One day she was talking to a social worker at the community center who suggested she look into an allied health career—perhaps medical assisting. That way, she could be working within a year and if she decided to pursue her education in the future, she could return to school to become a physician assistant or perhaps even a physician.

After talking everything over with her parents, Alyona enrolled in a medical assisting program at a local college. She was relieved to discover that there were other students whose native language was not English. Only a few of the other students spoke Russian, but she decided that was probably a good thing because this forced her to speak in English at school. She studied hard

and sought help from a writing tutor. Her parents were proud of her efforts and threw a party the night of her graduation.

"I really appreciate how much you've supported me," she told her parents. "I know things aren't that easy for you here, so it means even more to me."

"You know, Alyona, one of the reasons we came here was to ensure that you and your brothers had a good future," said her father as he gave her a hug.

"Well, I graduated. But I am really nervous about looking for a job. Do you think my accent and the problems I still have with writing and spelling will be problems?" Alyona asked.

"You will have to continue working on your English. But you passed your classes and the certification exam, so I do not know why you would have too much trouble with work," said her mother.

Alyona was able to get a job at a nearby clinic. One factor in her favor was that she spoke Russian. As the clinic director, Dr. McNeil, explained, "We have a large number of patients who speak Russian. I really want to be able to communicate with them, but learning another language just isn't something I have time to do while running the practice."

Alyona laughed. "I understand. I studied English in school in Russia, and I still spent months here learning and practicing."

Alyona sometimes struggled to understand and make herself understood when working with English-speaking patients, especially the younger ones who had interesting expressions she wasn't familiar with. But she found it really satisfying to help those who spoke Russian, especially the older people, who were worried about their health problems and found it comforting when the medical assistant spoke their language and understood their backgrounds.

Questions for Thought and Reflection

1. What factors helped Alyona succeed at learning English and completing her medical assisting program?
2. How did the attitude of Alyona and her parents influence her success?
3. Why was knowing a second language helpful to her employer?
4. What community resources do you have to help you with your English skills?

Beatriz grew up in the city of Curitiba in southern Brazil. Her native language, Portuguese, is different from Spanish. "No," she often has to tell people who know she is from South America. "I don't speak Spanish very well. In Brazil, we speak Portuguese."

Beatriz loved Curitiba, a bustling city with a year-round mild climate, beautiful parks and gardens, a variety of churches, and open squares. She enjoyed being outdoors, especially swimming, walking, playing tennis, and cycling on the city's many miles of bike paths.

When her father's multinational employer transferred him to Michigan, she was too young to stay in Brazil by herself. She tried to be positive and look on the move as an adventure. There were many adjustments: cold winters requiring more layers of clothes than she had ever worn; learning enough English to get by in school; making friends with other teens who didn't know much about Brazil; and getting along without her long-time friends in Curitiba. Life in the United States moved along at a faster pace than in Brazil where leisurely lunches and dinners, followed by conversation with family and friends, were common. There was no eating on the go, no one grabbing lunch and eating at their desk at work.

Beatriz had one year of high school remaining when the family moved. Fortunately, they arrived in early June, so she spent the summer taking English classes. Because school was not in session, she didn't have a chance to meet many teens her age and when the school year started in September, she shyly attended her first classes at the local high school. She took advantage of the tutoring her school offered for ESL students. Working hard, Beatriz was able to graduate with her class. She considered returning to Brazil, but her mother had recently been diagnosed with multiple sclerosis and Beatriz, as the oldest child, did not want to leave her.

After a few months of helping her mother at home, Beatriz began to think about her future. "Beatriz," her mother suggested, "why don't you think about a career in health care? You've done such a good job helping me, I think you'd be good at it."

The idea appealed to Beatriz. She wondered if she could combine her interest in sports and fitness with a career helping others. After exploring various options, she enrolled in a massage therapy program. She liked the hands-on nature of the work. She thought she might meet people who shared her interest in sports. Most important, she was still shy about speaking English and believed that with a career in massage, the need to speak and interact would be limited.

Beatriz passed her coursework. She found it difficult when she was assigned to do group work that involved discussing and contributing orally or when she had to answer a question in class or give an oral report. She declined invitations to join study groups or obtain extra help to improve her English, both because she was shy and she felt the need to return home to her mother as soon as the school day ended. However, she did manage to complete her program and graduate.

Beatriz is still self-conscious about speaking and feels fortunate that her younger brother is outgoing and unafraid to speak up. Whenever possible, she takes him along with her to do the shopping and other family business that her mother is no longer able to do. Her massage therapy school has offered to help her find a job after graduation. In fact, they are encouraging her to seek employment. But she is terrified about attending interviews. She not only worries that she may not understand a question, she doesn't believe she can think quickly enough and form a good answer in English. She spends the first month after graduation helping out at home, getting more nervous by the day. She finally decides that for now, seeking a job is something she just can't handle.

Questions for Thought and Reflection

1. What could Beatriz have done to increase her confidence speaking English?
2. What wrong assumptions did she make about the need to communicate in school, and in seeking a job and working as a therapist?
3. What suggestions do you have for Beatriz at this point?

Increasing Your Vocabulary

The English language has more words than any of us—even teachers and textbook writers—will ever know. However, to get along in English, you should know about 2,000 frequently used words. To succeed in college, this number grows to 10,000 to 15,000 words.[2]

Here are a few suggestions for increasing your vocabulary:

1. Set a goal of learning a certain number of new vocabulary words each week. While you are studying health care, you may want to concentrate on terms related to your future career.

2. In a notebook or on your computer, list new words as you encounter them. Write the word, its definition, and a sentence using the word. Write something personal to make the word your own.[1] Use the new words, in both oral and written forms, as often as possible.

3. Make posters of your new vocabulary and put them up where you will see them every day. Use pictures and drawings.

4. Record (or have a native English speaker record) your new words along with a sentence for each one. Listen to the recording often.

5. Study word lists such as vocabulary, key terms, and the glossaries in your textbooks.

6. Find other basic English word lists, such as those on the websites listed at the end of this chapter.

7. Try using Google Translate, available by simply typing "google translate" into your search browser. You can translate words and sentences between dozens of languages. The translations of complex sentences are not always correct but it works very well with vocabulary. Google Translate is also available as an app.

8. There are several online dictionaries for both everyday words and medical terms. Use the search terms "online dictionaries" and "online medical dictionaries." Good websites for everyday words include http://www.merriam-webster.com/dictionary and http://dictionary.cambridge.org. Try http://www.nlm.nih.gov/medlineplus/mplusdictionary.html for medical and health-related terms.

Prescription for Success: 5-2 Create Your Own Dictionary

Start a vocabulary list of your own. This can be a paper list in your binder or an electronic list on your computer, tablet, or phone. When you see or hear a new word, add it to your list. Include pronunciation hints (or record), the definition, and a sentence using the word.

Idioms

Idioms are phrases composed of words that when used together have a different meaning from the dictionary definitions of the individual words. Here are a few examples:

- You are pulling my leg = You are trying to trick me by saying something that is not true.
- I can't keep my head above water = I have so much to do that I can't manage this situation.
- She spilled the beans about Maria = She let out a secret about Maria.

Idioms exist in most languages and can be difficult for language learners to understand. Because these expressions are commonly used in English, consider adding them to your vocabulary learning goals. A list of the 66 most common idioms is available at http://www.smart-words.org/quotes-sayings/idioms-meaning.html. A much longer list is available at www.usingenglish.com/reference/idioms.

Prescription for Success: 5-3 Interesting Idioms

Idioms are commonly used in English. Learning them will add to both your comprehension and your speaking skills. Add them to your vocabulary list and practice using them each day.

Improving Your Pronunciation

Pronunciation can be a problem, especially if you learned English as an adult. Once our habits are established and the muscles in our tongue and mouth become accustomed to making the sounds of our first language, it becomes more difficult to form "foreign" sounds. It is a problem for some people to distinguish between similar sounds, so it is important to listen carefully.

If you can be understood easily, you may not need to worry too much about having an accent. Some people find accents interesting, even charming. However, if you are working on developing an "American accent," it is a good idea to model your speech after television newscasters. This is because they speak what is considered standard or neutral American English rather than one of the many regional ways of speaking found throughout the United States.

Perhaps even more important than the pronunciation of individual words is how they are combined into sentences and on which words and **syllables** (parts of words) the stress (emphasis) is placed. Using a rhythm that is different from the way Americans speak makes your speech difficult to understand. Therefore, listening carefully to native speakers and practicing entire sentences are important parts of pronunciation practice.

Combining Sounds

A common custom in spoken English is to link words together when there is a **vowel** sound between them. An example is the sentence "I want an apple." If each word is pronounced carefully and separately, this results in a "foreign" sound. Spoken by a native speaker, this sentence sounds like "I wannanappul." The words are run together, and the letter "t" disappears. Another example is "Would you like an apple?" which becomes "Wouldjuh likeanappul?" Consider the following examples:

1. "An elephant" sounds like "a-nelephant" or "uh-nelephant"
2. "An orange" sounds like "a-norange or "uh-norange"

You may not realize it, but many languages do this. French, especially, is full of linked sounds in which whole parts of words seem to disappear. When spoken quickly and naturally, Spanish does the same thing. We grow accustomed to understanding our own language. It's just more difficult when we don't know a language well.

Here are a few more examples of English pronunciation characteristics:

- The common use of the sound "uh" for vowels: mother—m*uh*ther; the—th*uh*; complicated—complicat*uh*d.
- The letter "t" pronounced as a "d" when the word requires a faster sound: little—liddle; anatomy—anaduhmy; thirty—therdy. (Note, however, that "thirteen" retains the "t" sound. This is because the word parts before and after the "t" in "thirteen" are longer than in "thirty.")
- Many words are pronounced differently from how they are spelled: have to—haffto; bright—brite.
- Some words are spelled the same but pronounced differently to convey different meanings: "read" is pronounced "reed" when meaning the present tense and "red" when meaning the past tense.
- Combinations of consonants. In many languages, there are vowels between consonants that give a kind of running start to the tongue. For example, the word just used—"start"—begins with two consonants, s and t. When first learning English, speakers of some languages may say "e-start"—they need that extra first vowel to get the word going.

As you can see, English pronunciation is not easy to learn by studying the language's written form. So just how do you learn to speak this language well? The answer is *by listening and practicing.* The best way is to spend time communicating with native English speakers who don't slow or simplify their speech.

They must also be willing to correct your mistakes. Their being too nice to say anything will not help you to learn. Practicing this way may sound challenging, but trying to learn English speech from rules is much more difficult. There is just no way to list and memorize all the different combinations of words and sounds. And it certainly is a lot more fun to work with someone else.

> **Prescription for Success: 5-4 Conversation Buddy**
>
> 1. Write a list of people with whom you can practice speaking English.
> 2. Choose someone on your list to be a "conversation buddy." Ask that person if he or she would be willing to talk with you regularly to help you with your pronunciation and vocabulary, when necessary. This will work best if you have scheduled times to meet. Write them on your calendar.
>
> *Hint:* If this person is also in your classes, you can talk about what you are learning and make even better use of your time.

Improving Your Reading Comprehension

Reading has the advantage of time—you can take your time and read a sentence over and over. You can also stop and look up new words in the dictionary. At the same time, this can create a problem because you may be tempted to look up every word you don't know and end up spending hours reading. English-language professor Kathy Flores recommends that students read an entire assignment first without stopping.[2] Your purpose during this first reading is to look for the main ideas. This can be difficult to do if you are constantly stopping to look up words. Here are some suggestions for completing this first reading[3]:

1. Ignore words that seem unimportant.
2. Use the **context** to guess the meaning.
3. **Scan** for specific information.
4. **Skim** for general information.
5. Read in units or chunks of words.

When reading textbook assignments, start by reviewing any key terms listed at the beginning of a chapter. This will highlight the vocabulary that the author considers to be important for understanding the chapter. Second, read the learning objectives. These will help you identify what is most important and what you should be looking for as you read.

Once you have finished the first reading, write a list of the main ideas as you understood them. Then read the chapter again, this time listing and looking up the words you don't know. Later, you can practice the words by writing sentences and using your preferred learning method, such as flashcards. Focus on learning key words for the subject you are studying.

Improving Your Spelling

Spelling is difficult for both native and non-native English speakers (including me!). In Chapter 8 there is a section on spelling written for native speakers of English. The spelling of English words is difficult for several reasons:

1. One letter can be pronounced in different ways, depending on the word. This is different from languages such as Spanish, in which the letters do not vary much in sound. Note the variations for the letter "o" in the following words:
   * *o*nce
   * *o*nly
   * w*o*man
   * w*o*men (These last two words can be really confusing! The words are almost identical, but in the plural form the "o" sound changes to "i"!)

   (If you are unsure of the differences in sound, ask a native speaker to read them aloud.)

2. The same combinations of letters can be pronounced in different ways, such as in l*ie* and rel*ie*ve. The letters "ough" have a variety of pronunciations, none of them including the letter g:
   * t*ough*—pronounced "tuhf"
   * thr*ough*—pronounced "throo"
   * d*ough*—pronounced "doe"
   * b*ough*t—pronounced "bawt"

3. Different spellings can be pronounced the same way. Consider the following examples with the sound "ee":
   * m*e*
   * m*ee*t
   * m*ea*t
   * ch*ie*f
   * p*eo*ple

   The following are a few more examples with the sound "oo":
   * f*oo*d
   * r*u*de
   * cr*ew*
   * gr*ou*p
   * thr*ough*
   * bl*ue*
   * sh*oe*

4. In some words, not all the syllables are pronounced when a native speaker talks quickly. See Table 5-2 for some examples.

These examples demonstrate why you have to memorize the spelling of many words. You may wonder why English has such a variety of vocabulary and spellings. It is largely because English has a number of different roots: Anglo-Saxon, Latin, and Greek. Other languages have contributed vocabulary to

TABLE 5-2
Examples of Words with Silent Syllables

Word	Syllables in Written Form	Syllables in Spoken Form
aspirin	as-pi-rin	as-prin
different	dif-fer-ent	diff-rent
temperature	tem-per-a-ture	tem-pra-ture
comfortable	comf-ter-ble	comf-ter-ble
vegetable	veg-e-ta-ble	veg-table

TABLE 5-3

Examples of Common English Grammar Challenges

Grammatical Point	Explanation	Examples
Using *a*	Use before words beginning with a **consonant**	*a* nurse *a* busy nurse
Using *an*	Use before words beginning with a vowel	*an* obstetrician *an* obstetric nurse
Using *the*	Use when you have a specific noun in mind	We need *the* nurse we saw this morning. (Not just any nurse but a specific one.)
The with plural nouns	Do not use *the* with plural nouns that mean "all" or "in general"	Incorrect: The physicians must study many years before they can practice medicine. Correct: Physicians must study many years before they can practice medicine.
Helping verbs	Do not use the infinitive (the "to" form of the verb: to study, to prepare) with helping verbs	Incorrect: I can to study in the library. Correct: I can study in the library. Incorrect: I must to prepare for the test. Correct: I must prepare for the test.
Verb forms that function as nouns	Certain verbs with –ing added function as nouns	I really enjoy *swimming* in the lake. Jaime will finish *studying* in about an hour.
Verbs + **prepositions** (phrasal verbs)	Many verbs can be combined with prepositions to create idioms in which the phrase has a meaning that is different from the meaning of the verb by itself	call off = cancel drop in = visit drop off = deliver get up = arise look up = visit, find run into = meet unexpectedly
Although and *but*	Certain word pairs are incorrect. Use one or the other, not both	Incorrect: Although the waiting room was full, but the office was running on schedule. Correct: *Although* the waiting room was full, the office was running on schedule. Correct: The waiting room was full *but* the office was running on schedule.
Using prepositions	These little words can be tricky. Even when the meaning is similar, different prepositions may be correct	To get to the workshop, Carla will travel *by* car. To get to the workshop, Carla will travel *on* the bus. To get to the workshop, Carla will travel *by* plane.

Adapted from Hacker D: *A writer's reference,* ed 6, Boston, 2007, Bedford St Martin's Press.

English, including Danish and Norman French. This is why we have so many different and overlapping spelling patterns. It also explains why English has such a large vocabulary: different words meaning the same thing were adopted from various languages.

There are some major spelling rules, and these are listed in Chapter 8 in Table 8-7. These rules can be helpful. However, as one author puts it, they are like weather reports. We can use them but cannot depend on them to be correct 100% of the time.[4] See also the lists of commonly misspelled words in Table 8-8 and commonly confused words in Table 8-9.

Improving Your Grammar

Grammar is a language's set of rules for constructing sentences, using verbs, punctuating, and so on. When using our native languages, we don't think too much about grammar. We just speak and write out of habit. When learning or improving our skills in another language, it can be helpful to learn grammar rules.

Rules help to organize a language to make communication easier and increase understanding. Some of the rules of basic English are contained in Tables 8-3, 8-4, 8-5, and 8-6 in Chapter 8. Certain points of more advanced English grammar present special problems for speakers of other languages. A number of these are explained, along with examples, in Table 5-3. The intention is not to offer a complete coverage of English grammar, but to present a review of some common challenges. If you find something you don't understand or that has been a problem for you, I suggest that you seek more complete explanations and practice exercises.

A word about grammar checkers: the grammar checkers included in word-processing software often do not catch errors. What is worse, their suggestions frequently suggest constructions that contain mistakes. This can be a problem for students who have limited experience with English. I suggest that you do not use them. There are highly rated grammar checkers online, such as Grammarly, but they are not free.

Many websites contain good explanations and examples of the grammar topics presented in this chapter. Choose topics you would like to learn more about and use a search engine or the website addresses listed under the "To Learn More" section. List five sites, along with each site's address and its contents that you will find useful for future reference.

Summary of Key Ideas

- English can be challenging but with study and practice, it can be mastered.

Positive Self-Talk for This Chapter

- I have the advantage of knowing more than one language.
- I am improving my English every day.

Internet Activities

ⓔ For active links to the websites needed to complete these activities, visit http://evolve.elsevier.com/Haroun/career/.

C hoose three websites in the "To Learn More" section to explore. Try the suggestions or do the exercises or activities you believe may be helpful and report on the results.

To Learn More

Activities for ESL Students

http://a4esl.org
The activities include grammar explanations, quizzes, and vocabulary practice.

E Learn English Language

http://www.elearnenglishlanguage.com
This site contains short grammar lessons, along with examples and diagrams.

English Club

http://www.EnglishClub.com
English Club provides help with all aspects of English, from reading to listening comprehension.

English Page

http://www.englishpage.com
Explore the online tutorials that teach English grammar and vocabulary. There are good practice exercises and links to dozens of other useful sites.

ESL Mania

http://www.eslmania.com
Contains information on topics ranging from grammar to writing a good e-mail message in English.

Flores K: What every ESL student should know: A guide to college and university academic success, Ann Arbor, 2008, University of Michigan Press

Flores shares tips for learning English gathered from her years of teaching English to college students from around the world who come to the United States to study.

Hacker D, Sommers N: A writer's reference, ed 7, Boston, 2010, Bedford/St. Martin's

This is an excellent, easy-to-use book that includes explanations and examples of grammar, sentence structure, punctuation, and organization of content. One entire section is devoted to special help for ESL students.

Hospital English

http://www.hospitalenglish.com
Vocabulary is grouped into families of health care words such as diseases, vocabulary for interaction with patients, and body systems. The site includes audio for pronunciation help and quizzes to check understanding.

Learn English Today

http://www.learn-english-today.com
This site has lessons on all aspects of English, including a good list of phrasal verbs.

Resources for English as a Second Language

http://www.UsingEnglish.com
This is a comprehensive site with lists of idioms, phrasal verbs, irregular verbs, grammar, and more. There are quizzes on all aspects of English, plus links to other useful websites.

Purdue University Online Writing Lab

http://owl.english.purdue.edu/owl/resource/678/01/
A section of this excellent Writing Lab is designed for ESL students.

References

1. Beare K. How to study English effectively. Available at: http://esl.about.com/od/intermediateenglish/a/study_english.htm.
2. Flores K: *What every ESL student should know: A guide to college and university academic success*, Ann Arbor, 2008, University of Michigan Press.
3. John's ESL Community: Reading strategies. Available at: www.johnsesl.com/templates/reading/strategies.php.
4. Norquist R, Top: 4 spelling rules. Available at: http://grammar.about.com/od/words/tp/spellrules.htm.

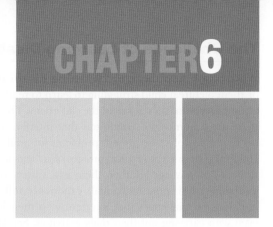

CHAPTER 6

Strategies for Students with Learning Disabilities

OBJECTIVES

1. Understand the nature of learning disabilities and common challenges associated with them.
2. Explore strategies and devices that help compensate for learning difficulties.
3. Identify your own learning difficulties and seek accommodations at school, during the job search, and on the job.

KEY TERMS AND CONCEPTS

Abbreviation Expanders Computer programs that allow a user to create, store, and reuse abbreviations for frequently used words or phrases.

Eye-Level Reading Ruler Plastic ruler especially designed to help individuals with visual and reading disabilities.

Guided Imagery Refers to various types of meditation and relaxation exercises that involve mental images of pleasant scenes and/or negative thoughts leaving the mind.

Learning Center A dedicated section of a school that offers help with academics and study skills.

Learning Disabilities General term for a variety of learning problems caused by differences in how the brain processes information.

Prefix Letter or group of letters attached to the beginning of a word to adjust its meaning.

Self-Advocacy Seeking solutions to your problems, taking steps to solve them, and asking for help when you need it.

Study Group A group of students who meet together on a regular basis to study, work, and support one another's learning.

Suffix A letter or a group of letters attached to the end of a word to form a new word or to alter the grammatical function of the original word.

Syllable The shortest part of a word that can be pronounced as a unit. For example, contamination has five syllables: con-tam-i-na-tion.

Tutor A person who helps others learn specific subjects or skills in a one-on-one or small-group setting.

White Noise Machine Device that produces random noise such as a rushing waterfall or wind through trees. (Used to block out irritating or disruptive noise.)

Yoga Practices for health and relaxation that include breath control, meditation, and the adoption of specific body postures.

The Challenge of Learning Disabilities

When people hear the term **"learning disability,"** many of them picture a child struggling to learn to read or perhaps a youngster who can't sit still in the classroom. The fact is that there are a number of conditions that interfere with learning and many of these present problems for adults as well as children. There are no typical profiles of a "learning disabled student" of any age. Rather, there is a variety of learning disabilities, and some individuals experience different combinations of challenges that interfere with their learning or even with carrying out their daily activities. See Box 6-1 for examples of common challenges.

You may have been diagnosed with a learning disability as a child or teenager. Or you may have simply wondered why you had, or are having, certain difficulties in school, on the job, or in your personal life. Learning disabilities are not always obvious, even to the person who has them, and for this reason they are sometimes referred to as "hidden" or "invisible" disabilities. Actually, it doesn't really matter if you "have" a learning disability. What matters is that if you have noticed you have more difficulty than other people with certain tasks, and if this often gets in the way of your learning and living productively, there are positive actions you can take. As an adult, you have self-awareness and can monitor your own behavior and work to make changes.

What Learning Disabilities Are—and Are Not

There are some things you should know about learning disabilities:

- They are *not* related to intelligence. In fact, some research indicates that individuals with Attention Deficit Disorder tend to have above-average IQs.
- They are not always obvious and can result in puzzling contradictions. (See Box 6-2 for examples.)
- They do not prevent people from having successful and high-level careers.
- Some people with learning disabilities are especially creative and able to come up with innovative ideas.
- Being learning disabled has *nothing* to do with a lack of effort or laziness.
- Having a learning disability does *not* mean you can't learn. It simply means you learn in different ways from other students.
- Learning disabilities are not a person's fault nor are they caused by a person's unwillingness to try to do better.

Learning disabilities are based on biological factors, mostly involved with certain specific brain functions. Scientific research has shown that they may be the result of one or more of the following: conditions present before birth; heredity; variations in brain development; neurological (pertaining to the nervous system) damage; or dysfunction of the central nervous system.[1] For example, different brain biology has been noted in the scans of the frontal lobes of the

BOX 6-1 Challenges Associated with Learning Disabilities

- Rarely completing projects you start
- Rarely meeting deadlines
- Being unable to manage time realistically
- Constantly feeling the need to move around or fidget
- Being unable to handle sequential or serial information
- Being unable to stay focused for more than very short periods of time
- Getting distracted very easily
- Seeing letters and numbers in the wrong order
- Having letters go blurry or jumping around when you are reading
- Experiencing great difficulty remembering oral instructions
- Having trouble judging distance and determining direction, such as left and right
- Always feeling disorganized and out of control
- Being unable to write legibly or neatly, even when you try
- Easily forgetting material that is presented visually
- Experiencing great difficulty in communicating thoughts orally or in writing
- Constantly losing your possessions

BOX 6-2 Contradictions in Performance

- You can think logically, but cannot write your thoughts in a paragraph.
- You are alert and skilled, but have trouble following directions.
- You understand mathematical theories, but get confused performing calculations.
- You practice for hours, but your handwriting is illegible.
- You have creative ideas, but cannot explain them clearly to others.
- You write beautiful stories and essays, but your spelling is very poor.

brain in individuals with Attention Deficit Disorder.[2] This is the area that controls executive functions. These include paying attention, focusing and concentrating, making decisions, planning ahead, and remembering what we have learned.

Strategies for Overcoming the Challenges of Learning Disabilities

There are many strategies you can use to overcome the challenges of learning disabilities. You are encouraged to try the strategies presented in this chapter. They are organized by academic and life skills, such as reading and time management, and presented in Tables 6-1 to 6-11. Choose strategies that correspond to the difficulties you are experiencing and that seem appropriate for you. Not all of them will work for every student. For example, let's look at the following suggestion: "Take notes as you read your textbook to increase your concentration." Now, if one of your problems is difficulty with your handwriting, this might not be good advice. In that case, you could place your book next to your computer and take notes on your word processing program. But if you are very slow at typing or very easily distracted, this might not work for you. So perhaps underlining key words in your text and making short notes in the margins might work best. Repeating the important points out loud may also work. Consider your own situation to determine what might work best for you.

If the suggestions don't work and you find yourself struggling with your studies, speak with your instructors and perhaps an administrator at your college. Don't wait until you experience feelings of desperation or panic. There is no need to miss achieving your academic and career goals when help is available.

You may also want to check with your physician. There are medications available for conditions such as ADHD (Attention Deficit/Hyperactivity Disorder), but deciding about their use requires a diagnosis and monitoring by a qualified health professional.

TABLE 6-1
Communication

Difficulties	Suggested Strategies
You find it difficult to follow what people are saying.	Keep your eyes on the speaker to avoid getting distracted. Ask the speaker to speak more slowly or to repeat things. If the person is the instructor, request a meeting outside of class. Ask if printed lecture outlines are available to help you follow along. Work on developing active listening skills (see Chapters 8 and 10).
You think you know what you want to say, but it doesn't come out right.	Practice speaking alone in front of a mirror. Use notes when engaging in an important conversation. Before speaking, take a few moments to think and be clear in your own mind about what you want or need to say.
You tend to ramble on and get lost in details when you are speaking.	Think about the purpose of your conversation: what do you want to get across? Practice being self-aware and observing your own behavior. When you catch yourself, use humor and say something like: "Oops, I'm rambling on again. The important thing is…" If appropriate, explain to your listener(s) that communication is difficult for you and that you may experience some problems.
You miss nonverbal signals that people give you during conversations.	Read about nonverbal communication. Practice observing others. Work with a friend who is willing to observe you and help you identify nonverbal language.

TABLE 6-2
Focusing

Difficulties	Suggested Strategies
You are easily distracted by extraneous noise.	When studying, wear headphones or earplugs or use a white noise machine. Sit near the instructor during lectures (if seats are assigned, request permission to sit up front). Avoid sitting near students who talk during class. Choose quiet places to study, such as the library. Turn off your phone when you are studying.
You are easily distracted by visual stimuli.	Choose a seat where there are minimal distractions, such as away from a window or an interesting wall display. Work in an uncluttered area. Minimize the number of items on your desk that might draw your attention.
You are distracted by your own ideas that come up, but are not needed at the moment. You are just bombarded with competing thoughts and ideas.	Keep a brainstorming log to note the ideas for consideration later. (I have 39 pages in a file on my computer containing writing ideas that have popped into my head while I was working on something else.) Try doing meditation, a practice that has been shown to increase focus and attention (Box 6-3).

Continued

TABLE 6-2—cont'd

Focusing

Difficulties	Suggested Strategies
It is very difficult to stay focused on a task for any length of time—even for a few minutes.	Try doing meditation, a practice that has been shown to increase focus and attention (see Box 6-3). Train yourself to keep focused on the task by deciding for how many minutes you will focus, even if it is just five or ten to start. Write down the time and keep bringing yourself back to your task until the stop time. Think about what you will gain by completing the task at hand.
You find it difficult to start or complete projects.	Think about your goal. Why is this project important to you? Build in rewards to encourage yourself to get things done. Break projects up into small steps with interim deadlines. Trying to do too much can be so overwhelming that you end up doing nothing.

BOX 6-3 Meditation, Yoga, and Guided Imagery

The following are purposeful relaxation and practices that clear the mind, promote calmness, and can increase our ability to focus and concentrate.

- *Meditation:* a process for quieting the mind. Meditation actually affects brain activity and has been shown to decrease blood pressure and offer other health benefits. It involves sitting quietly and clearing the mind of thought. This is not as easy as it sounds, especially for someone with ADD or ADHD. Some ways to benefit from meditation include choosing a quiet area; eliminating distractions and interruptions; and using a focusing technique such as repeating a word, counting, or focusing on your breathing in and out.

- *Yoga:* an ancient practice of assuming certain body postures and focusing on breathing. There are many types of yoga, and the postures range from easy to advanced.

- *Guided imagery:* a method of visualization that involves focusing mentally on peaceful, pleasant scenes. Some individuals imagine a brilliant white light entering the top of their head and flowing through their body, spreading positive feelings of peacefulness and calm.

TABLE 6-3

Hyperactivity

Difficulties	Suggested Strategies
You cannot sit still or refrain from fidgeting for any length of time.	Engage in regular physical exercise. Choose something you enjoy doing. When appropriate, move around when you study. Try relaxation exercises, yoga, or guided imagery to help you relax and slow yourself down (see Box 3-3 for a relaxation exercise). When you are attending gatherings where you must sit for extended periods of time, engage your hands in an appropriate activity such as taking notes or knitting.
You have trouble settling down at night and sleeping.	Thirty minutes before bedtime, turn off the television and computer to reduce the sensory stimulation. Instead, engage in a quiet, relaxing activity. Develop a "going to bed" ritual that signals to your body to slow down.

TABLE 6-4

Memory

Difficulties	Suggested Strategies
You cannot remember information given to you orally, especially things like multi-step instructions.	Ask the speaker to speak slowly, if necessary. Take notes. Ask if the instructions are available in written form. Ask the speaker to repeat anything you do not understand (it is very difficult to remember something you don't understand). Check your understanding of what people have said: "Let me make sure I've got this right," then repeat what you heard or read from your notes. See the suggestions for improving your memory in Chapter 3.

TABLE 6-4—cont'd
Memory

Difficulties	Suggested Strategies
You cannot remember what you have read or studied in class.	See the suggestions for reading in Chapter 7. Take notes of the main points as you read to increase your concentration. Writing also helps reinforce memory traces in the brain. Try the following to reinforce the material. Suppose you are studying diabetes. • *Visualize* how you might use what you are learning, such as in patient education. • *Associate* it with someone you know who has diabetes. • *Think* about the causes and the increase in diabetes cases in the United States. • *Create* a mental picture of the pancreas. • *Discuss* what you are learning with others. • *Explain* what you are learning to others, such as the effects of untreated diabetes. • *Read* other sources, such as information on the Web or brochures about diabetes. • *Review* the material periodically.
You cannot remember new vocabulary.	Create a word list that you review daily. Use some of the techniques above to visualize, create associations, and so on to "plant" the word in your memory. Try creating mnemonics such as the following: • Create a silly or interesting mental picture. Example: picture a *crane* lifting a large skull to remember *cranium,* the medical term for skull. • Link the new word to one with a similar sound and meaning. Example: *-stasis* is the medical word element for stoppage. It sounds like *stay.* If something stops, it stays in place.

TABLE 6-5
Note-Taking

Difficulties	Suggested Strategies
You cannot listen and write at the same time.	Request permission in advance to record class lectures. (Take care, however, to listen in class.) It is best if you use a recorder that has variable speed control so you can speed up or slow down the speech later as needed. Request permission to copy notes from another student. Ask your instructors if they can give you written outlines of their lectures. Try to copy down any information written on the board or screen.
You can listen and take notes, but what you write down doesn't make much sense.	See the sections on note-taking in Chapter 7.

TABLE 6-6
Numbers

Difficulties	Suggested Strategies
You have trouble copying strings of numbers in the correct order.	Break strings of numbers into groups of two or three digits. Write each small group, and check as you proceed. Cover part of the number as you read, especially if there are a series of zeroes. When copying two numbers, cover the one that you are not copying.
You find it difficult to read tables that contain lots of numbers.	Draw an extra thick line under every third row. Highlight the sections in different colors.
You have difficulty performing math calculations.	Read the section on math anxiety in Chapter 9. Go over the review material in Chapter 9. Request permission to use a calculator when doing your work. If you have trouble reading numbers and following your calculations, try a talking calculator. It may be easier for you to catch errors if you hear them.
It is hard for you to measure accurately.	Take a deep breath and work calmly and slowly. Write down measurements as you go along so you don't forget them. Double check your work. If in doubt, have someone else check your work.

TABLE 6-7

Organization

Difficulties	Suggested Strategies
You lose things all the time.	Designate a place for everything, especially items such as keys and eyeglasses. Figure 6-1 shows an example of an organized workspace. Store items close to where you use them. Set up specific places for important items such as bills to be paid and assignments you are working on. Keep your desk and work areas as free of clutter as possible so important items don't get buried. Keep items such as your cell phone attached to your purse or belt so they can't get lost.
Your desk is covered with piles of papers, folders, and notes, with many of their contents a mystery to you.	Work on clearing a small area at a time. Discard papers you no longer need. Create a simple filing system. Use colored file folders for different projects. (If you have trouble sequencing letters and keeping files in order, make an alphabet arc. This is a semicircle with the letters of the alphabet written from left to right along the curved portion. You may find it easier to read the letters than when they are positioned in a straight line.) Alternative idea: purchase a home filing system that comes with files, labels, and instructions for organizing papers and forms. Set up two accordion files: one with a section for each day of the week, and the other with a section for each month of the year. Place items that need attention in the corresponding file section. Be sure to check these files regularly. Alternative method: set up three trays labeled "This Week," "This Month," "This Term (or Semester)." Sort tasks accordingly; check the file labeled "This Week" daily and the other two weekly.
You frequently miss deadlines or appointments.	Keep a calendar or planner, either paper or electronic. Be disciplined about recording everything you need to do and checking your calendar frequently. Maintain a daily and weekly to-do list, either on paper or electronically. If on paper, use a small notebook, not little slips of paper that are easily lost.
You often find you don't have what you need for class, work, or household duties such as paying bills.	Create a list of things you must have each day and post it where you will see it, perhaps next to the front door. Each evening, set out what you will need for the next day. Do the same for your children to prevent the morning rush. See Chapter 3 for personal organization ideas.
You feel so overwhelmed by everything that needs to be done that you often become "paralyzed" and don't do anything.	Get an "organization buddy" who can help you get things into perspective, make a plan, and keep you motivated. Your buddy can be a family member, a friend, or even an organization professional. It just needs to be someone who is organized, patient, and sympathetic to your situation. Work on gradually clearing clutter that can cause an overload of stimuli, visual stress, and distraction. Think about what really needs to be done and what can be put off until later. Consider the consequences of your choices. Divide large projects that seem impossible to complete into small pieces; estimate the time needed to complete each; set deadlines for each piece and for the final project.

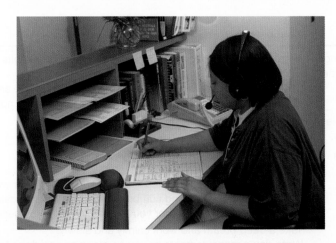

FIGURE 6-1 Working in an uncluttered area helps prevent distractions for individuals with Attention Deficit Disorder. *Is your study area conducive to concentration? If not, set up your desk in an organized manner. Try to keep it uncluttered by clearing it up regularly.* (From Bonewit-West K, Hunt S, Applegate E: *Today's medical assistant: Clinical & administrative procedures,* ed 2, St Louis, 2013, Saunders.)

TABLE 6-8
Reading

Difficulties	Suggested Strategies
You can't seem to remember anything you read.	Study the section on reading in Chapter 7 and try the methods suggested. The previewing and reviewing steps are especially helpful for students with retention problems. Use the following strategies, which are also listed in Table 6-4 (Memory). This time, let's suppose you are studying the process of digestion: • *Visualize* the path of a donut as it goes through the digestion system. Name each part of the anatomy it passes through. • *Associate* the digestive process with the energy you use going about your day. • *Mentally describe* the functions of the various digestive organs. • *Create* a mental picture of the digestive organs. Imagine each one in a bright color. Consider using an anatomy coloring book. • *Discuss* what you are learning, such as the causes of indigestion, with others. • *Read* other sources, such as illustrated material on the Internet. • *Review* the material periodically.
You have trouble keeping your place when reading.	Move your finger along the text as you read. Place a ruler or piece of paper under the line. Use an eye-level reading ruler, a special ruler made of opaque and transparent plastic in a variety of colors. Its serves to underline and highlight text in a colored tint, thus helping with both tracking and reducing the glare. Use a reading window, a slotted piece of plastic that shows one line at a time to reduce distraction from the surrounding text.
You have problems distinguishing letters and their order: 1. You see letters in the wrong order 2. You confuse reversible letters, such as *b* and *d, m* and *w* 3. You confuse words that look similar, such as *were* and *where* 4. You mistake the sequence of letters in long words, such as *conversation* and *conservation*	Pay attention to the context and meaning of sentences. If a word doesn't fit the context (doesn't make sense), examine it carefully to see if you have misread it. Practice seeing words as separate groups of letters (syllables) instead of as long strings of letters. Examples: presentation = pre-sen-ta-tion, terminology = ter-mi-nol-o-gy Learn common prefixes and suffixes. A prefix is a letter or a group of letters attached to the beginning of a word that partly indicates its meaning. Examples: • *anti-* means against: anti viral → antiviral • *mis-* means wrong or bad: mis diagnose → misdiagnose • *trans-* means across: trans plant → transplant A suffix is a letter or a group of letters attached to the end of a word to form a new word or to alter the grammatical function of the original word. Examples: • *-less* means without: pain less → painless • *-ment* means action or process: treat ment → treatment • *-ed* indicates past tense: inject ed → injected
You have difficulty reading print on a white background because it seems to glare. Letters are blurred and jump around on the page.	Copy written materials, such as class handouts, onto light colored paper (investigate to see which color works best for you). Use a colored overlay on your computer monitor screen, or change the background color on your screen, if possible. Investigate the use of colored overlays for placing on text or use colored eyeglasses.

General Suggestions

This section contains suggestions for dealing with a variety of learning disabilities. The first involves your physical health and fitness. Because learning disabilities are biologically based, it makes sense that maintaining good health habits is important. Physical exercise, which has been found to help prevent diseases of all kinds, is also helpful in relieving some of the problems that accompany learning disabilities. Some students report that they are more able to concentrate and learn if they engage in a little exercise each day.

At the same time, it is important to get adequate rest. This may seem like a contradiction for a busy student, but if you have a learning disability, it is quite important. This is because it takes effort to concentrate and learn, especially when you are overcoming learning difficulties. If you get overly tired, the brain simply cannot function as it should. It is recommended that students break up their studying into chunks of 20 minutes or so, taking short breaks between sessions. The emphasis here is on "short" because you may need only a few minutes to rest your eyes and your mind. Because you may have to spend more time studying than students without learning disabilities, good time management and teaching yourself not to waste time are especially important skills. For example, if you leave things until the last minute, you will find yourself rushed. This creates anxiety, even feelings of panic, and these feelings can prevent you from getting anything done at all.

TABLE 6-9

Taking Tests

Difficulties	Suggested Strategies
You misunderstand instructions and what the questions are asking.	Ask the instructor to privately explain the questions. State what you think a question is asking and ask for feedback to let you know if you understood it correctly. *Note:* If you believe you will need this extra help, advise the instructor *before* the day of the test.
You read and write so slowly that you don't have enough time to finish all the questions.	Request extra time to complete tests. *Note:* If you believe you will need this accommodation, submit your request *before* the day of the test.
You are too distracted by noises in the environment to focus on the test.	Request permission to take the text in a quiet environment. *Note:* If you believe you will need this accommodation, submit your request *before* the day of the test.

Note: See also the section on test anxiety and test-taking strategies in Chapter 8.

TABLE 6-10

Time Management

Difficulties	Suggested Strategies
You never come close to estimating the amount of time it will take to complete any given project or activity.	Keep a time diary for a couple of weeks. Write down the start and stop times for your daily activities. Then analyze them to see how long things really take. You may be astonished to discover that something you thought would take 15 minutes actually takes closer to an hour. Estimate how long it will take to complete an activity, then start by adding 50% to the time. For example, if you think a task will take one hour, budget 1.5 hours for it. You can adjust over time as you learn to set realistic goals.
You try to do too much during the time available and often end up feeling exhausted or burned out.	See the suggestion above for keeping a time diary. Try planning fewer activities than you usually would, and see how much you actually accomplish. Prioritize your tasks, and always do the most important ones first. Pace yourself. When doing something that requires concentration, work in blocks of 20 to 30 minutes at a time. Use a planner or calendar to mark final deadlines. Set interim deadlines for completing parts of the project, studying for a test, and so on.
You easily lose track of time. A 10-minute break becomes a 2-hour session of lost time.	Set timers or alarms when you go on a break, answer the phone, or look at your e-mail. Vibrating timers are available if these are more appropriate. Practice being aware of where you are, what you are doing, and the time.
You are rarely on time for appointments, classes, or social occasions.	Start recording how much time it actually takes you to get to places you commonly visit, such as school. Then add 10 minutes to your travel time. Resist doing "one last little thing" as you head for the door.

See also the section on time management in Chapter 3.

There are a variety of groups and services you might find helpful. These include the following:

- Services for learning disabled students that may be available at your college or in your community
- Support groups that consist of students with learning disabilities, in which they share their experiences and ideas for overcoming challenges
- **Study groups** with a variety of students
- **Learning centers** and **tutors** who help with specific academic skills and subjects

Lastly, what may be the most important advice of all: seek help from your instructors. Students with learning disabilities report that their greatest mistake was not getting help before they were struggling and feeling desperate. Your instructors want you to succeed. Give them the opportunity to help make that happen.

Prescription for Success: 6-1 Helping Yourself

1. Name five difficulties listed in the tables you believe to be obstacles to your academic and/or personal success.
2. From your list, choose one you want to work on.
3. Choose at least one strategy to try for a week and describe how you will use it.
4. Evaluate the strategy: how did it work for you? Why was it helpful or not?

TABLE 6-11

Writing

Difficulties	Suggested Strategies
You have serious problems with spelling.	Review the spelling rules and strategies presented in Chapter 8. Use the spell-check feature on your word processor. Carry a handheld spell-checker. Consider purchasing a medical terminology spell-checker. Investigate abbreviation-expander software. You can enter codes for words you use often so you don't have to continually reenter—and possibly misspell—them. Investigate proofreading software to supplement what came with your word processing program. This is available in medical report versions.
You make mistakes copying written material.	Work slowly and carefully. Copy onto colored, nonglare paper. Use paper with a slot cut into it or a reading window to cover the lines you are not copying.
You have difficulty organizing your thoughts and presenting them logically on paper.	Use a computer to do writing assignments so you can easily correct mistakes and move text around. When you aren't worried about the mechanics of writing, you can focus on the content and meaning. Ask your instructor to review your first draft to help you get on the right track. Have a qualified person critique and proofread your written work. See also the suggestions about writing in Chapter 8. Request extra time to complete long writing assignments. *Note:* If you believe you will need this accommodation, submit your request *before* the assignment is due.
You find that the white paper you are writing on seems to glare.	Request permission in advance to submit your work on colored paper (experiment with colors to see which works best for you).

Accommodations

Knowing yourself and your needs is the first step toward **self-advocacy**, which means seeking solutions to your learning difficulties, trying alternative ways of learning, and asking for appropriate and necessary help. You may need to explain the nature of your learning disabilities to people who don't understand them.

Accommodations are often available for students whose learning challenges prevent them from learning in traditional ways and who cannot demonstrate what they actually know through typical testing methods. The laws that protect individuals with disabilities apply to some people who have learning disabilities, depending on the nature and severity of the condition. These laws are *not* intended to excuse students from having to fulfill the requirements of their certificate or degree programs. Their purpose is to help students find ways to acquire needed knowledge and skills and demonstrate that they have mastered them.

It is important that if you do seek extra help or time to complete a test, you do so only when absolutely necessary. Taking advantage of the situation is unethical and unfair to other students. You must also consider carefully the possible effects of your learning disability on your work in health care. Using this time during your training to find solutions that you can apply to your working conditions will help ensure your future success.

Case Study 6-1

Overcoming ADD as an Adult

Marie has always had trouble staying organized and meeting deadlines. She struggled in high school and often found herself in class with the wrong notes. She was often late for class, missed appointments with her counselor, and was even late for social engagements with her friends. Sometimes she left the lunch she had packed on the kitchen counter in her haste to leave the house.

For Marie, this was normal. As a wife and mother, she lived her life in a flurry of activity and believed this was just how it was when you were a busy adult. Things got even worse after her divorce from Ted, her husband of ten years, as she tried to juggle a part-time job and raise two active boys. But again, she thought this was just how it was when a person had too much to do.

In spite of what seemed to be a frantic pace, Marie knew that her part-time job at a fast-food restaurant wasn't going to be enough. She didn't earn enough to cover the expenses even after the child support payments, and it wasn't enough to satisfy her desire for a meaningful career. After considering various career choices, Marie decided to enroll in a medical assisting program. She could finish the

Continued

program in less than a year and get into something she thought she would enjoy, as well as earning a better living.

However, Marie found it difficult to get to classes on time each day, complete her assignments, and take care of her sons' needs. The other students also seemed to have busy lives, but they appeared to be more in control than she was. One day in the school café, she decided to approach the subject with her classmate, Keisha.

"Keisha, you always seem to have it together. I'm always at loose ends."

Keisha laughed and said, "Well, I don't know about having it together. There's always so much to do."

Marie commented, "You seem so organized—always prepared for class."

"It wasn't always this way," Keisha responded. "In high school I felt out of control. It seemed like I was always getting distracted, didn't finish anything I started. And my bedroom! My mom was always after me to clean up the mess."

"So, do you still feel out of control?" asked Marie. "You sure don't look that way."

"Thanks! These days, only sometimes," said Keisha.

Marie is intrigued. "So what's your secret," she asks.

"No secret, really. I just finally discovered some things about myself and then did some research to see if there was anything I could do to improve—if there was hope for me!" Keisha laughed.

"It certainly looks like there was," said Marie.

"I learned that I have a mild form of adult ADD—you know, Attention Deficit Disorder," explained Keisha.

"No kidding!" exclaimed Marie. "I thought just kids had that—the ones who can't sit still, who can't pay attention in class."

"Actually, it's pretty common among adults. Sometimes it just looks different—being late, losing things, trouble focusing—that kind of thing," explained Keisha.

"Wow—that pretty much describes me. It seems like I'm always struggling to get things done—let alone get them done on time!"

"I realized that if I was going to start a new career, especially one in health care that required organization, I'd better see if there was anything I could do about it. Turns out there are books especially for adults—they helped me understand what was going on. It was a relief to know that I wasn't a little crazy," said Keisha.

"Well, I could sure use some help," said Marie.

"There are lots of strategies you can try. I'll get you the titles of some of the books I found helpful. You can also go online and use key words like 'adult ADD books.' There are also some good Web sites," said Keisha.

"I'd really like to take a look at those. I'll take some time this weekend," said Marie. "But now, I guess I'd better get going or I'll be late again for class! Keisha, I really appreciate what you've shared with me. Thanks so much."

Questions for Thought and Reflection

1. What do you think of Keisha's willingness to share her own situation with Marie?
2. What is your opinion of the advice she gave Marie?
3. Do you think Marie will follow up and research adult ADD? Why or why not?
4. If you had been at the table with Keisha and Marie, what advice would you have offered?

Trouble Ahead? 6-1

John didn't do well in high school, but did manage to graduate by taking summer school between his junior and senior years. He found his classes tedious and had trouble sitting still, but he didn't want to drop out like his older brother, Jim, who hadn't been able to find work and now was stuck living at home with their parents. "Stuck" was a good word for it, John thought. His parents didn't get along very well. They argued a lot and John really didn't know why they stayed together.

This situation at home was what motivated him to think about a future that would enable him to get a job that paid enough to move out on his own. He talked it over with his friend, Steve.

"I see your point, John," said Steve. "I know I've been at your place a few times when it was pretty tense."

"Yeah," said John. "I really need to get something going for myself. How do you like the program you started at BeWell College. What is it you're studying?"

"Pharmacy tech. It's pretty interesting and won't take forever to finish—less than a year," Steve said.

"I really need something where there are jobs. Know anything about that?" John asked.

"Well, it sounds pretty good. Lots of people are getting older and some of them take a lot of drugs—prescription, that is!" Steve laughed. "So the projections for jobs in pharmacies are pretty good."

"I think I'll stop by the school and look into this," said John.

"Good plan. You might want to look into medical assisting, too. It sounded like a good career, but I'm not a fan of blood—or any other body fluids!" said Steve.

After visiting with the admissions counselor at the college and reading over the material she gave him, John thought it over. He thought medical assisting sounded interesting—more physically active than working in a pharmacy. And he didn't think he'd mind the blood and "stuff." He was eager to get going, get done, and move on.

The first couple of days of class went okay, but then the daily assignments and quizzes started. The classes moved along quickly and contained a lot of information. Students were expected to be on time, wear clean uniforms, complete all reading assignments, and complete worksheets and other homework. It was more than John expected and he felt overwhelmed. This was worse than high school!

At the end of the second week, his instructor, Ms. Dawkins, asked to see him after class. "John," she started, "you don't seem to be off to a very good start. Your assignments are either missing or incomplete, your quiz scores are low—and you're late for class more often than not."

"I didn't expect so much work—reading and stuff. I thought this would be more hands-on. Reading and homework aren't really my thing," John replied.

"Can you be a little more specific when you say, 'reading and homework aren't my thing'?" asked Ms. Dawkins.

"Yeah, reading is dull. I have to sit there and that's really hard for me. I'd rather be up and about, *doing* something, not just looking at the pages," John explained.

"Well, reading shouldn't be just looking at pages. But I hear you saying you have a problem settling down and concentrating," said Ms. Dawkins. "Have you ever been told you might have a learning disability? Or maybe Attention Deficit Disorder?"

"Is that the ADD thing?" asked John.

"Yes, that's the abbreviation," Ms. Dawkins said.

"It kind of sounds familiar. I think someone at my high school said something about that to my mom, but she had her own stuff to worry about," said John.

"Well, it might be something you could check into now. It could explain why you're having trouble doing what's necessary to succeed in your program," said Ms. Dawkins.

"I don't know," said John reluctantly. "It sounds like something kids have. I'm just an active person. And honestly—and I don't mean to hurt your feelings—I think the classes here are kind of boring. Who needs to know a bunch of medical words to work with patients? They don't know these words. I wouldn't be using them."

"John, you use these words with the doctor and with your coworkers. It's the language of the health care field," explained Ms. Dawkins. "Let me explain that there are ways you can learn to deal with any learning problems you might have and succeed in your program."

"I don't know. It sounds like a lot of trouble. I already have homework and quizzes—and now I have to spend more time seeing about some kind of learning disability. Sounds like more work to me," said John. "You know, I appreciate your time, but I don't think this is for me."

Questions for Thought and Reflection

1. What do you think about John's reasons for studying medical assisting?
2. What is your opinion of Ms. Dawkins? Do you think she is a good instructor? Why or why not?
3. Do you think John will drop out of school?
4. What advice would you give John?

Learning Disabilities During the Job Search

Personal organization and good oral and written presentation skills are important for a successful job search. You may want to seek assistance from qualified helpers to work with you as you look for a job. These might include the following:

- The career services personnel at your school
- Your organization buddy
- Your instructors
- Your mentor, if you have one (see Chapter 3)

If writing is a problem, have a qualified person proofread your resume and any letters you send out. See if potential employers have applications you can fill out online; if not, ask if you can take the application home to fill out so you can check it over carefully. If you are called for an interview and communicating orally is difficult for you, ask for help from your school's career services personnel or an instructor. Perhaps they could spend some extra time helping you prepare. (See Chapter 14 for detailed information about job interviews.)

A question many students have is whether they should disclose their learning disability to a potential employer. The opinion of experts is that if your disability does not affect your job performance, then it is not necessary to mention it. If, however, you plan to request accommodations, you must disclose it to be eligible. (Do note that if you are not legally defined as "disabled," you may not be entitled to accommodations.)

Once on the job, there are things you can do to work more effectively, as follows:

- Ask your supervisor to help you prioritize tasks.
- Ask for oral directions to be repeated or given to you in written form.
- Apply the strategies you used in school. For example, if you used an eye-level ruler to help with reading, keep one with you at work.
- Request permission to take notes or recordings at employee orientations, workshops, or important meetings.
- Copy material you must read onto colored paper.
- Keep a timer at your desk or work area—or a small one in your pocket—to limit phone calls and conversations with co-workers.

As discussed previously, the important thing is to identify your own weaknesses and work to find ways to overcome them. People with learning disabilities can have successful careers and productive lives.

Summary of Key Ideas

- There are various learning disabilities, but most can be overcome by using specific strategies.

Positive Self-Talk for This Chapter

- I am learning what I need to know about health care.

- I am successfully using strategies to accomplish what I need to do.
- I know my strengths and weaknesses and am a good self-advocate.

Internet Activities

For active links to the websites needed to complete these activities, visit http://evolve.elsevier.com/Haroun/career/.

Explore at least three websites listed in the "To Learn More" section. Try the suggestions you believe might be helpful and report on the results.

To Learn More

ADDitude Magazine

Available at: http://www.additudemag.com

The emphasis of this website is "living well with ADD and learning disabilities." It contains useful articles for adults with ADD, including career advice.

Children and Adults with Attention Deficit Disorder (CHADD)

8181 Professional Place, Suite 201, Landover, MD 20785, Tel, 800-233-5050.

Available at: http://www.chadd.org

This organization provides helpful information and support as well as publishing *Attention!* magazine. The website contains questions to help adults identify the signs of ADHD.

Kolberg J, Nadeau K: *ADD-friendly ways to organize your life*, New York, 2002, Routledge

This book contains dozens of practical tips, presented in an easy-to-read format.

Crossbow Education

http://www.crossboweducation.com/shop-now/visual-stress/reading-rulers

Although this is a British website, it has good visual presentations of useful products to assist people with dyslexia and reading problems, such as eye-level rulers and reading windows.

Learning Disabilities Association of America

http://www.ldaamerica.org

Here you will find comprehensive information that includes help for adults with learning disabilities in postsecondary education and in the workplace. It includes explanations of specific learning disabilities and strategies for dealing with each.

Moody S: *Dyslexia: surviving and succeeding at college*, New York, 2007, Routledge

Dyslexia is a specific learning disability that affects one's ability to read. This book provides practical information to help students succeed.

National Attention Disorder Association

1788 Second Street, Suite 200, Highland Park, IL 60035, Tel. 847-432-5874, e-mail mail@add.org

Available at: http://www.add.org

This organization is specifically for adults with Attention Deficit Disorder. It publishes newsletters and brochures, holds conferences, and maintains a helpful website.

National Center for Learning Disabilities

https://www.ncld.org

This organization provides useful information for adults as well as children with learning disabilities.

National Resource Center on ADHD

http://www.help4adhd.org

Information and resources for all ages

National Resource Center on AD/HD: Succeeding in the Workplace, 2003. Available at: www.help4adhd.org/en/living/workplace/WWK16.

This article discusses dealing with ADD in the workplace.

Sarkis S.M.: *10 Simple solutions to adult ADD: How to overcome chronic distraction and accomplish your goals*, Oakland, Calif, 2011, New Harbinger Publications

This book provides tips for personal organization to help adults cope with Attention Deficit Disorder.

References

1. Horowitz S: The neurobiology of learning disabilities. National Center for Learning Disabilities. Available at: https://www.understood.org/en/learning-attention-issues/getting-started/what-you-need-to-know/learning-and-attention-issues-and-the-brain.
2. Maloff J: The biology of ADD. Internet Special Education Resources. Available at: http://www.iser.com/resources/ADD-biology.html.

CHAPTER 7

Developing Your Paper Skills I: Intake of Information

OBJECTIVES

1. Understand the importance of developing good note-taking skills.
2. Use effective listening techniques to take advantage of learning opportunities.
3. Have proper note-taking materials and understand the Cornell system and the importance of advance preparation for taking good notes.
4. Get more out of class lectures by using all of your senses, knowing the organizational pattern of lectures, knowing what to write down, and listening for clues from instructors.
5. Develop note-taking techniques that work for you in class, including the use of outlines, recording devices, and shortcuts with symbols and abbreviations.
6. Convert your class notes into powerful learning tools and review them often.
7. Realize the importance of note-taking skills on the job, including taking phone messages, medical record documentation, and charting.
8. Understand the importance of reading to learn, and be prepared to:
    a. Use pre-reading activities to make reading easier and beneficial.
    b. Understand the anatomy of a textbook.
    c. Use previewing when reading.
    d. Ask questions and highlight the important information.
    e. Review the material and use techniques to increase your recall and retention of the information.
9. Locate reliable sources of information to use in school and on the job.

KEY TERMS AND CONCEPTS

Active Listener One who listens purposefully and attentively, focuses on what the speaker is saying, and asks questions when necessary for clarification.

Appendix Section at the end of a book that contains supplementary information. (Plural form is *appendixes* or *appendices.*)

Charting Making written entries in a patient's medical record.

Concept A general idea or reference to a unit of knowledge.

Cornell System A method for taking notes in which space is left on each page for writing follow-up notes, questions, and summaries.

Documentation Placing information into a patient's medical record or creating reports about their condition, treatment, etc.

Glossary An alphabetical list of words with their definitions, usually located at the end of a book.

Internet A system that connects millions of computers, providing access to all kinds of resources and services.

Key Terms In note-taking, words that identify the most important concepts and ideas in a lecture.

Logical In an order that makes sense, following some sort of pattern and showing relationships.

Objective Statement of what students should know or be able to do as a result of a given learning activity.

Preface An introduction for the reader, placed at the beginning of a book.

Preview To look over a written selection, noting new vocabulary and content headings, before reading it carefully.

Rationale An explanation or reason for something.

Research To gather information from reliable sources.

Websites The specific "places" you see on the computer screen when you are connected to the Internet.

Note-Taking for School Success

Taking good notes combines the art of listening and the act of selective writing. Many students report having trouble taking good notes, but it is a skill that can be mastered. You actually have a big advantage because you can take in words much faster than your instructors can speak!

There are a number of important reasons for taking notes in class in addition to learning to take good notes because it is an important health care skill:

1. Taking notes forces you to attend class, pay attention, process the material mentally, and selectively write down what you hear. It converts you from a passive to an **active listener**. Increasing the number of ways you interact with new material greatly increases your chances of understanding and remembering it, so hearing and writing it down in class give you a head start in learning.

2. Your instructors are likely to present more information than what appears in your textbook. They may have examples and additional techniques from their work experiences or new information from a seminar they have just attended.

3. In the fast-changing field of health care, there is a continuous flow of new developments, and your instructors can provide you with the latest updates.

4. The scope of practice of health care professionals varies across the country. For example, some states allow medical assistants to take an active role in taking x-ray films. Therefore many textbooks on medical assisting include information about positioning patients when taking x-rays. In some states, however, only graduates of approved x-ray programs who have also passed a state exam are allowed to perform these procedures. Classroom instructors will give you the rules and regulations of the area in which your school is located.

5. Your instructors can help you understand difficult material, presenting the material in a way so you understand better. They may break it down into manageable chunks, provide examples, or explain it using different words.

6. Health care programs cover vast amounts of information. Your instructors' lectures can help you identify the most important points and give you clues about what will be included on a test.

7. Notes serve as powerful tools for studying and mastering important information needed for school and job success. In this chapter, you will learn techniques for converting your notes into study aids.

Personal Reflection

1. Are you satisfied with your current note-taking skills?
2. Why or why not?
3. What would you like to improve?

Active Listening: A Prerequisite for Good Note-Taking

Good note-taking requires good listening habits. You can't record what you don't hear, and listening is one of the most essential skills for the successful health care professional. Patient surveys report that the failure of the health care professional to listen is a major cause of dissatisfaction.[1] The classroom provides the perfect opportunity to learn information and an essential professional skill at the same time (Figure 7-1).

Success Tips to Develop Good Listening Skills

- Develop a positive attitude toward listening. Listening well increases your chances for success in life. Review your goals and think about how being a good listener will help you achieve them.
- Leave your mental baggage at the classroom or health care facility door. Try to go in with a clean slate for listening

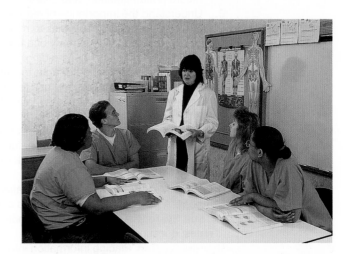

FIGURE 7-1 **Listen Up.** Listening in class is the first step in taking advantage of your instructor's knowledge and in taking good notes. *In what ways do these students appear to be listening? If this were a large classroom lecture rather than a small group, what might you do to help yourself actively listen for a sustained period of time? If this were your supervisor giving you directions, what would be the possible consequences of not listening actively?* (From Birchenall J, Streight E: *Mosby's textbook for the home care aide,* ed 3, St Louis, 2013, Mosby.)

and learning. If you are having a bad day or your mind is distracted, look at the class as an opportunity to focus, learn, and have a productive experience.

- Sit where you can both see and hear the instructor. Avoid sitting near people who talk or continually ask you questions during class. The distraction will disrupt your attention and can make you tense. (And don't you be the talker!)
- Concentrate on the content of the lecture, not the way it is delivered. It's easy to let the appearance, mannerisms, and voice of the instructor distract you from what is being said. Learning to focus on content is an important health care skill because patients will come to you with all kinds of physical and emotional conditions, and each patient merits your full attention.
- Reel in your wandering mind. Do your best to stay with the instructor mentally. If you think of something important, jot a quick note to yourself so you can take care of it later. Then return to concentrating on what you are hearing.
- Keep your mind open and suspend judgment. It is common to stop listening when we disagree with something we hear. A better strategy is to write down the point of disagreement. After listening to the remainder of the presentation, ask the instructor to clarify the point. There may be several "right answers" or ways to perform a technique. Perhaps you heard or interpreted the information incorrectly. If the instructor did make a mistake, show respect. Enjoying "being right" in front of the class is unacceptable classroom conduct. On the job, being disrespectful to a supervisor is generally not tolerated.

Prescription for Success: 7-1 My Listening Habits

You can start to improve your listening skills by practicing awareness. One way is to listen to the news or other program on the radio for several minutes at a time. Pay attention to when your mind wanders or you lose track of what is being said. (You can try the same technique in your classes if you don't have time to listen to the radio, but only if it does not further distract your attention from the lecture.)

1. Think about your listening habits. Is there a pattern to the breaks in your concentration? (For example, you are distracted by something visual or your private thoughts, you don't understand everything being said, or it is difficult to follow long periods of speech.)
2. What can you do now to start improving your listening habits?

Note-Taking Materials

Loose-leaf binders receive the highest marks from instructors for keeping notes together because they are the most flexible and the easiest to organize and keep in order. You can add new information in any order you wish, something you can't do with spiral notebooks. Binders allow you to insert class notes, revisions of your notes, handouts, assignments, reference sheets, and skills check-off sheets. Binders also offer the best protection against the weather and keep papers flat and neat. Portfolios and other types of folders with pockets tend to tear and get messy.

You can purchase several binders with thin vinyl covers and use one for each class. Or you can divide a large binder with indexed dividers. The section for each course can also be subdivided for class notes, handouts, reading notes, and assignments. Periodically review and tidy up your binder as needed.

Regardless of how you organize your binder, the important thing is to keep your notes for each class together and in order. Label the outside cover with the name of the class or classes. If you are using more than one binder, color-code or mark them in such a way that you never arrive at your anatomy class only to discover you have your pharmacology notes! Label the individual pages with the name of the class and the date.

Electronic devices, such as laptops and tablets, are gaining in popularity for taking notes in class. These are especially useful for students whose handwriting is illegible, as discussed in Chapter 6. However, a study at Princeton showed that students who take notes by hand retain material better than those who take notes electronically.[2] This may be because students using electronic devices tend to take down too much of what the instructor is saying without processing it mentally. Therefore, if you choose to use an electronic device, take care to continue paying attention to and mentally processing what the instructor is saying.

The Cornell System

The **Cornell system** is a method for laying out, editing, and studying from your notes to get the most benefit from them. It was devised by Professor Walter Pauk, who wanted to help his students improve their study habits. A key feature of the system is leaving enough blank space on the page to add specific kinds of information when you review and edit your notes. Set up each page on which you will take notes by drawing a line about 2.5 inches in from the left side. Then draw a line about 2 inches up from the bottom. Figure 7-2 shows this page layout.

The large space in the center is for recording notes during class. Use the left side after class to write key words, headings, questions, and other notes. The bottom space is for writing short summaries of the contents of the page. We will discuss how to use these spaces later in this chapter.

Advance Preparation for Taking Good Notes

"By failing to prepare, you are preparing to fail."

—Benjamin Franklin

Preparing for classes is an important part of listening and taking good notes. Advance preparation, according to many instructors, is the key to benefiting from class sessions. If you forget about class between meetings and just show up each time as the instructor begins to speak, you will lose out on a good part of your educational investment. To obtain the maximum benefit from your in-class experiences, try the following suggestions:

- Complete any assigned reading and other homework. Knowing something about the topic, rather than starting

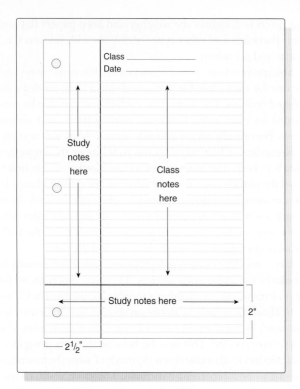

FIGURE 7-2 Cornell Format. This page layout enables you to turn your class notes into effective study aids. Rather than simply taking notes and putting them in your binder, you are encouraged to interact with the material. *Set up several pieces of notebook or other lined paper in the Cornell format: 1. Measure in about 2 inches from the left edge of the paper and 2.5 inches from the bottom; draw lines as shown in the diagram. 2. Use these pages to take your class notes for the next few days in the right-hand section.*

out cold, gives you a framework to guide your listening—and learning.

- Write out questions, based on your reading, and listen for the answers during the lecture. Here are some sample questions:
  - Why is this important?
  - How does it work?
  - What are the main parts?
  - Why is it done this way?
  - How is it done? How will I do this? When will I do this?
  - How will I apply this in my work?
  - How will this knowledge help me be a better health care professional?
  - How will it help me to help patients?
- Review your notes from the previous lecture. This sets the stage for a continuation of the subject and helps you recall questions or points you want to have clarified.
- Arrive at class a few minutes early so you can choose an appropriate seat, quickly look over your notes from the last class, and prepare yourself to take notes.
- Set your attitude for learning. Be positive and expect to acquire useful information.
- Take all the necessary supplies to class: a binder with extra paper, a pencil or pen, (or an electronic device for taking notes), your textbook, and handouts. (Make sure they're in the "big bag" discussed in Chapter 3. If books and binders get heavy, consider using a flight bag on wheels to prevent stress to your shoulders.)

Getting More Out of Class

Once you are in class, use as many senses as possible to help you understand the lecture and take better notes:

- If you are distracted by things you can see, such as a window with an interesting view or pictures and displays, try to avoid sitting where you can see them.
- Watch the instructor. Watch expressions and gestures that reinforce the lecture.
- Pay attention to anything shown on the board or other visual aids.
- Ask the instructor to write any words or phrases you don't understand or don't know how to spell.
- Think about the practical applications for what you hear during the lecture.
- Imagine yourself interacting with the topic: performing procedures, operating a machine.
- If you find it difficult to sit quietly for the entire class, make slight movements that don't disrupt others: count off the steps of a procedure on your fingers, stretch your legs, take deep breaths, move your pen or pencil with your fingers. Some students find that doodling helps them maintain their attention.

Organizational Patterns in Lectures

Most lectures follow an organizational pattern. Recognizing some of the ways that instructors present information can help you improve your note-taking.

1. **Clusters of information:** Topics are divided into chunks of related material, and the instructor covers one chunk before moving on to the next. Examples: the human body parts and functions are usually grouped by systems—skeletal, digestive, and reproductive. The topic of scheduling appointments for the medical office is usually organized by the different methods used to set them.
2. **Procedures:** These are often explained in a step-by-step sequence. Examples: how to measure an infant; how to perform one-person, adult cardiopulmonary resuscitation (CPR).
3. **Concepts or procedures with rationale:** Material is introduced followed by explanations and the reasons why it is important. Examples: laws followed by the legal reasons for maintaining patient confidentiality or why standard precautions must be followed.
4. **Definitions:** In addition to medical terminology, each area of health care has its own vocabulary. Lectures may be organized around explanations of new terms. Example: discussion of terms related to medical insurance billing.
5. **How things work:** Descriptions and explanations are given. Examples: the parts and operation of the microscope; the safe use of the autoclave.

6. **Lists:** descriptions and/or explanations of a number of items of equal importance. Examples: the purpose and interpretation of a series of lab tests; different medications and their use.
7. **Patterns:** These are created by instructors to present material in a specific order. Example: Anatomy and physiology course in which information about body systems is always presented in the same order, such as (1) names of parts, (2) purpose and function of each part, (3) common disorders of the system, (4) causes of the disorders, (5) diagnostic tests, (6) treatments, and (7) prevention.
8. **Verbal signals:** Certain words tell you where the lecture is going. Examples: "Let's go on to…" signals the transition to a new topic. "Therefore" and "In conclusion" let you know a summary statement is coming. "First," "second," and so on tell you there will be a list of items of equal importance.

Deciding What to Write Down

Instructors can say a lot during a lecture, and sometimes it's difficult to decide what to write down. If this happens to you, you're not alone. Students report this to be the hardest part of note-taking. This is especially true when a subject is new and you don't have the background to help sift the "must-know" from the "interesting-to-know." You need to write down enough to understand your notes later. But if you try to record every word, you're likely to miss half of what the instructor says.

As mentioned before, do the reading and assignments *before* going to class—even if it is not required. This will give you an overview of the topic. Your textbook has headings and other ways of emphasizing the major points of a subject. If you find the subject especially difficult and have the time, prepare a written outline of the chapters, along with any questions you have, before the lecture.

In class, listen for the main ideas. Your prereading will help you identify what these might be. Listen carefully to your instructors. They may list important points, introduce them and provide details and examples, and/or tell you what is most important. As you become familiar with the material and health care topics in general and take the quizzes and tests, you will find it easier to identify the major points.

Clues from Instructors

Many instructors provide clues, both consciously and unconsciously, about what is important in their classes. Here are some common instructor behaviors during lectures that say, "Write this down!"

- Saying, "This is important" or "You must know or be able to do this when you are working in the field" or "Write this down" or "This will be on the test." (They really do say these things. This is what you might miss if you are absent from class or daydreaming when you *are* there.)
- Emphasizing certain words or concepts by saying them loudly, writing them on the board or overhead, or repeating them. (It is a good idea to copy everything the instructor writes down.)
- Expressing extra interest or enthusiasm. This may indicate an area the instructor believes to be especially important.
- Illustrating points with stories and anecdotes.
- Asking questions of students during the lecture. These are usually points that the instructor considers to be important.

If you continually miss the major points of lectures, see your instructor outside of class. Ask for suggestions to improve your listening, follow the style of lecturing, and take better notes. Ask if the instructor has lecture outlines you can have to follow along in class. If English is your second language and you have difficulty understanding spoken and/or written English, seek help from your instructor or school advisor.

□ **Prescription for Success: 7-2 Applying What You've Learned**

1. Review the notes you have taken for this or another class. How effective are they in identifying the key points and helping you prepare for tests?
2. Practice listening for organizational clues in your classes during the next week. Choose two lectures and take a couple of minutes afterwards to record how they were organized. Were the lectures organized in clusters, procedures, concepts with rationale, definitions, how things work, presentation patterns, or something different?
3. Do your instructors give clues about what they consider to be most important in their lectures? Choose two lectures (from different instructors, if possible), listen and observe carefully, and note any of the behaviors below that you notice:
   - Tells you directly that something is important
   - Emphasizes words
   - Says words louder
   - Writes on board or overhead
   - Shows enthusiasm
   - Asks questions
   - Other (explain)

Note-Taking Method

The most common and recommended method for taking notes is the informal outline. Unlike a formal outline, you don't use letters and numbers or worry about perfect organization. Rather, focus on recording the important content. Write down the important ideas, then record the supporting information. Figure 7-3 illustrates notes based on information about working with anxious patients from *Today's Medical Assistant* by Bonewit-West, Hunt, and Applegate[3] as if it were presented as a lecture. (The "lecture segment" appears in Box 7-1.)

Note-Taking Guides

Some instructors distribute preprinted outlines to help their students focus on the important points of their lectures.

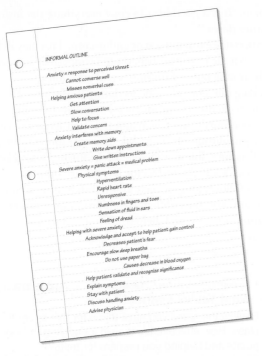

INFORMAL OUTLINE

Anxiety = response to perceived threat
   Cannot converse well
   Misses nonverbal cues
Helping anxious patients
   Get attention
   Slow conversation
   Help to focus
   Validate concern
Anxiety interferes with memory
   Create memory aids
   Write down appointments
   Give written instructions
Severe anxiety = panic attack = medical problem
   Physical symptoms
   Hyperventilation
   Rapid heart rate
   Unresponsive
   Numbness in fingers and toes
   Sensation of fluid in ears
   Feeling of dread
Helping with severe anxiety
   Acknowledge and accept to help patient gain control
   Decreases patient's fear
   Encourage slow deep breaths
   Do not use paper bag
   Causes decrease in blood oxygen
Help patient validate and recognize significance
   Explain symptoms
   Stay with patient
   Discuss handling anxiety
   Advise physician

FIGURE 7-3 Informal Outline. Examples of notes taken using an informal outline. The source for the notes is from the material about anxiety in Box 7-1 as if it were being presented as a lecture. Take a look at Box 7-1 to see how each heading in the notes is followed by a list of definitions, examples, or supporting facts. Don't worry if your notes are not as neat as the ones in the example. The important things are to record the important information and be able to read your handwriting! *Try practicing taking notes in outline form by having someone read a selection you haven't read yet from one of your textbooks. Then compare your notes with the material. Did you capture the important points?* (Adapted from Bonewit-West K, Hunt S, Applegate E: *Today's medical assistant: Clinical and administrative procedures*, ed 2, St Louis, 2013, Saunders.)

These can be very helpful, but should be used with caution. It can be tempting to go on auto pilot during lectures and listen only for the points listed on the guide. Another habit students sometimes fall into is copying down exactly what the teacher says. This is appropriate for recording definitions, formulas, and rules. However, you increase your chances of learning the material when you use your own words to take notes.

Using a Recording Device

There are conflicting opinions about the value of recording lectures to listen to later. Some educators believe that students who record their lectures pay less attention in class. And recordings don't include important nonverbal language and visual aids. Also, listening to recordings later is time-consuming. On the other hand, recording can be useful if listening is an effective way for you to review. It can also help students who have trouble understanding English or who cannot write legibly and/or write what they hear. If you decide recording is a good idea for you, be sure to obtain your instructor's permission. Some schools and/or individual instructors don't allow lectures to be recorded.

Anxiety is a response to a perceived threat. A person who is moderately to severely anxious is not able to converse coherently and will not pick up on nonverbal cues that he or she would normally notice. When working with a patient who is anxious, the medical assistant must first get the person's attention, slow down the conversation, and then help the person to focus on the conversation. It is important to validate the patient's concern, which reduces his or her anxiety level. This allows the patient's energy to be channeled in a more productive way. When patients are anxious, they may not remember what they are told. The medical assistant can help the patient by creating memory aids. For example, the medical assistant can prompt the patient to record a follow-up appointment in his or her appointment calendar. It is also a good idea to write the instructions down or provide the patient with a preprinted instruction sheet.

Severe anxiety can be medically problematic. Physical symptoms occur with a full-blown anxiety attack, often termed a *panic attack*. An overly anxious person hyperventilates, has an extremely rapid heart rate, and becomes unresponsive. Some people experience numbness in their fingers and toes; others feel a sensation of fluid in their ears. Some people become intensely fearful and have an overpowering sense of dread.

An anxiety attack must be dealt with as a medical issue first. Helping the patient acknowledge the anxiety is important. Acknowledging the anxiety helps a person gain control. In addition, having strong emotions accepted by another person decreases the sense of fear that many people have about their emotions.

If the patient is breathing rapidly, the medical assistant should encourage the patient to take slow, deep breaths. Experts no longer recommend having a patient breathe into a brown paper bag because this may cause blood oxygen levels to fall dangerously low.

If possible, the medical assistant should encourage the patient to validate that anxiety is present without minimizing its significance. If the patient has not experienced severe anxiety before, he or she may not realize the effects it can cause. The medical assistant can explain that any physical symptoms are the result of anxiety and stay with the patient until the symptoms begin to subside. With most patients, the symptoms begin to diminish after 1 or 2 minutes. After the person has returned to a level of relative calm, it may be possible to discuss how the person handles anxiety. The physician may also refer the patient to a counselor to work on strategies to manage it.

From Bonewit-West K, Hunt S, Applegate E: *Today's medical assistant: clinical and administrative procedures*, ed 2, St Louis, 2013, Saunders. Figures 7-3, 7-4, 7-7, and 7-8 were taken from this material as if it were given as a lecture.

Shortcuts with Symbols and Abbreviations

Creating your own symbols and abbreviations helps you to take notes more quickly and can make the notes more useful. Here are some ideas for symbols:

T = test item (instructor announced or hinted)
?? = got lost and need to fill in later
P = personal thoughts: your own ideas or questions about the topic. You can also bracket [xxxx] these to distinguish them from what the instructor says
J = important for job success, something employers look for

Try standard abbreviations such as those suggested in Table 7-1 for a list of suggestions you might find useful. If you create your own set of abbreviations, it's a good idea to put together a directory to keep with your notes in case you forget your coding system. Because you can't anticipate all the words you might shorten during a lecture,

write out potentially confusing abbreviations as soon as possible after class. Figure 7-4 shows how the informal outline notes, from Figure 7-3, would look if symbols and abbreviations were used. (IMPORTANT NOTE: On the job, using personal abbreviations when charting or creating notes for others is unacceptable because of the risk of confusion.)

> **Prescription for Success: 7-3 Create Your Own Abbreviations**
> Create 20 abbreviations to use in your note-taking.

Success Tips for Taking Great Notes

- Be there! Do your best to be present for both the beginning and end of class. Introductions and conclusions often contain valuable information about what the instructor

TABLE 7-1

Symbols and Abbreviations for Note-Taking

Standard Abbreviations	
Word	**Standard Abbreviation**
And	&
And so forth	etc
equals, same as, means	=
for example	eg
Less than	<
greater than	>
negative	–
not the same as, does not equal	≠
number	#
of, per	/
positive	+
regarding	re
therefore	∴
times	×
to, toward, leads to, goes to	→
versus	vs
with	w/ or C̄
without	w/o or S̄

Spell Words as They Sound Leaving Out Silent Letters

Examples	**Phonetic Spelling**
although	altho
through	thru

Standard Abbreviations	
Shorten Words by Leaving Out the Vowels	
Word	**Shortened Form**
blood	bld
book	bk
homework	hmwrk
learn	lrn
patient	pt
Make Up Your Own Short Forms of Common Words	
Word	**Shortened Form**
anatomy	anat
appointment	appt
because	bec
determine	det
important	imp
information	info
introduction	intro
necessary	nec
procedure	proc
psychology	psych
venipuncture	venip
Learn Common Medical Abbreviations	
Word	**Abbreviation**
cardiopulmonary resuscitation	CPR
electrocardiography	ECG
medical assistant	MA
occupational therapy	OT

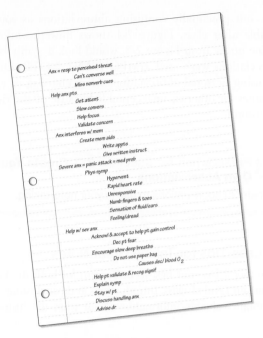

FIGURE 7-4 Using Abbreviations and Symbols. Using "shorthand" in the form of abbreviations and symbols can help you take notes faster and more efficiently. You may be able to capture more of what your instructor is saying. *Compare this example with the more complete outline in Figure 7-3. Do you think you would remember after class what you intended to say if these were your notes? If you decided to use abbreviations and symbols, what could you do to ensure that you understood your notes after several weeks when studying for an exam?* (Adapted from Bonewit-West K, Hunt S, Applegate E: *Today's medical assistant: Clinical and administrative procedures*, ed 2, St Louis, 2013, Saunders.)

considers to be most important. Conclusions may clarify points that seemed fuzzy or unrelated earlier in the lecture.

- Leave some blank space on your pages between the major ideas or clusters of related information so you can make additions when you edit and review. If you get lost and have gaps in your notes, leave extra space to fill in later.
- Write out examples, definitions, formulas, and calculations.
- Write on only one side of the paper so you can lay the pages out and see all your notes at once. You can also use the blank facing pages to create additional study notes. Figure 7-5 illustrates how this works.
- Do your best to write down words you don't know. Guess at the spelling and circle the words so you can look up their meanings later or ask the instructor.
- Write as neatly as possible. If necessary, practice improving your handwriting or try printing if it doesn't slow you down too much. Aim for a balance between speed and legibility. On those occasions when your notes are a total disaster, it may be worth your time to rewrite them.
- Erasable pens are good for taking notes, although regular pens can be used if you make corrections neatly. Pencils can break or need sharpening, and the writing tends to fade and smudge over time.

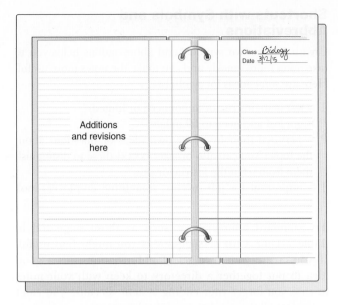

FIGURE 7-5 Use Space to Your Advantage. Take notes on only one side of the paper (that you have set up using the Cornell format). Use the clean reverse side of each previous page for adding to and revising your notes. *Set up a section in your binder for each of your subjects. Place several sheets ready for note-taking in each section. Refer back to the notes you have taken recently in class. Is there anything you want to add, using the reverse sides of these pages?*

On the Job

Using Abbreviations on the Job Abbreviations are used in health care work, so learning to apply them is an important skill. The following is an example of notes on a patient history form.[3]

Chief complaint: Ⓛ shoulder pain p̄ playing basketball this AM.

Present illness: Soreness and immobility Ⓛ shoulder × 8 hours; strained on collision w/another player.

Important note: Abbreviations used on medical records *must be standardized* (the same for everyone who adds information), so be sure to use only those that are approved by the facility in which you work. Also, some abbreviations are no longer allowed because they lead to confusion and medical errors. The Joint Commission and the Institute for Safe Medication Practices have both published lists of abbreviations that should not be used on the job.

Make Your Notes Work for You

It takes work to take good notes in class. Now let them work for you. Start by reviewing them as soon as possible after class. Try not to wait more than 24 hours because the average person forgets more than half of what was said during a typical class lecture within that time. Even a quick review will help create memory pathways for the new information.

Read over your notes and fill in any missing words or abbreviations with meanings you might forget. Next, fill in

Figure 7-6 (handwritten notes)

Class: Interpersonal Relations   Date: 10/19/15

Barriers to commun.

① Phys. impair.
  Vision   Pain
  Hearing   Medication
                  Dev. disabled
  To help
  Face pt.
  Speak clearly — don't speak
  Use description   loudly

See websites
• Alex. Graham Bell
• Natl. Fed. for the Blind

Hearing impaired may deny
  Careful – elderly pts. not
    nec. hard of hearing

② Language
  Limited Eng.

Children — Use words they understand

  To help —
  Use gestures   See ch. 4 in
  Good body lang.   text for
  Ask for feedback   suggestions
  Learn med. phrases

Ask about classes or books.
See appendix w/ phrases in MA text

③ Prejudice = opinion before facts are known
  ✻ Discrimination   ✻ (key concept)
    Limits effect. commun.
    Can neg. affect care given

④ Stereotyping   ✻ (key concept)
  Preconceived assumpt.
  Get to know indiv.
  Unfair to label

Speaker
Message
Listener's perception
What listener hears

⑤ Perception   ✻ (key concept)
  Receiver's percept. can interfere w/ message
  Ex. "all lawyers are corrupt"

  Often from experiences w/ group

  Treat all as indiv.
  Try to underst. other points/view
  Be willing to discuss

M E S S A G E

FIGURE 7-6 Make Your Notes Your Own. This is an example of personalizing your notes and turning them into real learning tools. Note how Emily wrote in additional information, referenced her textbook, created a flow chart, and stated key concepts. Use a colored pen to better highlight your additions. *Take a look at the notes you have taken recently in class. Is there anything you need to ask your instructor? Are there important points you should highlight? Any abbreviations you want to expand so you won't forget what they stand for? Any points you want to explore further?*

Figure 7-7 (handwritten notes)

KEYWORDS	LECTURE NOTES
Anxiety / Resulting behaviors	Anxiety = response to perceived threat / Cannot converse well / Misses nonverbal cues
Helping pts.	Helping anxious patients / Get attention / Slow conversation / Help to focus / Validate concern
Effect on memory	Anxiety interferes with memory / Create memory aids / Write down appointments / Give written instructions
Panic attacks / Symptoms	Severe anxiety = panic attack = medical problem / Physical symptoms / Hyperventilation / Rapid heart rate / Unresponsive / Numbness in fingers and toes / Sensation of fluid in ears / Feeling of dread
Helping with severe attack	Helping with severe anxiety / Acknowledge and accept to help patient gain control / Decreases patient's fear / Encourage slow deep breaths / Do not use paper bag / Causes decrease in blood oxygen / Help patient validate and recognize significance / Explain symptoms / Stay with patient / Discuss handling anxiety / Advise physician

FIGURE 7-7 Studying with Keywords. A proven learning method is recalling facts from your notes. List keywords in the space to the left of your notes. Then cover the right side and recall—out loud—what you remember about the concepts represented by the keywords. *Write keywords for the notes you took in a recent class. Review by quizzing yourself looking at only the keywords. Check your knowledge against your notes. How did you do?* (Adapted from Bonewit-West K, Hunt S, Applegate E: *Today's medical assistant: Clinical and administrative procedures*, ed 2, St Louis, 2013, Saunders.)

---

ideas or reorganize your notes, as needed. If there are gaps, look in your textbook, ask a classmate, or make a note to ask the instructor for help.

Use a highlighter or colored pen to mark key words and phrases. Personalize your notes with drawings, arrows to show relationships, pictures from magazines, or anything else that helps you focus on and better understand the material. See Figure 7-6 to see how Emily personalized and added to the notes she took in her Interpersonal Relations class. Consider recording if listening helps you to retain information better.

Using the Cornell System

Refer back to Figure 7-2 to see the Cornell page layout for taking notes. The space in the left column on each page is for writing key words or phrases (Figure 7-7) or your own quiz questions (Figure 7-8). The space at the bottom of the page is for writing summaries, in your own words, of the material on the page. (If you have trouble writing a summary, this is a good indication that you may not fully understand the material.) If you don't have enough room on the page containing your notes, use the back of the previous page, as discussed earlier and illustrated in Figure 7-5.

Reviewing Productively

The most important thing you can do with your notes is to review them often, at least twice a week. If your classes last for less than one month, review your notes even more often. As we discussed in Chapter 3, the key to long-term memory is *repetition over time.* Your review sessions don't have to be long, but make them a regular part of your study schedule. Keep in mind you are not simply learning to pass a test, but are accumulating knowledge to apply when you are working as a health care professional.

Engage your mind actively when you review. Passively reading and rereading your notes will not store them in your mind. Use the review column to the left of your notes to prompt recall of the information. Cover the notes you took in class, and explain the key words or answer the questions you wrote. This is *the most effective part* of the review because it forces you to think and helps transfer the content of your notes into your long-term memory.

You can use study techniques that take advantage of your preferred way of learning. Here are a few suggestions:

- **Visual:** Picture the words and concepts in your mind as you review; label drawings from memory; draw sketches of the material and the relationships between concepts. Rough sketches are fine—no one is grading the art!

YOUR QUIZ QUESTIONS	LECTURE NOTES
What is the definition of anxiety?	Anxiety = response to perceived threat
How can anxiety affect patient behavior?	Cannot converse well Misses nonverbal cues

What are ways the health care professional can help anxious patients?	Helping anxious patients
	  Get attention
	    Slow conversation
	    Help to focus
	    Validate concern

What can the health care professional do to help anxious patients remember important information?	Anxiety interferes with memory
	  Create memory aids
	  Write down appointments
	    Give written instructions

What is a panic attack?
What are the physical symptoms associated with severe anxiety?
	Severe anxiety = panic attack =
	        medical problem
	  Physical symptoms
	  Hyperventilation
	  Rapid heart rate
	    Unresponsive
	    Numbness in fingers and toes
	    Sensation of fluid in ears
	    Feeling of dread

What actions can the health care professional take to help patients who are experiencing severe anxiety?	Helping with severe anxiety
	  Stay with patient
	  Acknowledge and accept patient's feelings
	  Help patient validate and recognize significance of anxiety
	  Explain symptoms
	  Discuss ways of handling anxiety
	  Advise physician

Why is breathing into a paper bag no longer recommended for patients who are hyperventilating?	Do not have patient's breathe into paper bag Causes decrease in blood oxygen

FIGURE 7-8 **Testing Yourself.** Even more effective than studying from keywords is creating test questions based on your notes. In fact, using recall has been proved to be *the* most effective way you can learn from any written material. *Write test questions for the notes you took in a recent class. Review by answering the test questions—best if done orally—without looking at your notes on the right side of the page. Check your knowledge against your notes. How did you do?* (Adapted from Bonewit-West K, Hunt S, Applegate E: *Today's medical assistant: Clinical and administrative procedures*, ed 2, St Louis, 2013, Saunders.)

- **Auditory:** Review out loud, even if you must speak in a soft voice. Have someone read aloud your key words and questions and check your answers as you give them out loud. Record and then listen to your notes.
- **Kinesthetic:** Stand up, move around, recreate the lecture. Or teach someone else by explaining the information. Use movement and gestures to emphasize important points. If the content is about a procedure or something that involves movement, act it out or actually perform it as much as possible.
- **Interactive:** Exchange notes with a study partner or group. Discuss and quiz each other.
- **Global:** Write out concepts, then create a list of supporting facts.
- **Linear:** Look for **logical** patterns in the material.

Taking tests is a proven powerful learning tool. Create your own practice tests based on your notes. Write your questions to the left of your notes or on a separate page. You can also record them. Don't take your "test" for at least 3 days. Here are some suggestions for questions:

1. What is the definition of _____?
2. What is the meaning of _____?
3. What are the steps in performing a _____?
4. What is important to remember about_____?
5. Why must you _____?
6. What are the principal parts of _____?
7. How does _____ function?
8. What is the purpose of _____?

Finally, think about your own past experiences and how what you are learning relates to them and to what you already know about the topic. This gives you reference points and makes new information more meaningful.

Note-Taking on the Job

Note-taking is a skill that health care professionals use on many occasions. Figure 7-9 shows some common examples. A medical assistant, for example, may be called on to take notes as the physician examines a patient. And when the patients themselves explain their health background, symptoms, and reasons for seeking care, the information must be recorded correctly. A physical therapist assistant documents the treatment given. And nurses must record their assessments and care plans. Patient records serve as the basis for giving appropriate and consistent care; therefore, it is critical that they be both accurate and legible. In addition, they can serve as legal documents and are used in court cases to defend the actions of health care providers.

Good handwriting is important on the job because the quality of patient care depends on the ability of other health care professionals to read your written documentation. In spite of jokes made about doctors' chicken scratches, there is nothing funny about illegible medical records.

Taking Phone Messages

The telephone is often the first means of communication between patients and health care providers. Recording phone messages is an important form of note-taking. Even if your job does not normally require answering the telephone, there may be times when it is necessary. The following information is essential when taking a message for a nonemergency phone call:

1. The caller's name
2. Date and time of call
3. Who the message is for
4. The business they're calling from, if applicable
5. The caller's telephone number
6. A brief write-up of the message

Legibility is especially important when taking phone messages. And be sure the person to whom the message is directed receives it in a timely way.

Documentation

Recording information about patients in their medical chart or other types of report, called **documentation,** is part of many health care occupations. Here are a few examples:

- Athletic trainer: detailed records of athletic injuries; training-room treatment logs; athletic medical referral forms
- Nursing assistant: notes describing changes in a patient's condition; records of vital signs
- Dental assistant: enter descriptions of treatments on patient records
- Massage therapist: create client records that include the current medical condition, contraindications, cautions for

PATIENT HISTORY

Soc Sec Number: 203-46-7809

Patient Name: Sean D. Austin — DOB: 03/03/83
Address: 1234 Crown Ave. — City: Dayton — State: Ohio — ZIP: 24354
Home Phone: (937) 123-4567 — Work Phone: — Emergency Phone: (937) 545-4415
Status: M (S) W D — Spouse's name: — Referring Physician:
Occupation: student — Employer: — Phone:
Primary Insurance: Anthem BC/BS — Policy Holder: John Austin — Policy No. AN232435545

Chief Complaint: (L) shoulder pain p̄ playing basketball this AM.
Present Illness: soreness and immobility (L) shoulder x 8 hours; strained upon collision w/ another player

HT	62"	Sc Fever	—
Weight	112#	Rheum Fev	—
Past yr + −	8#	Measles	+
Temp	98.4°F	Mumps	—
Pulse	72	Rubella	—
Resp	12	Chicken Pox	+
BP	108/64	Asthma	—
LMP	NA		

FAMILY HISTORY

	Father	Mother	Brother	Brother	Sister	Sister	MGM	MGF
Heart	−	+	−	−			+	−
Bld Pressure	−	−	−	−			−	−
Diabetes	−	−	−	−			−	−
Bld Diabetes	−	−	−	−			−	−
Asthma	−	+	−	−			−	−
Epilepsy	−	−	−	−			−	−
Stroke	−	−	−	−			−	−

SURGICAL HISTORY

Surgery	Year	Physician	Surgery	Year	Physician	Surgery
Adenoidectomy	1986	Smith				
BTTI	1986	Smith				

REVIEW OF SYSTEMS

HEENT

Head	Acne	—					
Eyes	Vision	—	Glasses	—	Pain	—	
Ears	Hearing	—	Pain	—	Discharge	—	Tinn
Nose	Obstruction	—	Discharge	—	Epistaxis	—	Sinu
Throat	Teeth	—	Tongue	—	Gums	—	Thro
NECK	Swelling	—	Stiffness	—	Hoarseness	—	
BACK	Pain	—					
LUNGS	Cough	—	Hemoptysis	—	Sputum	—	Pain
HEART	Chills	—	Fever	—	Nightsweats	—	Whe
GI	Pain	—	Dyspnea	—	Edema	—	Palp
	Appetite	good	Diet	"normal"	Nausea	—	Vomit
	Diarrhea	—	Constipation	—	Jaundice	—	flatulence
GU	Belching	—					
	Frequency	—	Dysuria	—	Burning	—	Nocturia
MENSES	Incontinence	—	Hematuria	—	Discharge	—	Vaginal irritation
PREG HX	Menarche	—	Regularity	NA	Duration	NA	LMP NA
LIBIDO	Cramping	—	Menorrhagia	NA	Metrorrhagia	NA	
EXTREM	#Pregnancies		Miscarriages	NA	Abortions	NA	Live births NA
ENDO	Frequency		Satisfaction	NA			
SKIN	Joint pain	—	Weakness	—	Varicose veins	—	Swelling
NEURO	Hair	—	Nails	—	Sensitivity to temp	—	
HABITS	Dryness	—	Perspiration	—	Itching	—	Eruption —
STRESS	Paralysis	—	Tingling	—	Numbness	—	Tremor —
	Faint	—	Dizziness	—	Memory loss	—	Convulsion —
	Sleep	8hr/night	Caffiene	16oz/day(pop)	Smoking	—	Alcohol —
	Home	some	Work	—	Finances	—	General disposition "easy going"

WHILE YOU WERE OUT

FOR: Pt Billing — DATE: 05/04/15 — TIME: 10:20 am

FROM: Bonita Henderson

OF: (Dr. Arewells Pt)

PHONE NUMBER: (771)- 423-6740

FAX: ( )-

RX REFILL: — PHARMACY: — RX#:

REMARKS:
[X] telephoned [ ] needs to talk to you
[ ] will call back [ ] will call again
[ ] stopped by [ ] needs to see you
[X] please return call [ ] urgent

MESSAGE:
Questions about her April bill and insurance

taken by: G. Chester (AAMA)

CHARTING NOTES

02/10/14 — 9am c/o sore throat. T—99⁴F, P—72, R—18, BP—120/68, Throat culture obtained. Amoxicillin 500 mg P.O. given to pt.

P. Dunham (AAMA)

FIGURE 7-9 Examples of Note-Taking on the Job. Taking accurate and legible notes is an important health care skill. *When might you be required to take notes in your future career? What are some possible consequences if the notes in these examples were incorrect or impossible to read? Consider both the patient and the health care professional.*

massage; following a massage, record the action taken, the client's response, and the therapist's evaluation

Charting is the process of making written entries in a patient's medical record. Follow these guidelines when entering data in a patient record:

1. Ensure that the patient's name is correct.
2. Use black ink to make entries.
3. Write legibly.
4. Record information accurately, clearly, and concisely. Two types of data may be recorded:
   a. Objective: can be observed, such as test results, marks on the body, measurements, and behaviors
   b. Subjective: reported by the patient, such as headache, nausea, pain, anxiety

5. If it is necessary to correct entries, draw a single line through the incorrect information, enter the correction, the date, and sign with your initials. Never erase or make an incorrect entry illegible.
6. Use standard abbreviations and/or those approved by your facility.
7. Check that your spelling is correct, especially for medical terms.
8. Chart immediately after performing a procedure.
9. Sign the entry, including your full last name.

Medical records can serve as legal documents. Often it is medical documentation that determines the outcome of a medical malpractice suit. And remember this important health care rule: if it isn't documented, it isn't done.

Case Study 7-1

Good Notes Make a Difference

Jan is excited about starting her practical nursing program. She dropped out of high school to get married and was happy raising her four children. She got her GED a few years ago, but she always regretted not getting more education. Last year, her husband Frank was in a serious car accident and spent time in hospital, followed by weeks in a rehabilitation facility.

During that time, Jan saw the work performed by the nurses who attended to Frank. She could see what a positive difference the good ones made to Frank's attitude and progress. Jan noticed that it was the practical nurses who seemed to have a lot of contact with him and this kind of career appealed to her—one in which she would have direct patient contact and could make a difference. Going into health care would also give her the training she could use to continue Frank's long-term care at home, as well as replacing the income that he could no longer earn.

Her first few days in school are almost a blur. There is so much to absorb: so many school policies and rules, classes to attend, people's names to learn. She feels a lot of pressure to do her best, because she had to take out a student loan and the last thing she wants is to have wasted the money.

Jan attends all her classes, but it's been many years since she was in school and she's beginning to panic. She never was a top student and is finding it difficult to always follow her instructors' lectures. When she gets home and looks over her notes, they don't always make sense. There are gaps, they are unorganized, and she's pretty sure many of the words aren't spelled correctly. At least she can't find them in her textbooks.

At first, Jan is afraid to say anything. She's older than many of the other students and believes that at her age, she should be able to do this. After all, her children did well in school and she would be embarrassed to admit she is having trouble. Instead, she works extra hard studying in the evenings and tries harder to concentrate in class.

Jan does not do well on her first quizzes and begins to question whether she can be successful in this program. She worries a lot about this and actually loses a few nights'

sleep. Finally, she admits to Frank that she believes she has made a mistake.

"Let's take a good look at this," he tells her. "You've been out of school for more than 20 years. That's a long time."

"You're right about that," Jan admits.

"So, remember when we first got married? Did you know how to cook? How to keep a house? Why no, you had no experience being in charge of a household. But you learned—and ended up being the best cook in the neighborhood!"

"Okay, so what's that got to do with the trouble I'm having in school?" Jan asks.

"I think it means that you have to learn how to learn this new stuff. There's probably some techniques—like when you learned to cook—that you just need to know about," Frank says.

"That does make some sense," Jan responds. "Maybe I should talk with my instructors and see if I can get some help learning to learn."

The next day, Jan made appointments to meet with her instructors. They asked her a lot of questions about how she was studying, did she read the assignments in her textbook, and finally—how were the notes she took in class? After looking these over, her anatomy instructor smiled and said, "I think I know where we can start working on your study skills." And over time with work and the help of her instructors, Jan learned to take notes that she could use to help her learn and succeed in her classes.

Questions for Thought and Reflection

1. How is Jan's situation a common one for students, especially those who have been out of school for a while?
2. What are some reasons why she waited so long to ask for help?
3. Why do you think she was having so much trouble taking notes?
4. How was Frank able to help Jan see her problems more realistically?
5. What suggestions do you think her instructors gave her?

Dan Abrams believed he was lucky. He attended school with his girlfriend, Ashley, to become a physical therapist assistant. If it weren't for her taking notes in class and helping him review for tests, he probably wouldn't have made it through to graduation. Ashley took great notes in class and always gave Dan copies to study. Taking notes just wasn't his thing. He attended many of the classes, but he wasn't interested in learning to take good notes. After all, he would be working with patients. When would he ever use note-taking again?

Dan got a job at a small physical therapy practice and really enjoyed helping patients with their exercises. He communicated well with his supervisor, Doug Anderson, and got along well with the patients.

After he had been on the job for a couple of months, the patient load declined and Doug had to let the administrative assistant go. He felt badly about this, but he needed to cut expenses to keep the office open. This meant there would be some cross-training among the employees. The PT assistants, for example, would have to take turns answering the phones, taking messages, scheduling appointments, and taking the histories of new patients.

When the time came for Dan to take on some of these new duties, he decided to give it his best. But after taking down a few phone messages incorrectly and recording patient data inaccurately, he began to panic. He just didn't seem to be able to focus intently on what people were saying. His mind tended to wander and he would lose track before he could get their words or information down on paper.

Doug's priority was on keeping his business going and he finally told Dan that if he couldn't get it together, he would have to let him go. Doug simply didn't have the time to correct the mistakes and take the losses they were causing.

Questions for Thought and Reflection

1. What does Dan's experience demonstrate about the relationship of study skills and job skills?
2. Did Ashley make a mistake by giving Dan her notes to study?
3. Do you think Dan will make it as a physical therapist assistant? Why or why not?

Reading to Learn

"To read without reflecting is like eating without digesting."
—Edmund Burke

Reading, along with listening and taking notes, is one of the most important ways you will acquire information as a student. Like effective listening, reading to learn requires you to pay attention and participate actively. It should be approached purposefully because you must work at understanding, remembering, and applying new material. If you were reading instructions about how to perform a medical procedure, you would ask yourself, "Do I understand this? What, exactly, am I supposed to do?" and then you would read carefully to make sure you got it right. The same is true when reading your textbook. You will spend a great deal of time reading textbooks, so it makes sense to learn how to gain the most benefit from your efforts.

Textbooks are important learning tools. There are many reasons to complete your reading assignments:

1. The more ways you take in information, the more likely you are to remember it. Paths are worn over time by many walkers. If no one uses them, they disappear. Your memory paths are also created and maintained by repeated use. Even if a subject is discussed in class, reading gives you one more encounter with it.
2. Reading gives you background information for class lectures. It also reinforces what you hear in class.
3. Textbooks provide a permanent means of storing information. You can refer back to them over and over as needed.
4. Books contain supporting details, examples, graphics, and organizational aids for the topics you are studying (Figure 7-10).

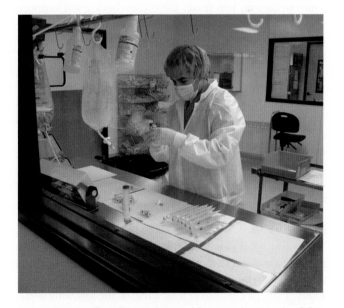

FIGURE 7-10 **Reading to Learn.** Many students today fail to understand the importance of reading and studying their textbooks. But working in health care requires mastering a lot of information, usually more than can be shared by the instructor in the classroom. To work safely and accurately, this lab technician needed to learn about bacteria, the proper storage of chemicals, the steps in test procedures, and many other topics. *Can you think of times after graduating that a health care professional needs to read technical literature? (Consider the fast pace of changes in health care.) Can you make a commitment to complete the reading assignments for the classes you are currently taking? Why or why not?* (From Hopper T: *Mosby's pharmacy technician: Principles and practice*, ed 4, St Louis, 2016, Saunders.)

Getting Ready to Read

There are several prereading activities you can do to make your reading easier and more beneficial. The first is to clear your mind of clutter. Reading requires concentration, and this is difficult when you have unfinished business on your mind. If something is bothering you that can be handled quickly, take care of it before you start studying. (But try not to let "urgencies" be an excuse to put off getting together with your books indefinitely.) If it will take more than a few minutes of your attention, write it down (your planner would be a good place) so you can deal with it later.

Next is to find a place that encourages reading rather than sleeping or daydreaming. Many people find that a straight-backed chair at a desk works best (you will be doing some writing as you read). Give your back good support, and make sure the lighting is adequate. An uncomfortable environment can tire you and cut your reading time short.

You need more than just your textbook to read actively, so gather your tools: notebook, pen or pencil, highlighter or colored pen, and a dictionary. Develop the habit of gathering the necessary supplies before you start studying. This is an important health care practice, too. You would not want to interrupt a patient procedure because you forgot to bring something from the supply room. Your study time is valuable, too, and should not be interrupted while you look for the dictionary.

Anatomy of a Textbook

When you get a new textbook, take a few minutes to look it over carefully. Don't wait until the end of the course to discover something that could have made your life easier. Every textbook contains at least a few of the following useful features:

1. **Preface:** An introductory section at the beginning of the book. It typically contains a statement of the author's purpose and an overview of the book's content and structure. Some prefaces include information of special value to students, such as how to use the different features, study tips, and career ideas.
2. Table of contents: Some books supplement the usual list of chapter titles with a complete listing of chapter sections. This detailed format gives you a good overall view of the topics covered.
3. **Appendices:** Extra materials placed at the back of the book. Their contents are based on the book's subject and

vary widely. Look these over when you first begin using the book, because you may discover valuable resources to help you understand both the textbook and the subject. There may also be sources of career information and reference guides. Examples from recent editions of health care textbooks include guidelines for infection control, important abbreviations, a metric conversion chart, Spanish translations of common health care phrases, laboratory test values, and a Celsius to Fahrenheit conversion scale.

4. Index: An alphabetical listing of all the topics in the book and the page numbers on which they appear. The items included are much more specific than those listed in the table of contents. The index is located at the back of a book and is very useful when you need specific information or are reviewing.
5. Bibliography and/or references: A list of source materials used by the author and/or recommended readings for students who want to learn more about the subject. Each chapter may have its own bibliography, or there may be one list at the end of the book.
6. **Glossary:** An alphabetical list of words with their definitions, usually located at the back of the book.
7. Vocabulary or **key terms:** Lists of new words, often placed at the beginning of each chapter. Because reading is based on understanding words, learning new vocabulary before you begin to read is essential for comprehension. Take a few minutes to study the terms listed before you read the chapter, marking any words you find difficult. Word lists may also contain clues about what the author considers to be most important.
8. **Objectives:** These are statements telling you what you should learn or be able to do as a result of studying and applying the information in the chapter. Knowing the chapter objectives gives structure and purpose to your reading. Use them to check your understanding after reading the material. Here are some examples of objectives:
   - Describe the steps in the communication process.[3]
   - Identify key differences between law and ethics.[3]
   - List and describe the three stages of a fever.[3]
   - Explain the advantages of outpatient intravenous (IV) therapy.[3]
9. Chapter introductions: In addition to giving an overview of the chapter content, these often contain explanations of why the material is important and how it relates to your career.
10. Section headings: Words or phrases that divide and identify sections of text. Headings give you an idea of the content that follows. An important part of previewing is going through the assigned reading page by page and reading the headings. You will see they are organized like an outline, often with several levels of subheadings. Some books distinguish the levels with different colors and lettering styles. The following

example of headings comes from a chapter entitled "Interacting with Patients" in *Today's Medical Assistant*[3]:

Communicating with Patients

- Verbal and Nonverbal Communication
- Interference with Communication
- Listening Skills
- Nonverbal Measures to Facilitate Communication
- Interviewing Techniques
    - Closed Questions
    - Open Questions
    - Keeping the Conversation Going
    - Drawing Out Patients
    - Avoiding Responses That Inhibit Communication

Headings provide a logical structure to guide your reading. In the example, you learn three things before even reading the chapter: (1) interviewing techniques are used when communicating with patients; (2) there are at least two kinds of questions; and (3) some types of responses interfere with good communication.

Prescription for Success: 7-4 Book Report

Look over your current textbooks. Which of the following features do they contain?
- Preface
- Detailed table of contents
- Appendices
- Index
- Bibliography
- Glossary
- Vocabulary or key terms
- Objectives
- Chapter introductions
- Headings
- Other

Previewing

"Advice worth repeating: Work smarter, not harder."

Many methods have been developed to help students gain maximum benefit from their reading assignments. Some methods have many steps and others just a few, but they *all* recommend that you **preview** the material before you start reading. Using a medical procedure as an example, you would never perform a treatment on a patient without taking a few preliminary steps: (1) identify the patient, (2) introduce yourself, (3) verify the procedure, (4) gather the necessary supplies, and (5) put on gloves.

Previewing in reading means that you:
1. Read the chapter or section introductions.
2. Study the vocabulary list at the beginning of the chapter.
3. Read the objectives for the reading selection.
4. Skim through the material to see the headings and subheadings, reading the first sentence of each.
5. Read the conclusion of the chapter or section.
6. Read the tables, figures, and charts.
7. Based on the information gathered, identify the main ideas.

You may be thinking that previewing is a waste of time and that it would be better to just jump into the reading and get it done. Not true! You are not "just reading." You are engaging in a learning activity and previewing increases your ability to comprehend and remember the information presented in your textbooks. Previewing is an excellent investment of your time.

Getting the Most from Your Reading

Two activities to help you interact with your textbooks are asking and answering questions and marking or highlighting. These actions focus your attention and serve as comprehension checks as you proceed through the text.

To use the question–answer method, change each section heading into a question and look for the answer as you read. When you find it, stop and answer the question aloud or quietly to yourself. This technique was developed almost 60 years ago when methods to increase the speed of learning were researched for World War II soldiers.[4] To this day, it has proved to be one of the most effective ways to master written material. See Table 7-2 for examples of study questions based on a few of the headings from "Communicating with Patients."

To benefit from questions, it's usually not necessary to write out the answers, although you may find it helpful with difficult material. (You must, however, say the answers, either silently or out loud.)

Prescription for Success: 7-5 Increasing Your Learning with Questions

Using this or any other textbook, list 10 chapter objectives or 10 section headings within a chapter. Then convert each into a study question.

The second interactive reading activity is marking your book by highlighting or underlining the most important information. Do this *after* you finish reading each section. If you highlight as you read, you may end up marking just about everything in the book. This defeats the purpose of highlighting. Highlight only the key words and phrases, rather than whole sentences. This will draw your attention to the important points when it's time to review.

In addition to highlighting, you can further increase your learning by writing in your book. This can take the form of key words, short summaries, questions, or responses. Use logical and easy-to-remember symbols, like the ones suggested earlier in the chapter for taking notes:

T = the instructor has indicated you will be tested on this material
?? = "I don't understand this and need to ask about it"
* = this information is important
** = this information is very important
circled word = this is a new word and I need to learn it

Many students like to use colored highlighters to mark their books. If this is your preference, avoid very bright colors because they can cause eye strain. You might want to use a

TABLE 7-2

Examples Using the Question–Answer Study Method: Try Using Questions You Create to Test Your Recall from Reading

Section Headings	Study Questions
Verbal and Nonverbal Communication	What is the difference between verbal and nonverbal communication? How are the two types of communication used by health care professionals when working with patients?
Interference with Communication	What are some example of factors that can interfere with effective communication?
Listening Skills	How can good listening skills be developed? Why are good listening skills important when working with patients?
Nonverbal Measures to Facilitate Communication	What is meant by "nonverbal measures"? When should the health care professional employ nonverbal measures?
Interviewing Techniques	When do health care professionals use interviewing techniques when communicating with patients?
Closed Question	What is an example of a closed question? When should closed questions be used when one is interviewing a patient?
Drawing Out Patients	What are two ways to draw out patients during the communication process?
Avoiding Responses That Inhibit Communication	What is meant by "responses that inhibit communication"? What are responses that a health care professional should avoid when communicating with patients?

pen or pencil to underline and make notes. A tool that combines the features of the highlighter and pen is a colored pen. When it is used to underline, the color draws your attention for easy review. Use the same pen to write in your book. This saves time because you don't have to switch back and forth between a highlighter and a pen.

Success Tips for Reading

- Look up unfamiliar words as you come to them by using the book's glossary, a general dictionary, or a medical dictionary. You can write the definition in your book, in your own glossary that you keep in your notebook, and/or on flash cards.
- Take advantage of illustrations, charts, lists, and boxed text. These give you examples and additional opportunities to master the material.
- Read through procedures carefully, paying special attention to the rationales. It is important for health care professionals to understand the reasons behind their actions because nothing in health care is routine. You must think through every action and know why you are performing it.
- Read in short sessions. Depending on the difficulty of the material, you may find you are able to read and absorb for only 20 to 30 minutes without a short break. Experiment to see what works best for you. Just don't wander off too far or get involved in a two-hour movie on TV!
- Don't worry about your reading speed. Health care textbooks contain lots of technical and detailed information. Your goal is not speed; it is comprehension. Read at a rate that keeps your attention and also allows you to understand the material. One way to prevent getting bogged down is to avoid saying each word, even if you are only doing this mentally. Try to read in phrases. When you drive a car, you see and act on many things at once. The same is true for reading, and with practice, you can see and process several words at a time.

TABLE 7-3

Converting Chapter Objectives into Quiz Questions

Chapter Objectives	Quiz Questions
List and describe the parts of the medical office.[3]	What are the various parts of a medical office? What is the purpose of each?
List and describe the seven sections of the health history.[3]	What are the seven parts of a health history? What is the content of each?
Explain the purpose of OSHA.[3]	What does OSHA stand for? What is the purpose of OSHA? How does OSHA affect the work of the health care professional?

Reviewing and Recalling

Reviewing soon after your first exposure to new material is the key to ensuring its storage in your long-term memory. Effective review techniques for material you have read are similar to those suggested for reviewing your class notes. A good habit is to review within 24 hours. Start laying down memory paths before you forget most of the information. What a waste to spend an entire evening reading an assignment, only to forget most of it by bedtime the next night! Even a quick review is helpful.

Reading to learn requires actively engaging with the material. Quiz yourself on the material you have read without looking at the text. This forces you to think and checks your understanding, and has been proved to be the most effective way to retain what you read. Try converting the chapter objectives into questions. Table 7-3 contains a few examples. If you have difficulty remembering, review the section and try again. If you continue having trouble, this is a sign you don't understand the material.

Self-quizzes are recommended for all students. In addition, there are a variety of other learning activities, based on various learning preferences, you might want to try:

- Use text illustrations to reinforce the material.
- Create stories about the illustrations to help anchor concepts in your mind.
- Attach significant concepts to people in a photograph.
- While looking at a picture of a piece of equipment, recall the name and function of each part, as well as how and for what purpose the equipment is used.
- Cover the labels on drawings and say or write down the names.
- Read the text aloud.

- Explain what you are reading in your own words.
- Create a dialogue to discuss the material.
- Have someone ask you questions.
- Record important points you can listen to.
- Go through explanations or procedures as realistically as possible in your mind. Or trying acting them out. For example, open and close your hand as you read about how the heart pumps blood.
- Draw mind maps or concept maps of the material.
- Write short summaries of the principal ideas.
- List the important facts that support the major ideas.
- Make flash cards with facts on one side and explanations or definitions on the other.

On the Job

Reading on the Job Reading is an important skill in your professional life. Directions for the proper use of medications and medical equipment, as well as for performing procedures, come in written form. Your ability to understand and follow written directions has an impact on patient well-being.

Reading is also necessary for keeping up with the rapidly advancing field of health care. Discoveries about how the body works, such as in the field of genetics; the development of new medications and treatments; and the invention of new machines and devices, such as computerized robots

that perform surgery, will make your current knowledge outdated in only a few years, if not months. Literally thousands of journals are devoted to medical and health care topics, and reading at least some of them will be an important way of staying up-to-date in your field.

Most health care certifications and licenses require continuing education credits for renewal, and this presents another need for reading and comprehending written material. Credits can often be earned through self-study, such as reading an article, and then answering questions or taking a test.

Case Study 7-2

To Read or Not to Read

Emily Hasbrow didn't really know what to do with herself after graduating from high school. After reading an article in the local paper about careers in massage therapy, her mom had an idea. "Emily," she said, "you're a perfect fit for this occupation. You've spent the last year moping around the house, not knowing what to do with yourself. You're really good with your hands, you like people—and maybe someday you can get a job on one of those cruise ships. That could really be fun."

When her mother agreed to let her continue living at home rent-free as well as helping her with school expenses, Emily finally decided to go ahead and give the program a try. She passed the school's entrance exam, bought the necessary books and uniform, and started attending classes the following week.

Emily thought the classes were okay, although not as interesting as she had hoped. And the homework—good grief! Did the instructors really expect the students to do that much reading? After a few days of slogging through her assignments, Emily decided that since she was going to class and taking decent notes, she couldn't see any reason to waste her time reading the textbook. When her mom asked about homework, Emily explained that there really "wasn't any." All the work was completed in class.

Emily was able to pass, with C's, the short weekly quizzes in her classes. But she had a surprise when the class had their mid-term exam. Where did the instructor get these questions? Emily couldn't remember having heard anything about some of this information. She had attended every class—had she fallen asleep or something?

When the tests were returned and Emily had earned a D, she went to see her instructor, Ms. Shepherd, to find out what had happened. Had Miss Shepherd given them the exam intended for a different class?

The instructor explained, "Emily, looking over your test, it appears that the questions you missed were on the information contained in the readings I assigned—the ones in your textbook as well as the supplementary reading material. Didn't you ever look at these?"

Emily looked down. She didn't want to admit that she hadn't been doing the reading because she thought it was a waste of her time. All she could say was, "Well, I guess I goofed up. I thought you were covering everything we needed to know in your lectures."

Ms. Shepherd smiled. "There's no way I have the time in class to cover everything you'll need to know on the job. That's why I give the reading assignments."

"Okay," said Emily. "I get your point. I'm going to have to decide how I want to spend my time and how much my education means to me."

Questions for Thought and Reflection

1. Do you think Emily is really interested in becoming a massage therapist?
2. What mistake did she make when deciding how to spend her study time?
3. What kind of attitude does Emily have about school?
4. Do you think she will stay in school and pursue this career? Why or why not?

Megan is glad to be finished with school—well, almost finished. She is now working at her externship site, a pharmacy located in a large grocery store, where she is practicing what she learned in her pharmacy technician program. Megan is glad to be working because, as she told her friend, Amy, "I'm just so tired of reading boring books and doing homework assignments every night."

Amy, who is studying to be a nurse, agreed that studying could become tiring, but it seemed necessary if they were to learn all they needed to know for their careers.

Megan is not happy to learn that Ted, the pharmacist who is her supervisor, expects her to read the employee procedure manual before she can start working with customers.

"Oh, great," she tells Amy one night on the phone. "Now I have to do *more* reading. I thought I was done with that."

"Well," Amy replied, "there might be important things about the pharmacy that you need to know."

"I just don't think I have it in me to go through that stupid manual," Megan said. "I think I'll just pay attention to what the employees are doing and ask questions when I need to."

Amy didn't think this was a good idea, but she had her own studying to do and didn't want to argue.

Megan followed her plan. She paid special attention to the actions of the pharmacy technicians and asked them questions about things she was unsure of. She thought she was doing just fine and told Ted that "Yes," she had read the manual from "cover to cover" and was ready to work with customers. The first couple of days went smoothly, but on the third day it seemed that every customer had some kind of question that Megan couldn't answer. Those that she couldn't bluff her way through, she asked the experienced technicians.

At the end of the day, Ted called her into the office behind the pharmacy. "Megan," he said. "I need the truth. There were questions today you were asking the staff that you would have known if you had read the procedure manual. Did you read the manual?"

Megan answered, "The truth? No, I didn't. I thought it might be a waste of time—that I could learn in other ways."

Ted sighed. "If you had told me this in the first place—the truth, rather than lying about having read it, I could let you have a second chance to read and study the manual and try again. But in this case, I'm afraid I'm going to have to ask the school to end your externship."

Questions for Thought and Reflection

1. What do you think of Megan's decision to learn about the pharmacy procedures by observing and asking questions instead of reading the manual?
2. Should Ted have tested Megan on the material rather than taking her word for it that she had read it?
3. Do you think Ted was fair in terminating Megan's externship?
4. What do you think Megan should do now?

Doing Research to Learn

Research is not limited to finding information for a paper you have to write or something that scientists do. We all do research, such as when we investigate which car to buy, how to find the best auto insurance, and how to change a tire. Research simply means finding sources of reliable information and obtaining what you need from those sources.

Library

Your school's library may be large and contain thousands of books and loads of other material, or it may be small and focused on the specialized materials needed to support the programs offered at the school. You should get to know both your school library and your local public library. If there are other schools of higher education nearby, inquire whether they allow the public to use their libraries. Some give checkout privileges for a yearly fee. Hospitals and clinics often have libraries for employees. It is possible you will have access to these during your clinical experience.

Today's libraries have many resources in addition to books and journals. Most offer Internet services, videos, DVDs, and other multimedia materials. Every library is different. Walk around and explore. Look for informational brochures and how-to guides, and ask the librarian for help.

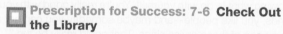

Prescription for Success: 7-6 Check Out the Library

Visit your school and/or local public library to learn about and create a list of the services offered.

Internet

The **Internet**, a connection of many millions of computers throughout the world, is a valuable source of all kinds of information. Literally anyone or any organization can create a **website** on the Internet. The following are a few examples of what is available:

- Articles from newspapers and magazines
- Informative articles by researchers
- Directories
- Dictionaries
- Up-to-date information on the latest research and innovations

- Opportunities to communicate with experts
- Job postings and applications
- Information about diseases and injuries for both patients and health care professionals
- Career advice from professional organizations
- Photographs
- Video presentations
- "Stores" from which you can order almost any product or service imaginable

If you don't own or have access to a computer, check with your school to find out what is available. A complete discussion on how to search the Internet is outside the scope of this book. However, it is easy to use and doesn't require a significant amount of computer experience. If you don't have much experience in searching the Internet, online tutorials are available and can be accessed by entering the key words "Internet tutorials" or "online search tutorials."

You can find information on the Internet in several ways. The first is by using a website address. All sites have one, just like houses. If you know the address, you simply type it in. If you do not know which sites have the information you are looking for, you can use a program called a *search engine*. You simply enter key words and the search is on! Here are the three general search engines recommended by the University of California (UC), Berkeley[5]:

- Google: www.google.com
- Yahoo! Search: www.search.yahoo.com
- Exalead: www.exalead.com/search

Google Scholar (scholar.google.com) is a specialized search engine that limits sources to scholarly literature, such as articles from academic publishers, theses and dissertations, and court opinions. The website contains search tips for more effective searching.

Evaluating Websites

A word of caution—the Internet is not controlled by any organization or agency that checks on the content or keeps the connections up-to-date. For serious research, be sure to check the credibility of the information supplier. Here are some questions you should ask about a website:

1. Who is the sponsor? Universities, government agencies, professional organizations, research institutes, and established publishers are usually good sources. (This is not to say that commercial sites do not contain excellent information. Just note whether their purpose is to inform or advertise a product.) The endings of the web address indicate sponsorship:

   university: .edu
   government: .gov
   professional organization: .org
   commercial enterprise: .com

2. Who is the author? He or she should have education and/or experience in the subject matter. Can you contact the author?
3. What is the purpose of the website? Many sites are designed to sell products or persuade viewers to believe in a cause. The material provided may be biased and/or not well researched.
4. How are claims supported? Check for statistics and references to original sources of information.
5. How current is the information? Are dates given? Advances and changes in health care and its delivery occur continually.
6. What is the purpose of the document? To present facts? To give an opinion? To sell a product or service?

Medical and Health Care Websites

The Internet is a relatively new technology. Websites close down, merge with others, or change their addresses, and this can be a source of frustration. The following are examples of reliable sites that have a wealth of information about health topics:

- Agency for Healthcare Research and Quality
  http://www.ahrq.gov
- Centers for Disease Control and Prevention
  http://www.cdc.gov
- Family Doctor
  http://familydoctor.org
- Healthy People
  http://www.healthypeople.gov
- Medicine Net
  http://www.medicinenet.com
- MedlinePlus, sponsored by the National Library of Medicine and the National Institutes of Health
  http://www.nlm.nih.gov/medlineplus
- National Institutes of Health
  http://health.nih.gov
- WebMD
  http://www.webmd.com

Health care professional organizations have their own websites. Appendix A contains a list of many organizations with their contact information.

Interviewing

The informational interview, described in Chapter 1, is a form of research. Many important studies are based on interviews, and interviews can help you find information not available from other sources. To interview effectively, you need to identify your purpose in advance and prepare good questions. You use note-taking skills to record all the key points given by the interviewee. Here are some examples of interviews that you might conduct as a student or health professional:

- Request career advice from a graduate of your school to learn how you can make the most of your education.
- Ask a medical specialist a series of questions about a health condition in which you have a special interest.
- Talk with personnel at community offices of organizations such as the American Heart Association and American Cancer Society to learn what information and services they have available.

Choose a topic in which you have an interest, and locate five different sources of reliable information. Briefly describe each source and state why you believe it to be reliable.

On the Job

Interviewing on the Job Providing good health care depends on the quality of information gathered from the patient. Asking good questions and listening carefully are used when collecting this important information. Nurses conduct assessments when developing care plans for their patients, and part of this assessment involves interviewing patients to learn about their health status. A common task of medical assistants is to interview patients and fill out the patient history (refer back to Figure 7-9 to see an example). And physical and occupational therapists gather the information needed to develop appropriate rehabilitation by interviewing their clients to determine their goals and needs. These are just a few examples of professionals who use interviewing skills to provide appropriate health care.

Summary of Key Ideas

- Class notes can be powerful study aids.
- Effective listening is one of the most valuable skills for academic and professional success.
- Repetition is the key to storing new information in your long-term memory.
- Reading to learn is an active process.
- Research is an everyday activity.

Positive Self-Talk for This Chapter

- I am an active listener.
- I take good notes in class.
- My notes are good study tools, and I review them regularly.
- I use techniques I enjoy to help me learn.
- I learn from my reading assignments.
- I use a variety of sources to conduct research.

Internet Activities

ⓔ For active links to the websites needed to complete these activities, visit http://evolve.elsevier.com/Haroun/career/.

1. Enter the key words "active listening," and find five suggestions for improving listening habits.
2. Use the key words "effective note-taking". Choose among articles you find to read and look for three tips you believe might help you.
3. The Academic Resource Center at Utah State University developed a series of over 40 Idea Sheets to help students. Review the list and choose five to read. Prepare a report on what you learned.
4. Search for tips on evaluating Internet sources. Begin with the information on the UC Berkeley website at www.lib.berkeley.edu. You can also locate information published by other universities by entering the term "evaluating internet sources." Develop a fact sheet of evaluation criteria.
5. Using one of the search engines or web addresses given in this chapter, conduct an Internet search for information about a health topic of your choice. Write a summary of what you find, including the source of your information and why you believe it is reliable.

Building Your Resume

1. Review Resume Building Block #5 in Chapter 2. Use the research skills described in this chapter to learn more about certifications and/or licenses, either voluntary or required, for your career.

To Learn More

Dartmouth College Academic Skills Centers

www.dartmouth.edu/~acskills/videos/index.html
The videos on note-taking and reading contain excellent information for all postsecondary students.

Study Guides and Strategies

www.studygs.net
This website has been a public service since 1998 and contains hundreds of helpful learning strategies categorized by topic.

UC Berkeley: Teaching Library Internet Workshops

www.lib.berkeley.edu
Click on *Guides*, then on *Finding Information on the Internet* for detailed information about how to get the most from popular search engines.

References

1. Anderson R, Barbara A, Feldman S: What patients want: a content analysis of key qualities that influence patient satisfaction. Available at: www.drscore.com/press/papers/whatpatientswant.pdf.
2. Take notes by hand for better long-term comprehension. Association for Psychological Science. Available at: http://www.psychologicalscience.org/index.php/news/releases/take-notes-by-hand-for-better-long-term-comprehension.html.
3. Bonewit-West K, Hunt S, Applegate E: *Today's medical assistant: clinical and administrative procedures*, ed 2, St Louis, 2013, Saunders.
4. Wahlstrom C, Williams BK: *The commuter student: being your best at college and life*, Belmont, Calif, 1997, Wadsworth Publishing.
5. University of California, Berkeley: Teaching Library Internet Workshops. Available at: www.lib.berkeley.edu/TeachingLib/Guides/Internet/SearchEngines.html.

CHAPTER 8

Developing Your Paper Skills II: Output of Information

OBJECTIVES

1. Explain why it is important for health care professionals to have good writing skills.
2. Identify the content of what you need to write and know how to gather and organize the information.
3. Determine the writing style that will best convey what you are writing and use writing tools and references to help you write effectively.
4. Describe how tests are part of the daily life of a health care professional and use them as incentives to learn rather than as instruments of torture.
5. Prepare effectively for tests and use techniques to help manage test anxiety.
6. Apply effective test-taking techniques to maximize your performance on classroom tests.

KEY TERMS AND CONCEPTS

APA American Psychological Association.

Audit To check an organization to see if it is following required laws, regulations, and/or professional standards. This is also a noun meaning the process of checking.

Auditor An individual who performs an audit.

Bibliography A list of information sources, including books, journal articles, websites, movies, and interviews, for any type of writing assignment.

Consonant All the letters in the alphabet except A, E, I, O, U, and sometimes Y.

Criteria Established standards used to measure performance.

Documentation Written records. In health care, it refers to detailed recordings, either on paper or electronically, of facts about and observations of patients and their care.

Draft The first version of a piece of writing.

Essay A short piece of nonfiction (based on facts and reality) that is meant to inform, persuade, or entertain the reader.

Fraud Dishonesty or trickery, especially in business.

Freewrite To record ideas as they come to you without worrying about perfect organization, grammar, and spelling.

Grammar A system of rules for putting words and sentences together.

MLA Modern Language Association.

Protocols Established ways of performing procedures.

Reimbursement Payments from a third party for services given.

Suffix A syllable attached to the end of a word such as *-ing* or *-ly*.

Syllable The shortest part of a word that can be pronounced as a unit. For example, immunization has five syllables: *im-mu-ni-za-tion*.

Text Written material, as contrasted with illustrations, drawings, graphs, and so on.

Vowel Any of the following letters: *A, E, I, O, U,* and sometimes *Y*.

Your Writing Ability: A Key to Professional Success

Good written communication is critical for the delivery of high-quality health care. Notes on patient charts, letters to insurance companies, and printed instructions for patients must be written clearly and accurately. Consistency of care, **reimbursement** for services, and good relations between health facilities and the public they serve depend on the quality of written documents. You may think you won't do much writing in your future work. Not true! Almost every job in health care today involves paperwork and some writing tasks.

Your writing is like a personal advertisement, representing who you are. It influences the opinions of other people about you and your work. Writing is a form of permanent communication. Unlike speaking which you can revise and correct as needed to help your listener understand your message, you have only one opportunity to express yourself in writing. Readers must rely on what they see on the page and may question your competence if you make grammatical and spelling errors or organize information poorly. How well you write makes an impression on potential employers when you are applying for jobs. Once you are hired, it reflects on your employer and the health care facility where you work.

Contrary to what you might think, the computer age has actually increased the importance of good writing skills. E-mail is replacing a lot of the communication that until recently was conducted over the telephone. Although e-mail messages tend to be informal and often use phrases instead of complete sentences, they must be expressed clearly and in an organized fashion to be useful to the receiver. The growing use of electronic health records also requires the ability to record information clearly and accurately. Technology is actually increasing, rather than decreasing, the need for you to develop your writing skills. The following suggestions will help you write more professional, effective e-mails:

- Include a meaningful subject line so the receiver has a clear idea of the content of the e-mail.
- Open with a greeting, such as "Dear Dr. Abrams."
- State your purpose in the first sentence: "I am writing to inquire about…" "I am writing in reference to…."
- Write short paragraphs using clear but polite language.
- Unlike texting in which abbreviations and acronyms are common, use complete words, standard spelling, capitalization, and punctuation.
- Do *not* write in all capital letters. This is the equivalent of shouting.
- Avoid sarcasm and take care with humor—these can be misinterpreted.
- *Never* write anything you wouldn't want your employer to see.
- Take care about sending confidential information.
- End with a closing.
- Proofread your message before sending.

- Reply to important and serious messages promptly.
- It is best not to send an attachment (due to the problem with computer viruses) the first time you contact a person.

Keep in mind that some people receive dozens—even hundreds—of e-mails each day. Write so that yours is one that gets read.

Writing is a skill you can learn, not a talent. And it is never too late to upgrade your skills. Although a complete writing course is beyond the scope of this book, this chapter contains information about the basics of good writing and includes suggestions to help you write more effectively. The main goal is to encourage you to care about your writing skills and motivate you to improve them, if necessary.

Prescription for Success: 8-1
Writing Effective E-Mails

Compare the following pairs of e-mails. Which of each pair do you think is written the most effectively? Explain why in detail.

Pair #1

Example 1

To: Staff

Subject Line: Tomorrow

Hey,

Don't forget tomorrow's mtg. Bring ideas for reorganizing file room & updating reception area, having your calendar to plan future meetings and someone volunteer to bring donuts.

Nan

Example 2

Subject Line: Tomorrow's Staff Meeting

Hello everyone,

This is to remind you of our staff meeting tomorrow at 10:00 in the conference room. Please bring the following:

- Ideas for reorganizing the file room
- Ideas for updating the reception area
- Your calendar to note future meetings

If someone can bring donuts, please let me know by 5:00 this afternoon.

Thank you,

Nan

Pair #2

Example 1

Subject Line: Job Openings

To whom it may concern:

I am writing to inquire about possible job openings at Bayview Hospital for lab technicians. Can you send me a list or refer me to a website where I can obtain this information?

Thank you,

Gerry Thomas

Example 2

Subject Line: Jobs

Hi,

Plz send me info about any jobs you have at your clinic.

Thx,

Gerry Thomas

Samantha Harris, a nurse administrator in a large Michigan clinic, held a meeting with her staff about problems with writing clearly and using abbreviations carefully. It seemed to be well received by the staff that attended. But she still had a problem that involved both attitude and writing clear messages—Janet Olson. Janet had not been at the meeting, and this was part of the problem: Janet's attendance in general. Although she was a competent medical assistant, when she was on the job, Janet had a multitude of excuses for being late or not being at work at all. If it wasn't a problem finding daycare for her young children, it was her car breaking down, or some other "crisis." Samantha understood that Janet's life as a single mother was difficult and that she very much needed the income from her job to support her children, but Janet's absences were getting too disruptive to the clinic and the other staff.

Samantha decided to call Janet into her office for a private talk. As usual, Janet became tearful when confronted about her absences and explained that it just "wasn't her fault" and unfair of the clinic to expect her to neglect her children or her own health. "After all," she snuffled, "I'm a mother first. And I see other people around here taking time off when they need it. I don't see why you're singling me out."

After Samantha showed Janet her attendance record and how it compared negatively to the average staff members record, Janet was ready with a number of excuses: her life was more difficult, the other staff had spouses who helped out at home, the last mechanic had ripped her off and not really fixed the car, and on and on. Janet always believed that her problems were out of her control.

At this point, Samantha decided to move on to the subject of the meeting Janet had missed. As it turned out, at least two of the examples she had presented for discussion had been Janet's errors. Because this was a private conference, Samantha described the examples and then asked Janet, "I'm wondering if you take the time to look over what you've written? Do you think about who is going to have to read your messages?"

Janet responded, "I'm really surprised you'd be upset about this. We're so busy around here, who has time to worry about being fussy about how they write their messages? Just get them down on paper and move on to the next thing."

"Janet, it's precisely because we are so busy that clear communication is so important," Samantha explained. "The staff doesn't have time to waste looking for the person who wrote something they can't read."

"Well, I can't understand how *they* can have so much trouble with this. I don't think what I wrote was *that* bad. It seems like they could figure out stuff that we handle every day," Janet said.

Samantha sighed. "Janet, this is really the biggest problem I see: your attitude. You fail to realize how important each of us is—including you—to the smooth running of this department. Even worse, you refuse to accept responsibility for your own actions. It's always someone else's fault or something beyond your control. I honestly don't see how we're going to work this out and keep you on if you continue with this attitude."

Questions for Thought and Reflection

1. Do you think Samantha fails to understand Janet's problems?
2. Should Samantha make more of an effort to help Janet? Why or why not?
3. What are possible consequences of Janet's sloppy writing?
4. What is Samantha's primary responsibility as a nurse administrator?
5. What do you think about Janet's attitude?
6. Do you think Samantha should fire Janet? Why or why not?

Write on! Developing Good Writing Skills

There are two components to good writing: content and form. Content refers to *what* you write: the information and ideas. Form is *how* you present it: grammar, spelling, and formatting. You must pay attention to both content and form in order for your reader to receive your intended message.

Content: Determine Your Purpose

The first step in writing is to think about what you want to accomplish. Your purpose determines what you say and how you say it, so it needs to be clear in your own mind.

The following list contains common writing goals of students and health care professionals.

1. **Demonstrate your knowledge and/or inform your readers.** This is one of the reasons why instructors ask you to write research papers (also called "term papers" or "reports") and answer essay test questions. They use these assignments to assess what you have learned about a subject. To do well on papers and tests, you must know about your subject, state information clearly, and provide accurate facts to support what you write. When your purpose is to show what you know, it is important not to pad your writing with repetition or statements that add nothing meaningful to the content. Although instructors often assign papers by numbers of words or pages, it is a mistake to use many words to make it look as if you've said a lot when you really have said very little.

2. **Persuade your readers or make a request.** You may be assigned to write a paper about a controversial topic in which you must convince the reader to accept your point of view or take certain actions. Outside of class, you might request a leave of absence or complete an application for a scholarship. When seeking employment, you will write cover letters to include with your resume. Their purpose

is to convince prospective employers to read your resume and call you for an interview. On the job, you might submit written requests to your employer for a raise, a promotion, or funding to continue your education. Other examples include submitting requests to vendors for information about their products, composing referral letters to physicians, or writing to insurance companies requesting action on unpaid claims.

There are various ways to persuade readers. One is to present facts that support your arguments. In the case of the letter to a prospective employer, you could list the ways you can be of benefit and can help provide great service to patients. Another method is to appeal to readers' emotions. For example, if you want to convince them to take action against cigarette advertising aimed at children, you could point out the need for adults to express their love for vulnerable children by protecting them from potential health hazards. It is generally most effective to use both facts and emotions so they support each other and strengthen your case. In the argument against cigarette advertising, you could cite the number and ages of children who start smoking each year, along with statistics about diseases and deaths caused by smoking.

3. **Provide an explanation.** Some school assignments, such as exercises in workbooks, ask you to explain the steps in a procedure or explain why something is done a certain way. Test questions that require short answers are often requests for explanations. On the job, you may write instructions for patients or directions for co-workers. It is important that this type of writing be very clear and organized in a logical order. Including information about why something should be done or why it should be done in a specific way strengthens your writing. This is because people tend to be more willing and able to follow instructions when they understand the reasons behind them.

4. **Narrate a story or event.** If you take an English or a writing class, writing an original story may be one of your assignments. Although stories are not commonly used in workplace writing, they can add interest and provide examples in persuasive or explanatory works. The main considerations in story writing are to use your imagination and to write good descriptions. An example of the use of creative writing in the workplace would be writing a story to help children overcome their fear of the dentist. A word of caution: stories used in the workplace should be directly related to the situation. And it is illegal to share work stories using the names of or personal information about real patients and events that take place at work.

Many pieces of writing have more than one purpose, and these can be combined so they reinforce each other. For example, when preparing instruction sheets for patients, they can be more effective if you include persuasive language that encourages the patients to follow their special diet or perform their exercises every day.

Content: Gather Information

Writing sometimes requires research and always requires thought. This may sound obvious, but many people simply start writing without any preparation or in-depth thinking. The result is a collection of words and sentences that don't say much. There are many sources of information, and the first one may surprise you—your own knowledge and experience. Start by writing down what you already know in whatever format you find most useful, such as lists of key ideas and facts, a mind map, or an outline.

After assessing what you know, identify what you need to find out. If the instructor has assigned a topic about which you know very little, consider developing a list of questions to help guide your research. For example, if you are to write about infectious diseases in the world today, your questions might include the following:

- What are the major infectious diseases?
- What are the symptoms?
- What causes these diseases?
- How are they spread?
- How are they treated?
- How widespread are these diseases? How many people are affected each year?
- What is the annual mortality rate?

Sources of Information

If you know very little about your topic, start your research with resources that provide definitions and general information. Examples include encyclopedia and journal articles, textbooks, nontechnical books for the general reader, and websites for the general public. Once you have an overall view of the topic, narrow your research to specific areas of interest. Your instructors may require you to consult certain types and numbers of resources beyond your textbook. They may also have good suggestions for additional sources of information.

As you consult each resource, record the important facts and ideas. Some people like to use note cards. Use a separate card for each topic or subtopic. If you need more than one card for each topic, number or mark them in some way to keep them organized. Another method is to take notes on sheets of paper (one side only), organizing by resource rather than topic. You may have several pages for each source. When it's time to organize, you can cut up the papers and sort the pieces by related information. Or you can leave the sheets whole and color-code the different topics or write key words in the margins to identify the various topics. This enables you to quickly scan the pages for needed information as you write. You can also take and organize your notes on a computer.

Creating a Bibliography

Whichever way you take your notes, you need a system to keep track of your resources so you can create your **bibliography** or reference list. This includes all the books, journal and magazine articles, brochures, websites, and any other resources you have used. See Table 8-1 for examples of what information to record about each kind of source. There are several standard styles you can use for creating your bibliography, so check with your instructor to find out which one you are to use. Table 8-2 contains examples of two popular formats, one from the Modern Language Association (**MLA**) and the other from the American Psychological Association (**APA**). Compare the examples and note that they contain almost the same information, just presented in a different order. Even if your project does not require a bibliography, it is a good idea to write down your sources so you can find them later if you need them. One way to keep track of your sources is to create a numbered list and then write the corresponding number on each card or page of notes.

Content: Organize Your Information

"Since it is not possible to think about everything all at once, most experienced writers handle a piece of writing in stages."
—Diana Hacker

When you are assigned a research paper or have a report to prepare for work, it can be difficult to decide how to get started and then how to organize what you want to say.

TABLE 8-1
Information Needed for Various Sources

Source	Facts You Need
Book	Author(s) or editor
	Title of the book
	Publisher
	Location of publisher (city)
	Year published
	Edition
Journal or magazine article	Author(s)
	Name of the journal or magazine
	Title of the article
	Volume number of journal
	Issue number
	Page numbers of the article
Newspaper article	Author(s)
	Name of the newspaper
	Title of the article
	Date of the newspaper
	Page numbers of the article
Website	Author(s) or creator(s) of site, if available
	Title of the site or "home page" if no title
	Name of any organization associated with the site
	Date site was created or latest update
	Date you accessed the site
	Complete site address

TABLE 8-2
Examples of Bibliographic Styles

Style	Book
Modern Language Association (MLA)	Young, Alexandra P., and Deborah P. Kennedy. *Kinn's the Medical Assistant*. 12th ed. St Louis: Saunders, 2014.
American Psychological Association (APA)	Young, A. P., & Kennedy, D. P. (2014). *Kinn's the medical assistant* (12th ed.). St Louis: Saunders.
Magazine	
MLA	Mattick, John S. "The Hidden Genetic Program of Organisms." *Scientific American* Oct. 2004: 60+.
APA	Mattick, J. S. (2004, October). The hidden genetic complex organisms. *Scientific American, 291,* 60-67.
Website	
MLA	Hopkins, M. E. "Critical Condition." *NurseWeek* 12 March 2001, 3 Jan. 2002 <http://www.nurseweek.com/news/features/01-03/shortage.asp>.
APA	Hopkins, M. E. (2001, March 12). Critical Condition. *NurseWeek*. [On-line] Available: http://www.nurseweek.com/news/features/01-03/shortage.asp [2002, January 3].

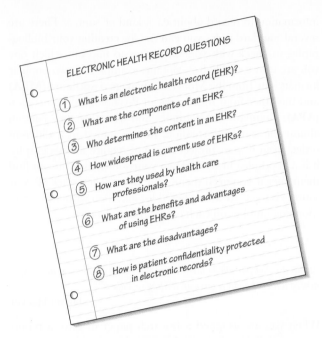

FIGURE 8-1 Organizing Information Using Captions. Think about what you'd like to know about your topic, then write questions you can use to guide your research. *Do you think this method might help you as you prepare to write a paper? Could you use this method for research to prepare a speech?*

Some instructors require students to prepare an outline as the first step in writing. If you find it difficult to think in outline form or you just don't know where to start, outlining can be as intimidating as writing the paper itself. Don't despair. There are other ways to organize your information. Suppose you are assigned to write a paper about electronic health records. Here are some ways you can gather and organize your information:

1. **Questions.** List questions you would like answered, such as the suggestions in Figure 8-1. Your information falls into place as you research and find the answer to each question.
2. **Idea sheets.** As you think of major ideas, write each one at the top of a separate sheet of paper. Then list all related and supporting ideas on the pages. To organize, lay the sheets out and move them around until you find the best way to order them. Figure 8-2 contains examples of idea sheets.
3. **Note cards.** Dave Ellis, writer of popular student success books, recommends the use of note cards for generating creativity and promoting organization.[1] List all your ideas, both major and supporting, on 3 × 5 cards, one idea per card. Sort the cards by topics or categories, and then arrange them in logical order. You can lay them out on a flat surface or pin them to a wall or large bulletin board as illustrated in Figure 8-3.
4. **Mind maps.** Mind maps, illustrated in Figure 8-4 for our topic, are diagrams drawn freehand that link and arrange words and ideas around a central key word or idea. Mind maps can be helpful if you don't have a clear idea of the

order you want for your material. Some people find mind maps useful when brainstorming because they don't require ideas to be organized in a linear way. The result is a "map" illustrating how ideas relate to and support one another. If you have several major ideas, you can make a series of maps.

Who Are My Readers?

Effective writers consider the needs of their readers. This is especially important in health care, where safe and consistent care depends on how well health care professionals communicate with patients and with one another. Whenever and whatever you write, take into account the readers' ages, cultural backgrounds, knowledge of health issues, and purpose for reading the material. Remember that you will not usually be present to clarify information, answer questions, or see from their facial expressions if they understand or agree with what you have written. This is why it is so important to write clearly and organize your **text** so readers can follow it easily. If you are addressing a mixed audience, plan your writing for the readers who are most likely to have difficulty understanding. When writing class assignments and tests, your instructor is the audience. He or she wants you to demonstrate what you know about a subject and how well you express yourself. There may also be specific requirements about the form of writing you are to use.

Prescription for Success: 8-3 Addressing Your Readers

1. Explain how instructions you write for a co-worker would differ from those you write for a patient.
2. Explain in what ways a letter asking for a job interview would differ from a letter you write to a friend.

Organize Your Content

Everyone prefers to read material that is easy to follow. Good writers achieve this by organizing material logically, and you can do this, too. How you organize your content is based on the type of document you are writing. Letters, research papers, and long essay answers are easier for the reader to follow if they are divided into sections:

1. **Introduction.** Present your major points. Tell what you are writing about. State your purpose.
2. **Middle or body.** Develop, support, and explain your ideas. Create a separate section for each topic or idea.
3. **Conclusion.** Show how everything you have written pulls together. Give your "final word" on the subject. Summarize your points. State what you have attempted to prove with your information. Tell the readers what action you hope they will take as a result of your writing. Figure 8-5 shows how a paper on electronic health records might be organized.

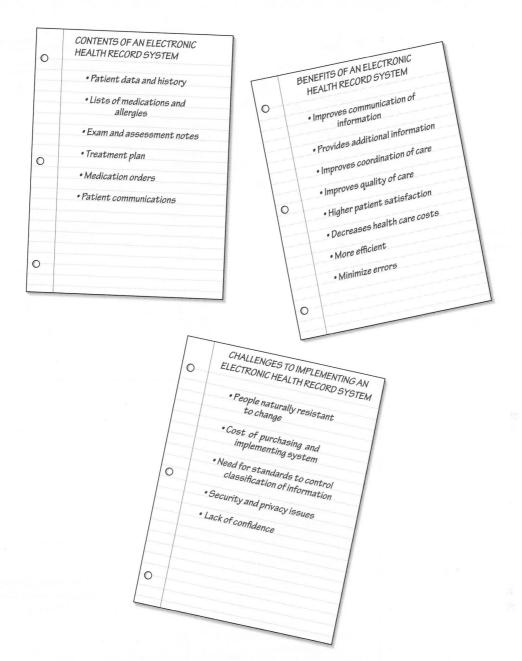

FIGURE 8-2 Organizing Information Using Idea Sheets. Using this method helps you organize material as you conduct your research. *Think of a topic and create at least five headings you could use for idea sheets.*

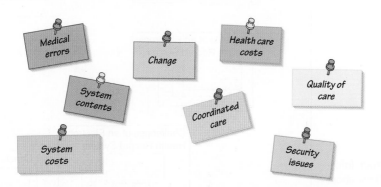

FIGURE 8-3 Organizing Information Using Note Cards. *Using the topic you used in Figure 8-2, list 10 sub-topics for your subject. Would the note card method help you organize and write about your topic?*

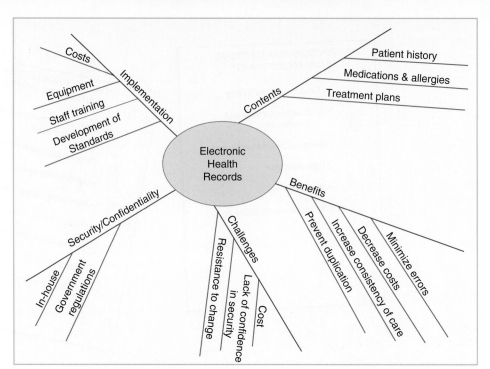

FIGURE 8-4 **Organizing Information Using a Mind Map.** This is generally most useful to visual learners, although it can help many of us brainstorm and relate ideas about a topic. *Again, using the topic you chose for Figure 8-2, think of everything you can about your topic and create a mind map relating the information.*

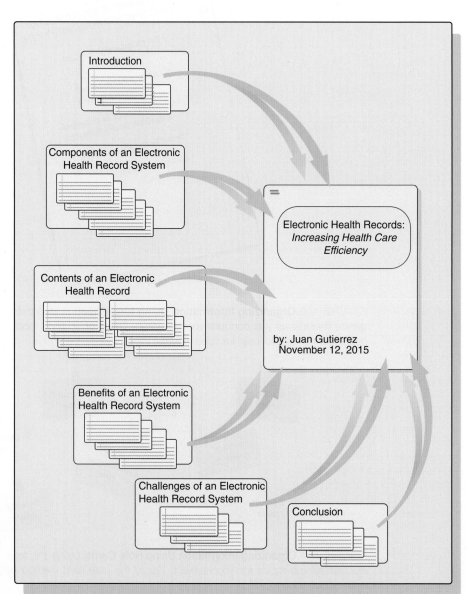

FIGURE 8-5 **Organizing Your Information for Your Readers.** Think about the flow of your information. *How should you introduce and then develop—support—your topic? What is the best way to conclude?*

Short answers to test questions and brief letters and notes require tight organization to cover all necessary material in a small space:

1. Give your answer or state your purpose or main point in the first sentence.
2. Give supporting details in one or two paragraphs.
3. Limit your conclusion to one or two sentences.

Instructions and directions can be organized into lists of steps or activities in the order in which they should be performed or in order from most to least important. Rationale or purpose (reasons why something should be done) can be included just before or after the step or action to which it relates. See Figure 8-6 for an example of how written instructions can be organized.

Trouble Ahead? 8-2

Ashley always enjoyed working with numbers and details, so when she was looking into career possibilities after graduating from high school, her friend Emily recommended medical billing and coding.

"It's a good career," Emily told Ashley. "And a great thing about it is you don't have to go to college for four years."

"I don't know," Ashley responded. "I want to be able to get a job—and one that pays okay."

"No problem," said Emily. "You know I chose medical assisting because I want to work with doctors and patients doing procedures and things. But I've heard that billers and coders are really needed so there are a bunch of jobs out there."

Ashley decided to look into the program at the local college where Emily was a student and ended up enrolling in the billing and coding program. "Why not?" she thought. "Sitting at home isn't getting me anywhere."

Although the college Ashley attended focused on the technical skills she would need on the job, it did include a few general education courses, such as writing, oral communication, and math. The writing class seemed okay to Ashley and she was able to keep up with the assignments and exercises on spelling and grammar. But one day a couple of weeks into the course, Ms. James, the instructor, announced that the students would be writing a research paper.

"Oh, great," thought Ashley. "I don't have enough to do without having to write a dumb research report!"

"I have a number of topics you can choose from," explained Ms. James. "They are all related to your future careers as billers and coders."

Ashley raised her hand. "Why can't we just read about these topics—or you can tell us. Isn't that why we're here in school?"

Ms. James explained that all health careers involve some type of writing and that research and collecting information would be a part of their careers, especially with the continual changes in laws and technology.

Although Ashley didn't say so, she thought these were just excuses to get the students to do what she considered to be busywork. For the next few days, she fumed about the "unfair" assignment and thought about how she would approach the task. The students had been required to choose a topic, so she chose electronic health records: benefits and challenges. She spent the next few days fussing about the project.

"I can't believe we have to spend our time on this," she complained to Emily the next time they talked.

"Yeah, it can be kind of a pain," agreed Emily. "But your topic sounds okay. Maybe it will be kind of interesting."

"What I really don't understand," said Ashley, "is why we can't just read something that's already been written." And as she spoke, she suddenly had an idea: reading—and using?—something that had already been written! Why waste her time repeating work that had already been done?

That evening, she looked on the Internet for papers on electronic health records. She found a number of websites that offered, for a price, to write the paper for her. Others had prewritten papers for sale. The prices were a bit high, so she decided to look for someone local who might be willing to just give her their paper—or sell it at a cheaper price.

She did some investigating and finally found someone who had written a similar paper two years earlier and was willing to share it. The best part was, the paper had earned an A grade and positive written comments from the instructor. Ashley paid the former student $25.00, made a few minor changes to the wording, wrote it up on her computer, and submitted "her work."

A week after the class turned in their papers, the instructor called Ashley into her office. "Ashley," she said, "I need you to tell me the truth. Did you copy your paper from someone else?"

Ashley looked down and thought for a few moments before she answered. "Well," she said, "it was mostly my work."

"I'm sorry, but I find that hard to believe," said the instructor. "I give this assignment each time I teach the course. I thought your paper looked familiar, so I checked my files. You see, I sometimes copy papers that are especially well written—and this was one of them."

"Okay, so I copied someone's paper. You know, some of us are really busy with school and part-time jobs. We just don't have the time to do assignments that take so much time."

"Well, Ashley," said Ms. James. "I have to tell you that I am less worried about your writing—or not writing—than I am about your attitude and lack of integrity. Even though that student voluntarily gave you his paper to copy, the fact is that this is plagiarism. It's a form of stealing—taking something that isn't your own. To make matters worse, you weren't truthful with me when I first asked you if you had copied the paper. This shows a lack of integrity."

"I really can't see that this is such a big deal. I'm doing okay in my coding classes, I won't have to write papers on the job ….," Ashley argued.

Continued

"Ashley, you're missing the point. You were dishonest in not doing your own work and then in not telling me the truth. Integrity is critical in health care work, especially in the career you've chosen. Billing and coding must be accurate and reflect what actually takes place with patients. There is no room for taking short cuts or dishonesty. I'm sorry, but I really don't think this is the right career for you."

Questions for Thought and Reflection

1. Why was Ashley's decision to copy another student's paper a serious offense?
2. What could she have learned if she had researched and written the paper herself?
3. How might coders and billers use research and writing skills on the job?
4. Do you think Ashley should be expelled from school? Why or why not?

Prepare an Informed Consent for Treatment Form

GOAL: To inform the patient adequately and completely about the treatment or procedure he or she is to receive, and to provide legal protection for the facility and the provider.

EQUIPMENT AND SUPPLIES
• Pen
• Consent form

PROCEDURAL STEPS

1 After the physician has provided the details of the procedure to be done, prepare the consent form. Be sure the form includes the following:
• Nature of the procedure or treatment.
• Risks and/or benefits of the procedure or treatment.
• Any reasonable alternatives to the procedure or treatment.
• Risks and/or benefits of each alternative.
• Risks and/or benefits of not receiving the treatment.

Purpose: To make sure the patient is fully informed about the procedure or treatment and the risks and/or benefits of having and not having it performed.

2 Personalize the form with the patient's name and any other demographic information the form lists.

Purpose: To correctly identify the patient and the procedure.

3 Deliver the form to the physician for use as the patient is counseled about the procedure.

Purpose: To prevent charges of practicing medicine without a license. The physician should explain procedures, risks, benefits, and alternatives and answer all of the patient's questions.

4 Witness the patient's signature on the form, if necessary. The physician also usually signs the form.

5 Provide the patient with a copy of the consent form.

Purpose: To ensure that the patient is fully informed about the procedure and has a copy of the information for his or her personal records.

6 Place the consent form in the patient's chart. The facility where the procedure is to be performed may require a copy.

Purpose: To keep a permanent copy of the signed consent form.

7 Ask the patient whether he or she has any questions about the procedure. Refer questions that you cannot or should not answer to the physician. Make sure all the patient's questions are answered.

Purpose: To make sure the patient has been fully informed by the physician before undergoing the procedure.

NOTE: The medical assistant does not explain the consent form to the patient; this is the physician's responsibility.

8 Provide the patient with the date and time of the procedure and any other instructions required.

FIGURE 8-6 Instructions, especially those dealing with important health care topics, should be clear and easy for the reader to follow. *List five characteristics that make these instructions easy to follow.* (Modified from Proctor DB and Adams AP: *Kinn's the medical assistant: An applied learning approach,* ed 12, St Louis, 2014, Saunders.)

Writing Style

The goal of writing is to communicate, so make it easy for your readers to follow you. "Short and simple" applies to both words and sentences. Avoid long, complicated words when simpler ones will do. See the examples in Box 8-1.

Avoid writing overly long, complicated sentences. They can be difficult to follow and your message can get lost. And to keep your writing lively, use active rather than passive constructions. This means starting sentences with subjects rather than direct objects. Here are some examples:

Passive: The lecture today was given by Dr. Appleton.
Active: Dr. Appleton gave the lecture today.
Passive: The book I liked best was written by Stephen King.
Active: Stephen King wrote the book I liked best.

Note that in the passive constructions, you have to read to the end of the sentence to see who the subject is—who is doing the action.

BOX 8-1 Examples of Using Simpler Words

INSTEAD OF:	USE:
in the near future	soon
make an adjustment in	adjust
at this point in time	now
in spite of the fact that	although
in the event of	if
take into consideration	consider
is in violation of	violates
make a statement saying	say

Source: The Health Care Communications Group: *Writing, speaking, and communication skills for health professionals.* New Haven, 2001, Yale University Press.

Even writing that is clear in meaning can be too wordy:

Wordy: Unpack the medical supplies. They are in the back room. After you have unpacked them, put them in the locking cabinet.

Better: Unpack the medical supplies that are in the back room and put them in the locking cabinet.

Wordy: I was late for class due to the fact that the car wouldn't start. I had forgotten to fill it with gas yesterday.

Better: I was late for class because I forgot to get gas yesterday.

A common error when writing long pieces is needless repetition. This is not always obvious to the writer, so put what you've written aside for a while, then look at it with fresh eyes. Have you stated the same idea more than once?

Starting to Write

Don't aim for perfection on your first **draft**. Many people, even professional writers, find a piece of blank paper very intimidating. A good way to beat the blank-paper monster is to just start writing. Begin with a rough draft, and don't worry about how rough it is. Writing creatively and writing perfectly and correctly require different intellectual skills that can actually cancel each other out. Peter Elbow, a professor who wrote a very helpful book about how to write, says that trying to write perfectly the first time is "dangerous writing" because you can't generate good ideas and be critical of your work at the same time.[2] He recommends that you spend half of the time on a project **freewriting** the rough draft and the other half revising. (This is a good argument for starting your writing assignments well in advance of the due date!)

When freewriting, don't worry about starting with the introduction because this can put unnecessary pressure on you to start out "just right" with good opening sentences. You may not even know at this point how your piece is going to turn out. Because writers develop and come up with new ideas throughout the writing process, you may add or delete topics. Go ahead and start with the middle section if that works for you. (An exception is when you are writing answers to essay questions on timed tests. State your answer at the beginning and spend the rest of the time supporting it.)

A technique called "brain dump" can work when you're really stuck getting started. It works like this: get out some paper and just start writing, using your ideas and the information you have gathered. This will be easier if you have used one of the techniques described earlier: outline, idea sheets, questions, and so on. Write quickly, and get as much down on paper as possible. Then go back and look for ideas and themes you can put in logical order. Although this is not always the fastest method for completing a paper or report, it can get you started when you find yourself with a bad case of writer's block. You may end up with a jumble of ideas that has to be unsnarled, but at least you have something on paper, and the chances are good you'll have something you can use. Many writers use brain dump to promote creativity and get ideas flowing.

Once you have completed your first draft, let it rest for a couple of days (or hours, if the due date is directly ahead). Then assume the role of your readers and try to imagine you are reading the piece for the first time. Read it aloud to hear how it sounds. Better yet, have someone else read it so you can listen for the following points[3]:

- Do you have an introduction?
- Is your purpose clear?
- Do your ideas flow smoothly, one to another?
- Have you supported your ideas?
- Is there enough information about each topic or idea?
- Have you included unnecessary details that should be left out?
- Do you repeat yourself unnecessarily?
- Does the conclusion summarize your information?
- Do you achieve your stated purpose?

Prescription for Success: 8-4 What Works for You?

1. Which of the organizational techniques presented do you think would work best for you?
2. Explain why.
3. Describe any other organizational or writing techniques that have worked for you.

Form: Attending to the Details of Writing

Your content may be important, interesting, and well organized, but poor **grammar** and spelling can cause your readers to misunderstand what you have written and even to question your competence. You may believe that worrying about grammatical details is unimportant. However, work in health care demands that you attend to details every day. Performing accurately and following exact procedures are valuable health care skills. In many types of written and electronic health care **documentation**, the contents and format are strictly controlled by federal and state laws as well as by nongovernmental regulatory agencies.

PROBLEM ORIENTED - PROGRESS NOTES						
Date	Time	Problem Number	FORMAT: Problem Number and TITLE: S = Subjective	O = Objective	A = Assessment	P = Plan
11/15/XX	9:30 AM	1	S: Mother states that her child has had a runny nose and her throat has been sore for 2 days.			
			O: Vital signs: T 98.8 P 96 R 24			
			Weight: 42 lb.			
			General: alert and active. HEENT: sclera clear. TMs negative. Positive clear rhinorrhea. Pharynx benign. Heart: regular without murmur.			
			Lungs: clear to auscultation and percussion. Abdomen: negative tenderness. Positive bowel × 4. GU: negative. Neuro: good tone.			
			A: Upper respiratory tract infection.			
			P: 1. A prescription for Rondec DM, 1/2 tsp q6h prn for cough and congestion.			
			2. Instructed mother to contact office if child does not improve.			

FIGURE 8-7 Problem-Oriented Progress Notes, a Common Use of Writing in Health Care. Notice how legibly and neatly the notes are written. *What would be possible consequences of incorrect or illegible entries on progress notes? What would you do if you were the next person working with this patient and couldn't read some of the entries?* (Modified from Bonewit-West K, Hunt S, Applegate E: *Today's medical assistant: Clinical and administrative procedures,* ed 2, St Louis, 2013, Saunders.)

On the Job

Writing on the Job Getting a job involves several writing tasks: your resume, cover letters you send to prospective employers with your resume, and thank-you notes you send after interviews. These written pieces demonstrate some of your qualifications, including your ability to write. They are a reflection of you, so it is important to use good organization and correct grammar and spelling.

An increasingly important task of health care professionals is accurately recording information about patients. The quality of this information can affect the consistency and quality of care patients receive. It also has an effect on reimbursement—that is, how much money the physician, hospital, or other provider of services receives from insurance companies. And something you may not know is that medical records can be used as evidence in court. For example, if a doctor is sued for malpractice, the clarity and completeness of medical records can help—or hurt—the case. See Figure 8-7 for an example of health care documentation.

See Box 8-2 for examples of documents you may be asked to write as part of your job.

BOX 8-2 Health Care Documents

- Letters
- Office memos
- E-mails
- Medical records
- Medical charts
- Phone messages
- Minutes of meetings
- Grant requests
- Promotional materials

Source: Villemaire D, Villemaire L: *Grammar and writing skills for the health professional,* ed 2, Clifton Park, NY, 2005, Delmar Cengage Learning.

care facilities. Even if your job does not include preparing insurance claims, your notes may provide the information on which the claim is based. Writing correctly and paying attention to details are skills that today's employers require.

First Aid for Grammar

All languages are organized into systems with rules that determine how words are organized. These systems and rules help listeners and readers make sense of what they are hearing or reading because they know what to expect. Comparing the structure of different languages is one way to illustrate the role grammar plays. Let's look at word order. In English, we usually place describing words (adjectives) in front of the words they describe (nouns). If a friend tells you, "I live in the house blue with the trim white," it might take you a few moments to figure out what she's talking about. You are not accustomed to this word order. But in Spanish, this would be correct. Spanish speakers expect to hear the noun before the adjective.

Written documentation is often the only proof to show that patients have received appropriate care. It is recognized in court and by **auditors** who perform compliance reviews of medical institutions. A standard rule in health care is "If it was not documented, it was not done." We might add "If it's poorly written, it's not documented properly and may not have been done properly!" Most patients have some type of insurance, and payment to the health care provider depends on clear and accurate claims submitted by health

Another example is the methods used in language to let you know who the subject is; that is, who is doing the action. In English, we use pronouns such as "I," "we," and "they" to tell who this is: I swim, we studied, they will graduate. Again, using Spanish for our comparison, these words are not always necessary because the last letters of verbs change to indicate the subject: estudio = I study; estudiamos = we study; estudian = they study.

There are many differences among the thousands of languages spoken the world over. The point is that each has its own grammar, the purpose of which is to help people communicate effectively. Mastering the grammar of the language(s) you use improves your ability to communicate.

Correct grammar is especially important in writing. Listeners may not notice the mistakes we make when we are speaking. If something is unclear, listeners can ask us to repeat or explain what we mean. Written material, however, must stand on its own. If it is unclear, the reader is not likely to have an opportunity to ask for clarification. Worse yet, readers may follow directions incorrectly, and this can result in costly mistakes when dealing with matters of health. In addition to helping ensure safety, proper grammar results in writing that reflects competence and professionalism.

Tables 8-3, 8-4, 8-5, and 8-6 contain grammar rules. They are not intended to be complete lists of "writing rules" for

TABLE 8-3
Parts of Speech

Part of Speech	What It Is	Examples	Sentence Examples
Noun	Name of a person, place, thing, idea, or process (such as a medical procedure)	Dr. Gutierrez, nurse, Texas hospital, microscope thought, urinalysis	**Dr. Samuels** is a **pharmacist** at the local **drugstore.** The **stethoscope** was lying on the **table.** The **technician** gave **Sarah** the **results** of the **test.**
Pronoun	Substitutes for a noun	*I, he, she, it, we, they, me, him, her, it, us, them, this, that, these, those*	**He** is the pharmacist at the local drugstore. **It** was lying on the table. **He** gave **her** the results of the test.
Verb	Expresses action or state of being	*study, graduate, work, enjoy, am, is, are*	Emily had to **work** hard to **finish** school, but after graduation she **got** a job she **enjoyed.** Now she **is** a medical assistant at a local clinic.
Adjective	Describes a noun or pronoun	*kind, little, active, intelligent*	The **kind dental** assistant* gave the **little** girl a **comforting** hug. *(kind describes the dental assistant; little describes the girl; comforting describes the hug)* * *It would also be correct to consider "dental assistant" as a noun.*
Articles	Three small words that are used with nouns	*the, a, an* Note: Use *an* before words that start with vowels *(a, e, i, o, u),* the letter *h* when it is silent, and words that begin with a vowel sound, such as M&M.	**The** physical therapist worked with **a** patient for more than **an** hour. Johnny asked **the** nurse for **an** M&M as **a** reward for getting **the** injection.
Adverb	Describes a verb, adjective, or other adverb	*quickly, gently, very, really*	The nurse **quickly** gave the injection. *(quickly describes "gave")* The veterinary assistant **very gently** picked up the kitten. *(very describes gently; gently describes "picked up")*
Preposition	Connective words that show a relationship between a noun or pronoun and other words	*as, at, between, of, on, out, since, than, to, with*	The road **to** the clinic was really crowded today. The medical biller placed the files **on** the table.
Conjunction	Joins single words or groups of words Different kinds of conjunctions are used to indicate different types of relationships between the words they join	*and, but, or, either...or, not only...but also, although, because, finally, however, meanwhile*	She took classes **and** worked in the dental office. You need to take **either** medical terminology **or** anatomy this semester. Janet originally wanted to be a nurse; **however,** she decided to become a respiratory therapist.
Interjection	Expresses surprise or emotion	*Oh! Hey! Wow!*	**Oh!** I'm so sorry. I didn't see you coming this way. **Wow!** I can't believe I did so well on that test!

TABLE 8-4
Common Sentence Ailments

Ailment	Example	Corrected
No subject	Said that his tooth hurts.	**He** said that his tooth hurts.
Run-on (no punctuation or connecting word)	He needed an x-ray exam the radiologist was called.	He needed an x-ray exam, **so** the radiologist was called.
Pronoun does not agree with the noun it replaces	Each patient should take their prescription to the pharmacy.	Each patient should take **his or her** prescription to the pharmacy. *or* All patients should take **their** prescriptions to the pharmacy.
Subject and verb do not agree	Both the nurse and the physician sees the fracture on the x-ray film. The equipment you need to perform an ECG are in the other room.	Both the nurse and the physician **see** the fracture on the x-ray film. The equipment you need to perform an ECG **is** in the other room.
Split infinitive (unnecessarily separating "to" and the verb)	After this type of surgery, it is good for patients to frequently walk around to avoid stiffness.	After this type of surgery, it is good for patients **to walk** around frequently to avoid stiffness.
Dangling modifier (when a subject is not named for an action)	While giving the patient a bath, it got cold in the room. (In this example, "it" appears to be "giving the patient a bath.")	While **the nursing assistant** was giving the patient a bath, it got cold in the room.
Incorrect pronoun	Jamie and me are working at the same dental office. Please give your urine sample to the nurse or to myself. The AARC has a special newsletter for we respiratory therapists.	Jamie and **I** are working at the same dental office. Please give your urine sample to the nurse or to **me**. The AARC has a special newsletter for **us** respiratory therapists.
Incorrect verb form	The patient already drunk the glass of water. Mr. Daley has broke the same leg twice.	The patient already **drank** the glass of water. Mr. Daley has **broken** the same leg twice.
Meaning is unclear because of the word order	When he hit his arm against the window, it broke. (Which broke—his arm or the window?)	When he hit his arm against the window, **his arm** broke. *or* He broke his arm when he hit it against the window.

TABLE 8-5
Cures for Capitalization Problems

When to Use	Examples
First word of a sentence	**T**he result of the test for strep throat was negative.
Proper nouns and adjectives: names of people, places, organizations, institutions, religions	**D**iane is working as a nurse in **K**enya on a **U**nited **N**ations project in a **C**atholic hospital.
Professional titles when used with the person's name	I understand that **D**r. Nguyen is a leading oncologist. (BUT: I understand that the doctor is a leading oncologist.) They are here to see **N**urse Edmonds. (BUT: They are here to see the nurse.)
The major words in the titles of books, articles, movies, software programs, etc. (Exception: only the first word is capitalized in some bibliography and reference lists. See Table 8-2.)	**C**areer **D**evelopment for **H**ealth **P**rofessionals is the title of this book. **S**teel **M**agnolias is a movie in which one of the main characters is a young woman living with diabetes.
The first word of a quotation	The physical therapist told the patient, "**I**t is very important that you do these exercises every morning and evening."
Days, months, and holidays	I think **C**hristmas was on a **F**riday last year.
Trade names of products and brand name drugs	The physician recommended **S**udafed for the patient's nasal congestion. The lab technician used **A**cetest to confirm the presence of sugar in the patient's urine.
Abbreviations	**AIDS** (acquired immunodeficiency syndrome) **CPR** (cardiopulmonary resuscitation) **ECG** (electrocardiography) **RDA** (registered dental assistant)

TABLE 8-6
Punctuation Remedies

Mark	When to Use	Examples
Period.	To end sentences, unless you use a question mark (?) or an exclamation point (!)	There are five patients waiting in the reception area.
	After some abbreviations	Dr. A.M.
Comma,	Connect two sentences (independent clauses) into one with a connecting word (and, but, or, nor, yet, for, so)	The surgeon performed the knee replacement surgery, and the physical therapist directed the patient's rehabilitation program. The patient was very nervous about the procedure, so the physician ordered a sedative.
	Separate items in a series	Encephalitis, epilepsy, meningitis, and multiple sclerosis are disorders of the nervous system.
	After introductory phrases	While the patient filled out the necessary forms, the dental hygienist gathered her supplies. When the EMT couldn't detect a pulse, he quickly began to perform CPR.
	Around optional information (nonrestrictive clause)	Mrs. Washington, who has been seeing Dr. Gonzalez for several years, is doing well on her new medication.
	After transitions (however, therefore, for example, in other words)	She is doing well with her diet; however, she needs to walk at least a mile each day. Alternative medicine is gaining popularity in the United States; for example, many patients have found pain relief with acupuncture.
	After the closing in letters	Sincerely, Very truly yours,
	With dates, addresses, titles, and numbers with more than four digits	The surgery is scheduled for August 12, 1999, at Grand General Hospital. Dr. Sally Halloway, M.D., will perform the surgery. There were 86,000 procedures performed in the United States last year.
Semicolon;	To connect two sentences (independent clauses) that are not joined with a connecting word	Occupational therapists help patients regain as much normal function as possible after a serious injury; they also help patients adjust psychologically to their disabilities.
	To connect two independent clauses that are joined by a transitional expression (examples: however, also, therefore, furthermore, meanwhile, as a result, in conclusion)	I believe that medical care should be available to everyone in the United States; furthermore, it should be affordable.
Colon:	After an independent clause that is followed by a list	There are several habits that contribute to heart disease: smoking, a high-fat diet, lack of exercise, and psychological stress.
	After the salutation in a formal business letter	Dear Dr. Chang:
	With hours and minutes	Your appointment is at 4:15 P.M.
	With proportions	The ratio of medication to water should be 2:1.
Apostrophe'	To show possession	The patient's cast needs to be changed today. Please get John Bergen's file out for the dentist.
	To substitute for missing letters in contractions	Let's see if we can find better prices for these supplies. You're doing well with your therapy. It's a good method for sterilizing instruments.
Quotation marks" "	Around direct speech	"You should eat at least five servings of fruits and vegetables each day," said the dietitian.
	Around titles of articles, poems, short stories, songs, TV programs	"The Rising Costs of Health Care" article that appeared in today's paper was interesting.
	Note: Put periods and commas inside quotation marks. Put colons and semicolons outside quotation marks.	"Nova," a public television program, had a good review of current AIDS research.
Dash—	To give emphasis or more information	Diseases that were thought to be conquered—tuberculosis, measles, and hepatitis—have once again become public health concerns.
	To show a change of thought	Mrs. Crawford—who reminds me of my grandmother—comes in every Wednesday for chemotherapy treatment.

English. If you need more help, ask your instructors about other resources. Your school may offer English classes and/or tutoring. There are many good books and websites with information about grammar and writing. (A few examples are listed at the end of this chapter.)

A couple of notes about grammar references: first, many professional organizations have preferred styles for writing. For example, some organizations prefer that abbreviations for time be written in lower case using periods: "a.m." for morning, "p.m." for afternoon and evening. Others suggest using uppercase to show time: A.M., P.M. Find out if there are style books or references for your profession.

Second, a word about grammar checkers on word-processing software. I am writing this book using a popular computer program. To my surprise, many of the suggested changes have been incorrect. In many cases, making the "corrections" would result in sentences that don't make sense. At the same time, many obvious errors are not caught. Although word-processing software has made writing and making corrections easier, the final judge is still the human writer.

Prescription for Success: 8-5 **How's Your Grammar?**

1. How would you rate your knowledge of English grammar? Is it excellent, very good, good, fair, or poor?
2. If you scored yourself "Fair" or "Poor," what of the following can you do to improve?
- Take classes at school
- Use special services at school, such as a computer lab or tutoring program
- Study on your own
- Workbooks
- Software
- Videos
- Other

First Aid for Spelling

Many people, even good writers, have difficulty with spelling. English is a combination of many languages and contains silent letters, different ways of pronouncing the same letter, different ways of spelling the same sound, and other irregularities. There are a few rules, but the spelling of many words simply must be memorized. Developing a good learning system for spelling will be helpful when you are learning medical terminology. Spelling medical terms correctly is critical because errors can negatively affect patient care. Some medical words look alike and can be confused. Here are a few common examples:

- ilium—part of the hipbone
- ileum—part of the intestine

- alveoli—tiny air sacs in the lungs
- areola—brown pigmented area around the nipples

Begin now to practice good spelling habits. Tables 8-7 contains spelling rules; Table 8-8 lists commonly misspelled words. In Table 8-9 you will find commonly confused words. You may have wondered about some of these yourself—words that are spelled the same with different pronunciations and those that are spelled differently but have the same pronunciation!

You can use these tables, along with other spelling aids, as a study guide. Make them even more useful by adding your own problem words. If the sample suggestions given in Table 8-9 for learning commonly confused words don't make sense to you or seem silly, you might want to create your own hints for remembering them.

Prescription for Success: 8-6 **How's Your Spelling?**

1. Quiz yourself by having someone read the words in Tables 8-8 and 8-9 for you to spell.
2. After correcting your quiz, separate out any words that you missed. (Didn't miss any? Congratulations! Skip the rest of the assignment and consider volunteering to help classmates who have difficulty with spelling.)
3. For those of you who missed a few words, make a commitment to learn them in the next few weeks. Devise your own study plan, and reward yourself when you reach your learning goals.

Success Tips for Spelling

- Try the memory techniques suggested in Chapter 3.
- If you have children in school, make spelling a family activity.
- Work on spelling in a study group: quiz one another, have contests, give small prizes, and make learning fun.
- Start your own dictionary and spelling list to keep in your notebook or on your computer.
- Make flash cards to quiz yourself.
- Put cards on the bathroom mirror and other places where you'll see them every day.
- Spell aloud.
- Create a "mental movie screen" on which you visualize the words spelled out in large colored letters.
- Create hints and associations.
- Write the words over and over. Try using colored pens and/or writing larger than you usually do.
- Record practice words to listen to at home or in the car.

Writing Is Important, Too

Angela, a recent graduate of a medical administrative assistant program, has been hired by Dr. Richard Crane to work in his front office. She has been on the job for a couple of months now. Angela has a warm, friendly personality and has been well received by Dr. Crane's patients. She remembers their names, asks about their families, and expresses caring in other ways. They feel at ease coming into the office, unlike in the past when the woman at the front desk was rather abrupt.

Dr. Crane is very appreciative of this pleasant change in the front office atmosphere. He is a popular doctor in town, but had been receiving complaints about the cool reception her patients received with his previous front office staff. It's been a welcome relief to have patients who are more comfortable when he sees them. As one long-time patient told him, "I really like Angela. I have to be honest and tell you that hiring her was a good change for your office."

But Dr. Crane has a dilemma. He is a one-physician office and can't afford many staff members. Angela covers the front desk, answering the phone, greeting patients, and entering data into the computer. But he needs her to do some tasks that involve writing. Unfortunately, he has some concerns about her skills, especially with spelling and punctuation. Although the documents are fairly short, he needs them to be done correctly. After all, they come from his office and therefore, reflect on him and his professionalism, along with that of his staff.

In many ways, Angela has become a valuable asset to his practice, so he really doesn't want to have to let her go. He decides to discuss the problem with her and see if she would be willing to take steps to improve her writing skills.

Questions for Thought and Reflection

1. What do you think Dr. Crane should say to Angela?
2. How might he best start the conversation?
3. What suggestions should he offer about how she can improve her writing skills?
4. How do you think Angela will respond to Dr. Crane?

TABLE 8-7
Spelling Prescriptions

Rules	Examples	Exceptions
I before *E* except after *C* or when the word sounds like *AY*, as in *SAY*	relieve receive neighbor weigh	either foreign height seizure
Drop final silent *E* when adding a **suffix** that begins with a **vowel** Keep final silent *E* when adding a suffix that begins with a **consonant**	achieve—achieving care—caring achieve—achievement care—careful	change—changeable argue—argument judge—judgment true—truly
When adding *-ING* to a word that ends in *IE*, replace the *IE* with *Y*	die—dying tie—tying	
Double the final consonant of a one-**syllable** word when adding a suffix that begins with a vowel *unless* there are two vowels or another consonant before the final consonant	trim—trimming look—looking test—testing	
Plurals		
Add *S* to most words	disease—diseases wound—wounds	
Words that end in a consonant + *Y:* change the *Y* to an *I* and add *ES*	laboratory—laboratories pregnancy—pregnancies	
Words that end in *S, SH, CH,* and *X:* add *ES*	crutch—crutches cross—crosses	
Words that end in *SIS:* change to *SES*	diagnosis—diagnoses urinalysis—urinalyses	
Words that end in a vowel + *O:* add *S*	radio—radios	
Words that end in a consonant + *O:* add *ES*	echo—echoes	

TABLE 8-8
Commonly Misspelled Words

absence	disease	leisure	receipt
absorption	efficiency	license	receive
accessible	eighth	loneliness	recognize
accidentally	eligible	magazine	recommend
accommodate	eliminate	maintenance	reference
accumulate	embarrass	management	resuscitate
achievement	emphasize	maneuver	rhythm
acknowledge	encourage	marriage	safety
acquire	enthusiastic	miscellaneous	satisfactory
address	entirely	necessary	schedule
affiliated	environment	negligence,	scissors
aggravate	equipped	negligible	secretary
analyze	equivalent	neighbor	seize, seizure
appropriate	especially	noticeable	sensible
assistant	exaggerate	obstacle	separate
association	exercise	occasion,	several
athlete	exhausted	occasionally	severely
beginning	experience	occur, occurrence	significance
behavior	extremely	often	similar
belief	fascinate	original	sincerely
beneficial	fatigue	pamphlet	strategy
bureau	February	parallel	strictly
business, businesses	fluctuation	particular	substantial
cafeteria	foreign	patience	succeed
caffeine	forty	perform	success
calendar	fourth	persistent	surprise
cancel, canceled	fragile	physically	sympathy
column	friend	physician	technique
coming	government	pneumonia	temperature
commitment,	handkerchief	possession	thorough
committed	harass, harassment	practical	though
committee	height	precede	tongue
communicate	hygiene	preference	transferred
comparative	impatient	prejudice	typical
competition	indefinitely	privilege	until
cooperate	infinite	probably	urgent
correspond	intelligence	proceed	useful
criticism	interesting	prominent	usually
criticize	jewelry	psychiatry	vacuum
decision	judgment	psychology	vague
definitely	knowledge,	qualified	vegetable
describe	knowledgeable	quantity	view
despair	label	questionnaire	Wednesday
develop	laboratory	quiet	weight
discipline	legitimate	quite	writing

Tests: Part of School, Part of Life

Taking tests is not limited to your life as a student. Much of what the health care professional does every day is a kind of test. Let's compare some typical classroom test questions with the performance of a procedure on a patient.

TEST FOR A CLASS	PERFORMANCE OF A PROCEDURE
Supply definitions	Know when to use the procedure
List items needed to perform a given procedure	Gather equipment and supplies for the procedure
Recall information	Create mental checklist of steps
Write explanations	Provide patient with clear explanation and instructions
	Perform procedure correctly
Write short answers to questions	Record results accurately on patient chart

TABLE 8-9
Commonly Confused Words

Words	Meanings	Sample Hints for Learning
accept	to take or receive	take—a<u>ccept</u>
except	excluding, all but	e<u>x</u>clude—e<u>x</u>cept
access	way of entering	
excess	too much	e<u>x</u>tra—e<u>x</u>cess
adapt	adjust	a<u>d</u>just—a<u>dapt</u>
adopt	to take as one's own	<u>o</u>wn—ad<u>o</u>pt
advice	helpful suggestions (noun)	
advise	to give advice (verb)	
affect	to influence (verb)	
effect	result; to bring about (noun or verb)	
allowed	permitted	
aloud	capable of being heard	<u>loud</u> sound
already	before now; so soon	
all ready	completely prepared	It's <u>all</u> done.
capital	official seat of government; form of wealth	
capitol	building in which elected members of federal or state governments meet	
choose	to select	
chose	selected (past tense of "choose")	
coarse	rough (adjective)	The dog has a rough <u>coat</u>.
course	class; path or track (noun)	<u>Our</u> class is on track.
conscience	part of the mind that determines right and wrong	
conscious	awake; aware	
council	governing body (noun)	
counsel	advice; to give advice (noun or verb)	
defer	delay	d<u>e</u>lay
differ	to be different; to disagree	<u>differ</u>—<u>differ</u>ent
desert	dry land area	1 rain <u>sh</u>ower in the desert.
dessert	eaten at the end of a meal	2 cups of <u>su</u>gar in dessert.
incompetent	unable to function properly and/or manage one's own affairs	
incontinent	unable to restrain the discharge of urine	
it's	contraction of *it is*	The apostrophe replaces the letter *i*.
its	possessive form of *it*	
later	after the usual time	
latter	the second of two	2 *T*'s = 2nd of 2
lay	put or place something (past = *laid*)	
lie	rest on a surface (past = *lay*)	
lead	(Yes, these words are confusing!!) type of metal; to guide; connecting wire	
led	guided (past tense of *lead*)	
loose	not tight (adjective)	Bigger word, like a shirt, is looser.
lose	to be unable to find (verb)	I lost one *O*.
maybe	perhaps	
may be	possible; permissible	
miner	mine worker	
minor	younger than the legal age	
overdo	to do too much	
overdue	late or past due	
patience	quality of being uncomplaining, unhurried	
patients	people under medical care	
passed	went by; earned satisfactory grade	
past	before now; ended	
personal	private	
personnel	employees	
principal	head of a school; main or most important	The princi<u>pal</u> is your <u>pal</u>.
principle	general truth or rule	A princip<u>le</u> is a <u>ru</u>le.
stationary	not moving	S<u>ta</u>y in one place.
stationery	paper for writing letters	<u>Le</u>tters are written on station<u>e</u>ry.
than	compared to	
then	at that time	

Continued

TABLE 8-9—cont'd

Commonly Confused Words

Words	Meanings	Sample Hints for Learning
their	possessive of they	
there	in that place	
they're	contraction of "they are"	Apostrophe stands for the letter *a*.
to	toward, for the purpose of	
too	also, very, more than enough	
two	2	
weather	climate conditions	Weather can be <u>wet</u> <u>a</u>nd windy.
whether	introduces alternatives	
who's	contraction of *who is*	Apostrophe stands for the letter *i*.
whose	possessive of *who*	
you're	contraction of *you are*	Apostrophe stands for the letter *a*.
your	possessive of you	<u>Our</u> is possessive; so is <u>your</u>.

Using Tests to Your Advantage

Classroom tests and work on the job both involve interpreting sets of instructions (questions and job tasks), performing within time limits (class session and appointment schedules), following given standards (instructor **criteria** and facility **protocols**), and being measured by indicators of the level of performance (grades, patient satisfaction, evaluations, and raises). In reality, performing on the job is more serious in terms of requirements and consequences than any classroom quiz or final exam. Students can repeat a test—or a class, if necessary—but correcting a medical error, winning back an unhappy patient, or reversing the poor opinion of your supervisor is more difficult. At the extreme is the possible damage done by an incorrect procedure or inaccurate medication dosage.

The intention here is not to terrorize the future health care professional, but to put the subject of tests in the classroom in perspective. Tests are a fact of life, and if approached with the right attitude, classroom tests can provide you with opportunities to increase your learning. For example, tests encourage students to study. Most of us perform best when there is a consequence for our actions. Scientists now believe that the process of taking a test, not just studying for it, is a powerful learning tool. They hypothesize that retrieving information from the brain when you answer questions alters how it is stored and makes it easier to remember in the future.[4]

In Chapter 3, we discussed how "good stress" can stimulate us physically and mentally to be alert and take appropriate actions. In the same way, you can harness the anxiety experienced when thinking about future tests to energize yourself and focus your efforts on learning. You can use tests to mark your progress toward achieving your long-term goal of becoming a competent health care professional—that is, after all, the real reason you are learning (Figure 8-8).

Tests also teach you to work under pressure, which is a daily reality for health care professionals. You can never take your tasks for granted, and classroom tests provide practice for working calmly and efficiently when it counts. Planning and preparing ahead, thinking about what you are doing, and

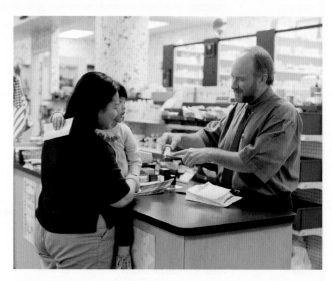

FIGURE 8-8 Prescription medications can effectively treat thousands of medical conditions. At the same time, medication errors take place up to one million times a year, killing up to 7000 people. Therefore, it is critical that everyone who works in pharmacies have the proper knowledge to work safely on the job. *What are possible consequences when pharmacy technicians pass their classes by cheating, rather than by learning the necessary information?* (From Hopper T: *Mosby's pharmacy technician: Principles and practice*, ed 3, St Louis, 2012, Saunders.)

performing to the best of your ability are habits that apply to both test taking and work.

Finally, test results give you opportunities to improve and advance your learning. Answer sheets and scores are not for the exclusive use of your instructors. Take advantage of them to help you as a student. They identify what you know and don't know. Review your answers to discover which material you haven't mastered. What did you not understand? What do you need to ask the instructor? What should you review again? Fill the gaps in your knowledge now, while you are still in school. Don't brush off wrong answers and hope the knowledge all comes together on the job. Remember why you are in school: to learn the basics

Dolores Michaels

Dolores, a nurse in a large California medical clinic, discusses the importance of good writing skills in the medical field.

Q Is being able to write well really that important for a health care professional?

A Absolutely! In fact, in our clinic written communication is central to everything. We have individuals who take phone messages from patients. These messages get passed on to doctors or to nurses like me who are responsible for reviewing them and getting back to patients. If we can't read or don't understand the message, we waste time checking back with whoever wrote it. In a fast-paced clinic, this can really create problems.

Q Do you have any examples of problems that resulted from unclear writing?

A Well, the other day I got a written message that said, "Patient has planteritis." This was a mystery because there's no such thing as "planteritis." I didn't want to call the patient without having some idea of the problem, so I had to take time to find the person who wrote this. Turns out the patient had "plantar fasciitis," which is inflammation of the tissue in the bottom of the foot. I have to say that good spelling is really critical. Another problem is with abbreviations. When we're in a hurry we tend to use them, but they can cause problems. The other day a nurse wrote on a chart, "Will call tom for a dressing change." The other staff then wasted time looking for someone named Tom who the patient was supposed to call. It turned out that "tom" was an abbreviation for "tomorrow." Totally different thing.

Q So abbreviations can really be a problem?

A Yes. You have to be really careful when using them. An interesting example is the shortcut for "shortness of breath." This is a common condition, but if someone simply writes "patient is sob," the meaning is open to interpretation. If this were the only sentence on a chart with no context, it could be really inappropriate! So you really have to be careful.

The idea is to save time, but if abbreviations aren't clear, they can waste time. One day a doctor wrote "brbpr." I had no idea what this was and had to take time to find the doctor. It turns out it meant "bright red blood per rectum," but there was no way I was going to figure this out.

Even when everyone agrees on a facility abbreviation, it can be confusing to personnel who move from one department or facility to another as fill-ins. Something like "mltcb" means "message left to call back." But lots of medical personnel work in various departments and facilities, and this can be confusing.

Q It sounds like we're not talking about the kinds of writing that students think of as assignments, like papers and reports.

A No, I'm referring to things like memos and electronic notes. These aren't long, but they're extremely important. They must be clear and accurate because we need the right information to give appropriate patient care. It's important to be precise and include all necessary details. If you're describing a wound, for example, you need to note the location, size, condition—all the things that the next person who sees the patient can use to see if the wound is healing or getting worse.

What students also need to understand is that these are legal records. If there's a malpractice suit, for example, they can be used in court as evidence.

---

of your profession. Sometimes you will make mistakes, a student right. Learning from your mistakes is a student responsibility.

Personal Reflection

1. What are some other similarities between classroom tests and working on the job as a health care professional?

What Tests Are—and Are Not

"Think of a test as a challenge instead of a threat."
—Walter Pauk

Tests can turn otherwise sensible individuals into quivering masses of anxiety. For many students, the grades earned on tests influence their feeling of self-worth. You may be worried about appearing stupid and wonder if you have the ability to learn. Or you may feel insecure about your test-taking skills. Although there is no denying that tests are used as indicators of progress by both instructors and students, understanding more about tests and their purpose can help you control them rather than letting them control you.

Good tests measure your knowledge and ability in specific areas. They can also measure how much you have packed into temporary memory as a result of last night's cram session, so they may or may not indicate the extent of true learning or your ability to perform effectively on the job. Tests, however, are never a measure of your value as a person. You can be an "A" in life even if you do not receive straight As in class.

Realities About Tests

Tests ask for only samples of what you are expected to know. Many students are disappointed when everything they studied does not appear on a test. They believe they have wasted their time and should have had to study only what was going to be on the test. But health care professionals must know a great deal of information. If instructors included everything on tests that students should know, there would be time only for testing and none left for teaching!

Samples are reliable indicators of overall knowledge. For example, if you are expected to learn 1000 medical terms, the instructor may randomly select 75 for a test. The percentage of those 75 that you know is a good indication of how many of the 1000 you know. Keep in mind that knowing more than what is on the test is a requirement for job success, not a waste of your time.

Tests provide instructors with feedback about their teaching. Student performance on tests helps instructors adjust their classroom strategies to ensure that their students have opportunities to master the subject and skills. If many students do poorly on all or part of a test, it may indicate to the instructor that the material needs to be re-taught in a different way.

Good tests are not easy to create. The truth is that poorly written tests do exist. Even instructors with good intentions can write questions that are unclear and confusing. The best strategy is to ask the instructor to explain the question(s).

▣ Prescription for Success: 8-7 Make Tests Work for You

1. Describe five ways you can use tests to your advantage as you prepare for a career in health care.

Preparing Effectively for Tests

The best way to prepare for tests is the same way you prepare yourself for career success: Start early and study to learn. Being prepared for tests means mastering the content of your courses. Let's review a few study techniques that lead to successful test taking:

- Manage your time so that studying is a priority.
- Identify and use study techniques that work best for you.
- Use learning techniques that help move information into your long-term memory.
- Take good notes in class and review them often.
- Read textbooks actively and review them regularly.
- Seek help early if you are having trouble.

In addition to practicing good study habits, there are specific steps you can take to prepare for important tests.

1. Find out as much as possible about the test. Suggested questions to ask your instructor: "What type of questions will be asked (such as multiple choice and true-false)?" "Will there be a time limit?" "Will it be given at the beginning or end of class?" "Will you review first?"
2. Review your notes, textbook, handouts, and any other class materials to check your comprehension. Is there anything you don't understand or can't remember, even after reviewing? Write a list of questions to ask in class. (This is why you start your review early, not the night before the exam!)
3. Make a schedule, and divide what you have to review over the time you have available so you won't run out of time.
4. Use the study tools you developed when you reviewed throughout the class—or create some now. Here are a few ideas:
   - Keywords or questions to prompt recall of notes and text.
   - Outlines, charts, or mind maps to help you organize the material and make it meaningful for you.
   - Flash cards to practice recall. Put aside the ones that you know well and concentrate on the ones you have

the most difficulty remembering. Your goal is to move all cards into the "know-these" pile.
   - Saying aloud or writing answers to your prompts and practice questions.
5. Identify and concentrate on the material you find most difficult and have the most trouble remembering. Don't keep restudying material that you know. (Except when you are deliberately overlearning, as discussed in Chapter 3.)
6. Use the practice questions and quizzes you created from your class notes and your reading. This may be the *single best way* to ensure you are prepared for classroom tests.

▣ Prescription for Success: 8-8 Studying for a Test

1. Choose at least three study techniques to use when you prepare for your next test.
2. Create a plan for using these ideas, including the actions you will take and a study schedule.
3. After you have taken the test, describe how the techniques worked for you.

On the Job

Test-Taking On The Job Many of the strategies that work for successful test taking have applications in health care work.

Follow Directions This is a big one in health care. Your ability to follow directions can affect the safety of patients and the quality of your work. Examples include being willing and able to take direction from a supervisor, reading and understanding the instructions for a piece of equipment, following the steps to perform a laboratory test, and staying within legal guidelines for your occupation.

Ask for Clarification of Directions You must be able to ask your supervisor questions about any aspect of your work that you don't understand.

Keep Your Cool Work in health care can be fast-paced. And you'll often be dealing with people who are frightened, in pain, and stressed out. Working calmly and carefully under all kinds of conditions is essential.

Check Your Work for Accuracy Checking your work is another health care skill to ensure safety and accuracy. For example, it is essential to always check the identity of any patient you are working with. And a medication is never given to a patient until the label identifying it has been checked *at least three times*.

The Anxiety Monster

You have studied throughout the class, you have reviewed for the test, and you feel pretty secure about your knowledge of the material, but you are panic-stricken by the idea of your final exam. You just know you'll freeze up and won't be able to remember a thing. You may even feel physically ill when you enter the classroom on test days. There just doesn't seem to be any way around it—you just "can't take tests." This is a real problem for many students, and solving it is an important step toward achieving your professional goals. Following is a list of actions to help you manage test anxiety:

- Evaluate your study habits and test-review methods. Can you improve them? Are you really using your study time efficiently? For example, some students spend a lot of time reading notes over and over but never actually quizzing themselves without looking at the written information. They think they know it, but without their book or notes, they can't remember very much.

- Think about your actual test preparation. It may seem like you are spending a lot of time reviewing because you feel worn out by it. In reality, if you engage in a marathon review session the last 2 days before the test, you may feel as if you studied a lot but are too tired to remember much of the material.

- Be honest with yourself. Do you have trouble understanding in your classes but don't ask for help because you are embarrassed? Remember that instructors are there to help you, and asking for help is not nearly as embarrassing as failing a test or finding that you lack information needed to perform your job. Have you been an active participant in class? Do you lack the time after class to stay for extra help? Is there another reason? If you are serious about achieving your career goals, you must decide to make school a priority and organize your life so that you can study when and as much as needed.

- Don't let your classmates freak you out. If you worry about competing with them, such as finishing the test first or earning a higher grade, you can get distracted from focusing on your own performance. Your education is not a race with winners and losers; the goal of a health care program is for everyone to win by graduating and becoming a competent professional. Although the awarding of grades tends to set up a competitive environment, modern health care is delivered by teams of individuals who must work cooperatively, not competitively. Some classmates are even more anxious about tests than you. These people often express their nervousness by talking a lot and predicting total gloom and doom. Be upbeat with them rather than letting their negative talk increase your own anxiety. Avoid participating in "ain't it awful" conversations around test time.

- Join forces with positive students. Organize a study group to review, share ideas, quiz one another, and cheer one another on. Have each person make up a few test questions and quiz the others. Seek out classmates who are dependable and will contribute to the group. Keep the number small (three to five) so that everyone can make a contribution. If the group is too large, it can be very difficult to plan meetings that accommodate everyone's schedule.

- Use visualizations and positive self-talk to promote learning and good test performance.

- Practice good health habits and the stress management techniques described in Chapter 3. Remember that physical exercise releases endorphins, the body's natural tranquilizers. Do your best to get enough sleep before tests so that you're not exhausted and more subject to anxiety. Finally, the relaxation exercise described in Chapter 3 is effective just before taking a test. Take deep breaths to help quiet the mind. Help your body work for instead of against you.

If you review thoroughly and try the suggestions for relieving anxiety, but still find yourself freezing up during exams and feeling as if even dynamite couldn't blast facts out of your brain, you can try a technique called "desensitization." This is a treatment developed for people who have anxieties that interfere with their daily lives. It works by providing exposure to small doses of the source of the fear and then gradually increasing the size and number of exposures.[5] Develop a plan to increase your exposure to tests. Have a friend or family member make up and give you tests, starting with short quizzes. Make them as realistic as possible. For example, set and stay within a time limit. Ask your instructor to give you practice tests. Find out if you can take these in a classroom under conditions as close to those of a real test as possible. Sponsors of professional exams may have sample tests you can take. These techniques may seem like a lot of work and even a little embarrassing, but if test anxiety is running your future career off track, desensitization is worth trying.

Don't Trip Yourself Up

Some students procrastinate in preparing for tests (and starting other projects, such as term papers) because they are afraid of failing. Their fear causes a kind of paralysis that prevents them from taking positive steps to prepare. For other students, not studying creates an excuse for failure. Another problem is feeling overwhelmed. Students who feel there is just too much to learn may decide to give up without really trying. If any of these behaviors sound familiar, make a deal with yourself to try something new. Study throughout the course, use the suggestions in this chapter on preparing for tests, ask for help, and work with a study group. The chances are very good you will experience success, and that can be habit-forming!

The Day Before the Test

It's the day before the test and you still have a little time to prepare. In addition to doing a final quick review of your notes and other materials, help yourself by taking care of the following:

- Get yourself organized—set out what you need to take with you the next day—so you don't have to rush in the morning.
- Plan ahead to eat a good breakfast.
- Drink some water to stay hydrated.
- Be rested—get as much sleep as possible the night before.

The Day of the Test

Okay, it's the day of the test and you feel reasonably prepared. You certainly don't want to perform poorly because you fail to follow some common sense test-taking guidelines. Here are some helpful hints you can apply to any test situation:

- You deserve a good start, so plan to arrive early. Don't stress yourself out by rushing in late, scrambling to find a seat, and missing the introductory instructions.
- Bring your supplies, including books, notes, and a calculator (if these are allowed). An erasable pen (blue or black ink) works well because it is darker than a pencil, but you can make corrections neatly.
- Read and/or listen to all instructions. Ask the instructor to explain anything you don't understand. This is not the time to be shy. You have a right to know exactly what is expected.
- Quickly review the *entire* test before starting. Read *all* directions on every page. If you have questions, quietly ask the instructor.
- If there are different types of questions, note which ones will take the most time to answer and/or are worth the most points. Then quickly plan how to divide your time among the different parts of the test.
- If the test is longer and/or more difficult than you expected, do *not* panic. Take a deep breath, follow the guidelines and focus on doing your best.
- Give yourself a boost by answering the easiest questions first. When there are different types of questions, it is usually best to move from the shortest to the longest answers: true-false, multiple-choice, matching, fill-in, short essay, long essay. This is like giving yourself a warm-up. Also, the questions that have the answers provided for you to choose from may give you ideas for questions in which you must supply the answers from recall.
- Limit the time you spend on questions you find very difficult or don't know. Mark them and return later after you complete the rest.
- Proofread your answers before you turn in your test. Did you answer all the questions? Mark the correct boxes on the answer sheet? Follow all directions correctly? Check for spelling errors, words left out, and other careless errors.
- Use all the time allowed if you need it. You don't earn extra points by finishing early, and hurrying may cost you a few correct answers.

Specific Test-Taking Techniques

A message repeated throughout this book is the importance of mastering the knowledge and skills presented in your classes. The well-being of patients depends on what and how well health care professionals learn. The purpose of studying is to learn for the future, not just to pass tests. And the *best* way to prepare for tests is to know your material well.[6] That said, it is also true that learning about commonly used test formats can help you be more effective in showing what you know. Students who are unfamiliar with question formats can waste time and energy figuring them out.

It is important to keep in mind that some of the techniques suggested for answering test questions would be downright dangerous if applied to work in health care.

For example, most study skills books recommend that if there is no penalty for incorrect answers, go ahead and guess. With true-false questions, you have a 50-50 chance; with most multiple-choice questions, the chance is 25%. But there is no room in health care for a 50-50 chance of correct performance. Some tasks, such as administering medications, must be 100% correct. There is no guesswork allowed here!

The suggestions given in the following sections are based on the experience of many students. However, they are only guidelines and do not substitute for knowledge.

True-False Questions

Purpose. Test your recognition of correct facts, statements, and cause-and-effect relationships, as well as your ability to distinguish fact from opinion.

Examples. *Read each of the following statements. If the statement is true, circle the T. If it is false, circle the F.*

T F 1. Classroom tests are always good indicators of how well students understand a subject.

T F 2. Test performance can be improved by cramming as much as possible the day before the test is given.

T F 3. Reviewing material regularly throughout the course is the best way to do well on tests.

Suggested Techniques for Answering

- Be sure that every part of the answer is correct. If any part of it is false, the entire answer is false.
- Watch out for words like "always" and "never." Few things in life are that final, and statements with these words are often false. (There are exceptions, however. For example, there are safety rules in health care that must *always* be followed and legal rules, such as those concerning the release of patient records, that can *never* be violated.)
- Carefully consider answers with middle-of-the-road words like "usually," "sometimes," and "often." They tend to be true.
- Do not spend a lot of time on true-false questions you really don't know, especially if they are at the beginning of a test that also contains more time-consuming questions.
- Guess only as a last resort (and only if there is no penalty).

Multiple Choice Questions

Purpose. Test your knowledge of terminology, specific facts, principles, methods, and procedures.

Examples. *Circle the letter to the left of the response that best answers each question.*

1. Which is the best reason for learning to spell correctly?
   A. Patients are impressed by correct spelling.
   B. Patient care can be negatively affected if words are misspelled on medical documentation.
   C. Students who spell correctly get better grades in school.
   D. It increases the chances of receiving a promotion at work.

2. The Cornell note-taking system has proven helpful to students because it:
   A. Prevents them from having to review notes after class.
   B. Helps them record everything the instructor says.
   C. Provides a format that encourages review.
   D. Teaches specific active listening techniques.

Suggested Techniques for Answering

- Read the instructions and questions carefully. If the question asks you to identify the "best" answer, it is possible that more than one is correct. In the first sample question, all answers are good reasons for spelling correctly. So you need to think about which is the most important reason, and that is patient safety. Therefore B is the correct answer.
- If the direction states to select the correct answer (as opposed to the "best," "most complete," etc.), consider each statement separately and ask yourself if it is true or false. (Many professional exams are multiple choice.)
- Read through all the answers before selecting one.
- Immediately eliminate answers that are obviously incorrect.
- If the answer requires a math calculation, do the problem yourself before you look at the answers.
- Match each answer to the question rather than comparing the answers to each other.
- If you are guessing, choose an answer that has information you recognize.
- You can sometimes eliminate choices by using logic. For example, if two answers say basically the same thing, they must both be incorrect. As with true-false answers, if any part of a statement is wrong, the entire answer must be wrong. If the answer is silly or farfetched (instructors sometimes like to have a little fun), eliminate it immediately.
- If you are allowed to write on the test, circle or underline key words in the question to focus your attention when you read the answers.

Matching Questions

Purpose. Recognize definitions of terms and identify correct facts based on simple associations.

Examples. *On the line to the left of each number in Column A, write the letter from Column B that explains one of its uses.*

COLUMN A	COLUMN B
_____ 1. Comma	A. Substitutes for letters that are dropped when contractions are formed
_____ 2. Semicolon	B. Indicates a change of thought within a sentence
_____ 3. Colon	C. Connects two sentences into one long sentence when a connective word is used
_____ 4. Apostrophe	D. Follows the greeting in a formal business letter
_____ 5. Dash	E. Connects two sentences into one long sentence without the use of a connective word
	F. Is placed at the end of a sentence

Suggested Techniques for Answering

- Read the instructions carefully. Note whether any item can be used more than once.
- Quickly count each column to see if both columns have the same number of items. Sometimes they do not. It is possible that an item may be used more than once.
- Read through both columns before you write in any answers.
- Do the ones you know first.
- Some students find it easier to read the longer answers first (usually placed in the right-hand column) and then look for the shorter match. See which method works best for you.
- Mark or cross out each item as you use it, if you are allowed to write on the test paper.

Fill-in-the-Blank Questions

Purpose. Test your ability to recall terminology, facts, and procedures and to interpret information.

Examples. *Fill in each blank with a word or phrase that correctly completes the sentence.*
1. _____ is a method for overcoming severe test anxiety that involves exposing oneself to testing situations.
2. An explanation of why a procedure is performed in a certain way is called the _____.
3. The best way to ensure you are prepared for a test is to _____ your notes and textbook regularly over time.

Suggested Techniques for Answering

- Read the entire statement before attempting to fill in the blank(s).
- Write answers that fit the form and content of the words around them. For example, if the last word before the blank is "the," you know the answer is a noun.
- It sometimes helps to convert the phrase into a question in which the answer is the correct fill-in.

Short-Answer Questions

Purpose. Recall facts and definitions or write explanations that demonstrate your understanding.

Examples. *Write a short answer to each of the following questions using the spaces provided. Some questions have several parts. Your answers do not need to be complete sentences.*
1. List three reasons why many educators recommend using a three-ring binder to keep your notes and class materials in order.
2. Explain why previewing is a critical part of the reading process.
3. Describe four ways of starting to write a paper when you are having trouble determining exactly what to write and/or how to organize it.

Suggested Techniques for Answering

- Read the instructions to find key words that tell you exactly what is expected in the answer. Are you asked to explain? Give two examples? List five reasons? Define? Give the steps?

- If you are asked to write several sentences, answer the question as directly and completely as possible without padding with unnecessary information.
- If you don't know the entire answer, write down as much as you do know. You may receive partial credit.

Essay Questions

Purpose. Demonstrate ability to select, organize, relate, evaluate, and present ideas. These questions provide an opportunity to show what you know about the topic.

Example. *Write a well-organized essay at least one-page long explaining the meaning of this statement: "Study skills are career skills." Support your answer with examples and references to SCANS and the National Health Care Skill Standards. You will be graded on how well you demonstrate understanding of the concept, as well as on spelling and grammar.*

Suggested Techniques for Answering

- As with the short-answer questions, read the instructions to find out what you are supposed to include in your answer. Provide evidence for your response? Give examples to illustrate? Give the sequence? Explain reasons and purposes? Defend your answer? Compare and contrast?
- Support your statements. Even if the question does not specifically ask for examples or evidence, you should fully explain or defend your answer.
- Don't spend time with a lot of words that don't really mean anything, such as repeating the question or writing a long introduction. Answer questions directly.
- If you have trouble organizing an answer in your head, quickly jot down a few key ideas, an outline, or a mind map.
- Use the rule journalists use when they write a newspaper article: state the most important information first by answering the question as quickly as possible. Use the rest of the time to develop your answer, write examples, provide evidence, and so on. This way, if you run out of time, you know you have included the most important information.
- Include the principal ideas of the course, as appropriate, especially ones the instructor emphasized.
- Apply the principles of good writing.

After the Test

Much as you'd like to forget about the test you just took, don't. Just like athletes who analyze each game to learn which plays worked and which didn't, use debriefing to your advantage. As soon as possible after finishing the test, review your notes and books to find the answers to the questions you were unsure about or just didn't know.

When the test is returned in class, try not to react emotionally. If you earned a top score, give yourself credit. Continue to review the material from time to time to reinforce and retain important facts and information. If you did poorly, don't lose heart. Instead, try the following:

- Listen to any review the instructor gives of the test.
- If you have to return it to the instructor, take notes on a separate sheet of paper.
- Pay special attention to the questions you missed and write down the correct answers.
- If the instructor explains information, be sure to take notes.
- Ask questions about anything you don't understand.
- If your instructor does not discuss the test with the class and you did poorly, make an appointment to discuss it privately.

At your earliest opportunity, review your notes and your textbooks. Did you miss some of the major points? Study the wrong material? Not really understand it? What can you do to improve your performance next time? See Table 8-10 for suggestions on dealing with common test problems.

TABLE 8-10
Common Test-Taking Problems

The Problem	What to Do
You didn't study at all or waited until the last minute and crammed.	You know what to do!
You studied but couldn't remember the information when you needed it for the test.	Check your understanding. Information you don't comprehend well can be very difficult to remember. Did you use prompts to study and review the material without looking at the answers? Or did you simply reread your notes and textbook? Passive review, simply looking at the material, is not an effective learning technique for most people.
You were extremely anxious during the test and froze.	Review the section in this chapter on anxiety and try using the techniques. If they don't work for you, seek additional help.
You made careless errors.	Allow time to proofread your test before turning it in.
You didn't understand what the questions meant.	When you are studying, be sure to look up any words you don't know. During the test, ask the instructor for clarification. If English is your second language, see your instructor for help.
The questions were not what you expected. For example, you memorized a list of facts and definitions, but the test asked you to apply information to new situations.	Review your notes or other information about the test to see if you misunderstood. Be sure to attend all classes so you will hear announcements about test content. If you believe the instructor was unclear about the format and/or content of the test, speak to him or her privately. Critical thinking and problem-solving skills, which involve applying information to new situations, such as test questions, are discussed in Chapter 9.

Learning to Study

Rosa Gonzalez is the first in her family to pursue studies beyond high school. She is enrolled in a dialysis technician program. Although she finds her classes interesting, they are also very challenging. They are much more difficult than those she took in high school. As she told her friend, Amelia, "High school classes were pretty easy. I didn't really have to study that much to get by."

Amelia, who is now working in her family's store, replied, "This is why I didn't go to college. I'm earning enough in the store and don't have the hassle of studying and tests to worry about."

Rosa told her friend that she really wanted something more out of life—that she thought health care would be really interesting and satisfying. "But," she said sadly, "maybe I've made a mistake."

After receiving a D on her first major exam, Rosa felt ready to give up. That evening, she said to her mother, "Mamá, I'm so discouraged. I'm thinking about dropping out of school." "But Rosa," her mother replied. "I thought this meant so much to you."

"I know," said Rosa. "It did—or I thought it did. But I'm afraid I'm too dumb or something. I'm just not getting it." Her mother thought for a moment. "Rosa, I know that you're not dumb. Listen, you're paying good tuition money for school. Why don't you talk with your instructor and see if she can give you some help?"

Later that night, Rosa thought over what her mother had said. It did make some sense. She had taken out loans to pay for school. Maybe she should do more than just sit in class. The next day, she made an appointment with her instructor, Ms. Santori.

As they talked, Ms. Santori asked about Rosa's study habits. "Well," Rosa said, "I really don't have a lot of time to study. And in high school, I just paid attention in class and did okay. I didn't have to do that much to get by."

Ms. Santori pointed out, "Getting by won't do here, Rosa. You're training for an important career that affects patient health and safety. The tasks you'll be performing must be done correctly and accurately. You've got to be prepared."

Rosa admitted that she hadn't thought about this. She asked Ms. Santori for suggestions about improving her time management and study habits to do better.

"Rosa," said Ms. Santori. "I like your attitude. I'd be glad to help you. We can get started today by looking at your out-of-class schedule and exactly what you do when studying for tests."

Questions for Thought and Reflection

1. Why is Rosa having difficulties handling college-level classes?
2. Do you think Rosa should consider getting a job like Amelia did rather than going to college?
3. What suggestions do you think Ms. Santori will give Rosa?
4. Do you think Rosa will complete her program and succeed as a dialysis technician? Why or why not?

Jed Stuart's parents always expected that he would attend college. They hoped he would attend the university where they met and became engaged, thinking he would enjoy living in a fraternity, attending parties and football games, and participating in other college activities. Jed, however, really didn't consider himself to be the "college type." He was never very social, but preferred staying home and playing video games and watching sports and movies on television.

During his senior year of high school, his parents insisted that he start making plans. "Jed," his father told him. "You've got to start thinking about your future." "Dad," Jed said. "I'm really not interested in going away to school and living in a dorm with a bunch of guys I don't know."

"Well," his dad said, "you know our house rules. After high school, you either need to go to school or get a job and pay some rent if you want to live here. You'll be an adult and you'll have to act like one."

Jed realized that the only jobs he would qualify for didn't pay much. And although he wasn't crazy about continuing his education, he knew he didn't want to be stuck in a dead-end job for the rest of his life. He knew from the

career exploration class that seniors were required to take that jobs in health care were pretty promising. And he had seen some ads for schools that were close by so he could continue living at home.

Jed talked with the admissions counsellor at a local college about the various programs offered. He decided to apply for the medical coding program. He liked the idea of mainly working alone, and the job prospects and salary sounded pretty good. He decided he would enroll in the program after graduation in June.

Once in college, Jed thought his classes were okay. The main thing he didn't like was having to work with other students when group projects were assigned. He also hesitated asking questions in class when there was something he didn't understand. Besides being shy, he believed it was the instructors' responsibility to explain the material well enough so that students could understand the material. This was his reasoning for not spending much time studying his textbooks. If the instructors didn't explain it in class, he figured that it must not be that important.

Jed passed the first few short quizzes in his classes, but failed the midterm exams in two classes. As he told

Continued

his parents, "The instructors in these classes really aren't that good. The students haven't worked with this stuff before—how do they expect us to learn it if they can't explain it well?"

Questions for Thought and Reflection

1. What do you think about Jed's reasons for selecting a medical coding program?

2. Do you think he will do well on future tests?
3. Do you think Jed will complete the program?
4. How is his attitude about working with others and speaking up in class likely affecting his academic success?
5. Is his opinion about the responsibility of instructors correct? Why or why not?
6. What responsibilities do students have for succeeding in their programs?

A Word About Professional Exams

Many health care professions have exams you must pass to work in the field. The purpose of professional exams is to ensure high standards for practitioners by testing for knowledge and competence. These exams may be administered by a governmental agency or a professional organization. Passing them allows the professional to use one of several special designations such as "licensed," "certified," or "registered." Most exams require a fee. Your school may have included this cost in your tuition or fees. The school may also assist you in applying to take the exam. Some exams are given year round, others only on certain dates. Find out whether professional exams are required for your occupation. Learn as much as possible about the exam(s) while you are still in school.

Some professions do not require formal approval (certification, licensing, etc.) for graduates to work. At the same time, voluntary testing is available and recommended for many careers. For example, many physicians prefer to hire only certified or registered medical assistants, designations earned by passing professional exams administered by the American Association of Medical Assistants and the American Medical Technologists, respectively. Some medical insurance companies require physicians to hire only credentialed professionals.

Success Tips for Passing Professional Exams

- Start preparing early (note the word is "prepare," not "worry"). This suggestion is not intended to add further stress to your already busy class and study schedule. It is a reminder that if you prepare over a period of time, you will learn more and experience less stress when the time comes to actually take the test.
- Keep your notes, handouts, and textbooks organized so you can find and use them for review before the exam.
- Pay attention to any information and advice your instructor gives you about the content of professional exams.
- Some textbooks refer to specific exams and requirements of professional organizations, and the authors of the textbooks design their content and review questions to help students prepare throughout their courses. Take advantage of these features!

- Find out if there are any review books available in your school library or for purchase or online materials to help you focus your studies on mastering the material likely to appear on the exam.
- Practice tests are available for many exams. Check with your professional organization.
- Find out whether review workshops are available in your area.
- Plan to take the exam as soon as possible after you become eligible. This is usually on graduation from your program, although some occupations also require work experience. You are less likely to forget information and lose your confidence if you do not wait too long.
- Think of the timed tests you take in school as opportunities to practice taking an important exam under pressure.

Some Honest Talk About Cheating

Health care professionals must follow high ethical standards. High-quality patient care and safety depend on their actions, and there is no room for cheating in any form. Furthermore, governmental regulations have increased, and **audits** of health care facilities are common. The consequences for **fraud**, taking shortcuts, and even trying to just "get by" are severe, including costly fines and closures of health care facilities.

You may believe that cheating on tests in school isn't as serious as cheating on the job, but this is not true. Health care graduates who cheat to pass their classes, instead of learning what they need to know on the job, may become dangerous practitioners. You are in the process of becoming a professional, and what you do now is setting the groundwork for your future actions. Integrity (honesty, sincerity) is an essential characteristic of the health care professional, and cheating undermines that integrity. Cheating is an unsatisfactory and potentially destructive way of approaching your education. It converts the opportunities offered by tests to develop effective study habits and to learn what you need to know into unacceptable behaviors.

Even if you do not cheat yourself, helping others to do so promotes incompetence in the health care system. Would you or one of your family members want to be treated by "professionals" who cheated to pass their classes? Do you want to carry the load at work for a co-worker who is used to taking the easy way out? Helping friends cheat allows them to avoid taking responsibility for themselves. This can lead to the habit of dependence and unsatisfactory performance on the job, resulting in negative consequences for everyone.

Personal Reflection

1. What are some possible future effects on the job for students who passed their classes by cheating instead of studying?

Summary of Key Ideas

- Good written communication contributes to good patient care.
- Your competence is often judged by your writing ability.
- Writing well is a skill that can be mastered through effort and practice.
- It is never too late to improve your spelling and grammar skills.
- Tests are part of life.
- Test anxiety can be conquered.
- The best preparation for a test is to know the material.

Positive Self-Talk for This Chapter

- I write clearly and effectively.
- I spell and use grammar correctly.
- I use the act of writing to help me learn new material.
- I use tests to motivate me to do my best in school.
- I prepare in advance for all my tests.
- I manage test anxiety effectively.

Internet Activities

For active links to the websites needed to complete these activities, visit http://evolve.elsevier.com/Haroun/career/.

1. Purdue University has an excellent online writing lab that includes information sheets and quizzes. Explore areas you find interesting or with which you have problems and write a short summary of what you learn.
2. The *Merriam-Webster Dictionary* website includes definitions, pronunciation, and word games. Choose 10 unfamiliar words from this book or any of your other textbooks. Find the definitions and write a sentence using each word.
3. Study Guides and Strategies has an extensive list of topics in its resources. Read about at least two of the topics listed under "Preparing for Tests" to find techniques you can use.
4. Western Washington University has a great booklet called "Academic Success" that contains useful information on study skills. The section on studying for

exams has excellent suggestions. Select three or four and try using them when preparing for your next test.

Building Your Resume

1. Review Resume Building Block #5 in Chapter 2. Learn more about any exams needed to become licensed or certified in your career. Are there strategies in the test-taking sections of this chapter you can apply to start preparing for these exams?
2. Consider how developing your writing skills will help you put together a well-worded resume.

To Learn More

Elbow P: Writing with power: techniques for mastering the writing process, New York, 1998, Oxford University Press

http://www.grammarbook.com.
This is one of the best books on writing I have found, considered to be a classic. It has many techniques to help you effectively put what you want to say on paper. Contains grammar rules with examples and has quizzes you can take to test your understanding.

Hacker D: A writer's reference, ed 7, Boston, 2010, Bedford/St. Martin's

This is an excellent, easy-to-use book that includes explanations and examples of grammar, sentence structure, punctuation, and organization of content.

Medical Assistant Practice Test

http://www.tests.com/practice/medical-assistant-practice-test

Pauk W: How to study in college, ed 7, New York, 2005, Houghton Mifflin

Professor Pauk developed many original and practical ideas to help students study more effectively.

Purdue University's Online Writing Lab

http://owl.english.purdue.edu
Purdue offers information on dozens of topics related to writing of all types in its award-winning writing lab.

Quizlet

http://www.quizlet.com/20284907/billing-and-coding-practice-test-flashcards/
This site contains study aids for billing and coding tests.

The Health Care Communications Group: Writing, speaking, and communication skills for health professionals, New Haven, 2001, Yale University Press

Good advice presented on how to write clearly and correctly.

Test Prep Review

http://www.testprepreview.com
This site has links to practice tests for a variety of occupations.

Villemaire D., Villemaire L: Grammar and writing skills for the health professional, ed 2, Clifton Park, NY, 2005, Delmar Cengage Learning

Excellent review of grammar. Includes many practice exercises, along with the answers, so students can study on their own. Each chapter contains examples of writing used in health care, such as letters, charting, and office memos.

References

1. Ellis D, Toft D, Mancina D, McMurray E: *Becoming a master student*, ed 12, Boston, 2009, Houghton Mifflin.
2. Elbow P: *Writing with power: techniques for mastering the writing process*, New York, 1998, Oxford University Press.
3. Palau SM, Meltzer M: *Learning strategies for allied health students*, St Louis, 2007, Elsevier.
4. Carey B: *Forget what you know about good study habits*. Available at: http://www.nytimes.com/2010/09/07/health/views/07mind.html?pagewanted=2&_r=0.
5. Fry R: *How to study*, ed 6, Franklin Lakes, Clifton Park, NY, 2004, Delmar Cengage.
6. Pauk W: *How to study in college*, ed 7, New York, 2005, Houghton Mifflin.

CHAPTER 9

Developing Your Practical Skills

OBJECTIVES

1. Apply strategies to help you get the most benefit from laboratory sessions and master hands-on skills.
2. Explain how to succeed when taking online courses.
3. Use critical thinking in your everyday and professional life.
4. Develop skill in using a problem-solving process to make good decisions in both your personal and your professional lives.
5. Plan and start putting together a personal reference guide to help you in school, during your job search, and on the job.
6. List the purposes and benefits of an externship.
7. Describe how to maximize learning and gain the most benefits from both on-site and simulated externships.
8. Explain the importance of knowing how to apply math skills in health care.
9. Approach the learning of math with a positive attitude and, if necessary, apply techniques to overcome math anxiety.
10. Evaluate your own math skills and, if needed, devise a plan to improve them by using appropriate tips to help you master math.

KEY TERMS AND CONCEPTS

Average (also called the *mean*) The result obtained by adding several quantities together and then dividing this total by the number of quantities.

Brainstorming A problem-solving technique in which you generate as many ideas as possible without judging them for quality or practicality.

Contaminate To make impure or infect by introducing organisms, such as bacteria, that can cause disease.

Critical Thinking A process of thinking purposefully in which you apply knowledge and use logic and reasoning to separate fact from opinion, guide your actions, make decisions, and select the best choice among the alternatives.

Dosage The amount of medication to be administered.

Evaluate To judge or determine the worth or condition of something.

Math Anxiety The fear of math. People with math anxiety don't believe they have the ability to learn math.

Metric System A system of measurement used throughout the world that is based on meters (length), grams (weight), and liters (volume).

Nursing Process An orderly approach to patient care that nurses use to identify and resolve patients' health problems.

Percentage an amount or number in each hundred (3% = 3 out of 100 items).

Protective Equipment Special clothing and accessories worn by health care workers to protect themselves against body fluids that may be infectious. Also referred to as personal protective equipment (PPE).

Role Play A way of practicing interpersonal exchanges in which students play the parts of health care professionals, patients, supervisors, and co-workers.

Learning Practical Skills

Most jobs in health care involve a lot of hands-on activity, and the level of your performance is critical to your success on the job. Future health care professionals must master a variety of skills. Depending on your specific occupation, these skills range from filling out forms accurately to performing a urinalysis to taking an x-ray film. Learning to apply the **theory** you learn in class to practical situations is one of the most important components of your education.

Hands-on practice builds a bridge between school and the world of work, as illustrated in Figure 9-1. There is a big difference between knowing about a procedure and actually being able to do it well. Performing a blood draw, for example, is very different from hearing about it. Practice sessions provide you with opportunities to take risks in a safe, monitored environment where you can learn from your experience—and from your mistakes.

At the same time, it is important to learn the theory and background information that support the procedures you will practice in the lab. For example, giving injections requires an understanding of the principles of infection control. Insurance coding requires knowing the terminology of basic human anatomy and medical diagnoses.

Learning in the Lab

Depending on your program of study, practice may include performing procedures, engaging in **role play**, working on the computer, and completing pencil-and-paper activities. You may solve problems, work with "patients," conduct tests, or do calculations. See Figure 9-2 for an example.

Being Prepared for Lab Sessions

Advance preparation will help you benefit fully from lab sessions. Lab time is often limited, and the instructor will expect you to get started on the assigned activities without delay. The first step in being prepared is to read your textbook. Don't depend on your instructor's explanations or on being able to "figure it out." Reading gives you time to think through the steps and, as we discussed in Chapter 7, gives you a framework for lectures and demonstrations. Many health care textbooks present procedures in recipe or how-to format. Read through each step. Note all hints and cautions that contain important safety information for you and the patient.

In addition to reading your textbook, study the illustrations. Are the health care professionals wearing gloves? How are they positioned in relation to the patients and equipment? What do the equipment and instruments look like? How are

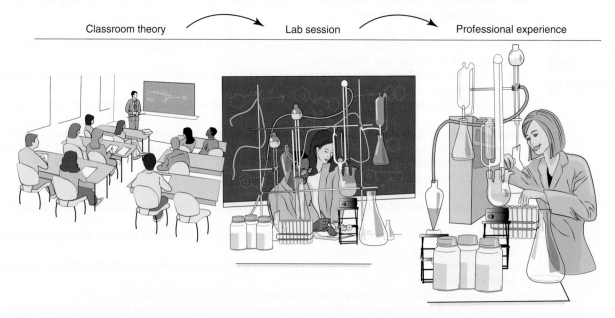

Classroom theory → Lab session → Professional experience

FIGURE 9-1 Lab sessions and your externship provide a bridge between what you learn in class and your work on the job. Do your best to apply and practice what you have learned. *What mistakes might the lab technician pictured on the right make if she had neglected to do her best in the lab classes she took in school?*

they held? In which direction should movements be made? For example, in disinfecting a surgical site on the skin, it is important for cleansing to be done in a circular motion, moving from the center toward the outside edges, so as not to **contaminate** the areas already cleaned. The effectiveness of a procedure is often based on details such as these.

If your instructor demonstrates a procedure in class, focus on the steps or actions involved. Take notes only if doing so doesn't distract you from watching and listening. If action is involved, mirror the instructor as closely as possible. For example, when watching a demonstration of the proper way to hold a syringe, use your highlighter or pen to copy the motion. Developing the ability to observe carefully is, in itself, a valuable health care skill.

Don't hesitate to ask questions about any point you don't understand. Get as complete an understanding as possible before going to the lab, to minimize mistakes and avoid wasting practice time.

Last—but very important!—pay special attention to learning safety rules. Your future job may require you to operate expensive and potentially dangerous equipment and to handle chemical and biological hazards. The human immunodeficiency virus (HIV) and the hepatitis B virus can be spread by mishandling blood and certain body fluids. Laws regulate the proper disposal of contaminated items. All health care professionals must learn and follow the **standard or universal precautions** developed by the U.S. Centers for Disease Control and Prevention. The time to start applying these precautions is in your lab classes.

Success Tips for Learning in the Lab

- Take along any study materials, reference books, supplies, or **protective equipment** needed to participate in the scheduled activities. Set them out the evening before if you have an early start on the day of the lab.

- Work with "real patients." Treat the students you work with in the lab as you would if you were on the job. Demonstrate courtesy and concern. (Remember, "Your career starts now.") If you are entering patient data on the computer or practicing patient scheduling, work as if the exercises involved real people who were depending on your ability to maintain accurate and efficient records and schedules.

- Aim for accuracy. All health care tasks depend on accuracy to ensure safe, high-level patient care. You will also be expected to comply with various laws and regulations, both in the lab and on the job. In many procedures, "almost correct" is not good enough. Only perfection is acceptable. For example, a sterile field is a germ-free area prepared to prevent infection during procedures such as minor surgeries. It is either sterile or it is not. Brushing an ungloved hand against an object in the sterile field may seem like a small error, but the field is no longer sterile. Work carefully in the lab. Never skip a step because this is "just practice" and these are not "real surgeries" or "real medications." When establishing your work habits, it is important that everything you do be done as realistically as possible. See Figure 9-3.

- Respect your instructor's time, but do ask questions as needed. If the instructor is busy observing or assisting other students, write down your questions so you won't forget them.

- Understand that there may be more than one correct way to perform a task. Your instructors, as well as future supervisors, may each have different ways of performing a

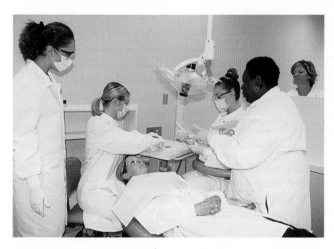

FIGURE 9-2 Put forth your best efforts when working in practice sessions with your classmates. These dental assisting students will apply what they learn on real patients in the future, so it is essential they learn and practice proper techniques. *How can you get the most from practice sessions and assignments in your classes?* (From Bird D, Robinson D: *Modern dental assisting,* ed 11, St Louis, 2015, Saunders.)

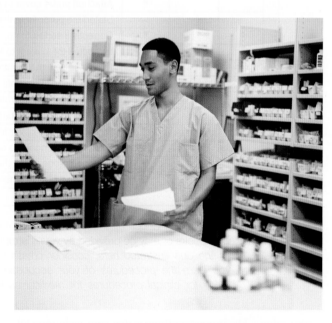

FIGURE 9-3 Working accurately and handling drugs safely is important in many occupations. There are other procedures that range from giving injections to billing insurance companies accurately that require following certain protocols. *What can you do now to develop good work habits you will apply later on the job?* (© Jupiterimages/Photos.com/Thinkstock)

Name: _____   Date: _____

Evaluated by: _____   Score: _____

Performance Objective

OUTCOME: Measure oral body temperature.
CONDITIONS: Given the following: electric thermometer and oral probe, probe cover, and a waste container.
STANDARDS: Time: 5 minutes. Student completed procedure in _____ minutes
Accuracy:
Satisfactory score on the Performance Evaluation Checklist.

Performance Evaluation Checklist

Trial 1	Trial 2	Point Value	Performance Standards
		•	Sanitized hands.
		•	Assembled equipment.
		•	Removed thermometer from its storage base.
		•	Attached oral probe to thermometer unit.
		•	Inserted probe into the thermometer.
		•	Greeted the patient and introduced yourself.
		•	Identified the patient and explained the procedure.
		•	Asked the patient whether he or she has ingested hot or cold beverages.
		▷	Explained what to do if the patient has recently ingested a hot or cold beverage.
		•	Removed probe from the thermometer.
		▷	Explained what occurs when probe is removed from the thermometer.
		•	Attached probe cover to probe.
		▷	Stated the purpose of the probe cover.
		•	Correctly inserted the probe in patient's mouth.
		•	Instructed the patient to keep the mouth closed.
		▷	Explained why the mouth should be kept closed.
		•	Held probe in place until an audible tone was heard.
		•	Noted patient's temperature reading on display screen.
		•	Removed probe from patient's mouth.
		•	Discarded probe cover in a regular waste container.
		•	Did not allow fingers to come into contact with cover.
		•	Returned probe to the thermometer unit.
		▷	Stated what occurs when probe is returned to the thermometer.

FIGURE 9-4 Check-off sheets can help you monitor your progress. These are often included in workbooks or may be provided by your instructors. *If your classes do not have forms such as the one illustrated here, consider creating some of your own to track your progress as you learn the procedures of your occupational area.* (Modified from Bonewit-West K: *Study guide for clinical procedures for medical assistants,* ed 9, St Louis, 2015, Saunders.)

procedure. The important thing is that your technique follows accepted practice and is safe for both you and your patients.

• Keep up with your lab assignments. Many health care classes give out "check-off" sheets to students that the instructor uses to observe the students' performance of each

required procedure. Figure 9-4 shows an example for taking a temperature. Note how each step is listed separately. This is because health care procedures must be done in a certain way (called a *protocol*), with many of the steps essential for the success of the procedure. When the procedure is completed satisfactorily, it is checked off on the sheet.

Lab Follow-Up

It is important to follow up and review what you learn in lab sessions, just as it is in note-taking and reading. You can do a number of things to help move what you learn in the lab to your long-term memory.

1. Join or organize a study group to practice procedures and quiz one another on the rationale, safety concerns, and supporting theories.
2. Write out the steps of each procedure from memory. Include any safety concerns or rationale.
3. Make flash cards to help you remember important facts—rules and regulations, normal values (blood cell counts, body temperature, the purpose of various lab tests, and so on).
4. Make charts, using color and illustrations to highlight the important points about each procedure.
5. Recite the steps out loud, or record them and review by listening.
6. Rehearse the steps for each procedure in your mind. Act them out. Develop mental checklists of the steps. Some students find it helpful to use mnemonics (techniques to help the memory). For example, RICE is a popular way to remember the immediate first aid treatment for sprains:

   R = rest
   I = ice
   C = compression
   E = elevation

Prescription for Success: 9-1 Making the Most of Lab Assignments

1. Describe any previous experience you have had with lab courses. How well do you learn from practical sessions?
2. Which study and learning techniques do you think will work best for you in the lab?
3. Describe how you think working on the job will be different from the practice sessions you do in school.

Taking Online Courses

Many schools now offer online courses that students can complete at times and locations of their choice. Online courses are convenient for busy adults who find it difficult to attend on-campus classes while working and carrying out family responsibilities. In some cases, students take both on-campus and online courses to obtain the credits they need to graduate.

In spite of the advantages, students must take care not to get tripped up by the seeming ease of online classes. Students sometimes have unrealistic expectations; they discover after starting that these classes can take even more time than classroom courses. Common problems are not scheduling enough time to complete the required work and not taking advantage of help from the instructor or the various computer resources. If you are taking both on-campus and online courses, be sure to give each the needed attention to learn the subject matter and pass the classes.

Success Tips for Online Classes

- Become familiar with the computer and software tools needed to complete the course.
- Print a copy of the syllabus and refer to it often.
- Record tests and due dates for assignments on your calendar.
- Schedule time to "attend" class and take it as seriously as you would an on-campus class.
- Let friends and family members know when you'll be "in class".
- Keep up with the work and meet all the deadlines.
- Be persistent: you may encounter challenges, such as technical problems or not understanding an assignment.
- Be careful not to get distracted by computer games or online surfing during your study time.

Critical Thinking

Every day we are confronted with situations that require us to solve problems and make decisions, both large and small. The quality of your life depends to a great extent on your ability to make good decisions. On the job, this ability also affects the lives of your patients and co-workers.

Critical thinking is a term you will hear used a lot in health care. There are many definitions. In this book, it means paying attention to what you are doing; considering whether what you hear or read makes sense; using logic and reasoning to make choices and decisions; and applying what you have learned in class to new situations. An important part of critical thinking is separating facts from opinions. Facts are based on evidence, experience, and observation. Opinions are based on feelings, emotions, and unproven beliefs. Distinguishing between the two requires a foundation of knowledge and the ability to research and find the facts. Gaining this knowledge is a major reason for studying and mastering the information you are presented with during your health care studies. See Figure 9-5 to see the various components of critical thinking.

On the Job

Critical Thinking on the Job I observed good examples of critical thinking when my husband was in the hospital. The entire hospital had started converting to a new computer system a few hours before he was admitted. All patient information, charting, records of medications—everything—was now being entered on laptop computers the staff wheeled around on small stands.

One problem with the new system was figuring out how to delete information entered by mistake. We observed the physician struggling with medications he wanted to delete from his orders. After he left the room, we commented to the nurse about the increased risk of medication errors for the next few days until everyone learned to use the new system. She responded that the staff would have to pay even more attention than usual to medical orders and double check anything that didn't seem correct. They would have to think critically and apply their knowledge about drugs.

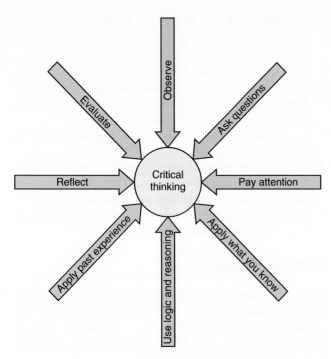

FIGURE 9-5 Thinking critically is an active process. It is necessary for making sound decisions and taking the correct action in a given situation. *Why is critical thinking an essential skill for the health care professional?*

A Six-Step Plan for Problem Solving

Having an organized way to approach problems makes it easier to find effective solutions. Many helpful methods have been developed. Some are specific to certain health care occupations. For example, Box 9-1 contains the steps that make up the **nursing process**. The more general problem-solving method presented in this chapter is organized into the following six steps:

1. Define the problem.
2. Gather information.
3. Develop alternative solutions.
4. Consider the possible results and consequences.
5. Choose a solution and act on it.
6. **Evaluate** the results and revise as needed.

Step One: Define the Problem

"A problem well stated is a problem half solved."
—Charles F. Kettering

You may be faced with what seems to be an obvious problem, but sometimes what we believe to be the problem is only a symptom of a deeper underlying problem. For example, suppose that Kathy, a nursing student, is earning Ds and Fs in her pharmacology class. She may define the problem as "getting low grades in class." Grades, however, are only a symptom of the problem, not the problem itself. Asking questions is one way she can start to identify the real problem.

BOX 9-1 The Nursing Process

1. *Assessment*: Systematically collecting data about the patient.
2. *Nursing Diagnosis*: Describing actual and potential health problems based on the data collected.
3. *Planning*: Setting goals for the patient and establishing a nursing care plan to achieve them.
4. *Implementation or Nursing Interaction*: Carrying out actions to assist the patient to promote, maintain, and restore health.
5. *Evaluation*: Measuring the patient's progress toward achieving the goals set in step 3. Determining ways to assist patients who do not reach their goals. Setting new goals for patients who are progressing as planned.

Adapted from: http://www.nursingprocess.org/Nursing-Process-Steps.html

---

- Do I understand the textbook? The lectures?
- Do I use good study habits?
- Do I put off studying for this class? If so, why?
- Do I attend all the class sessions?
- Am I able to follow the instructor's presentations?
- Does the subject require background knowledge that I don't have?
- Am I having difficulty understanding what is asked for in test questions?
- Do I complete all the homework assignments and projects?
- Do I have the math knowledge and skills needed to understand and perform the necessary calculations?

Suppose that Kathy identifies the problem as a weakness in math. She makes lots of mistakes when calculating **dosages**, converting between systems of measurement, and working with proportions. Her poor grades are a symptom of her problem, which, now identified, she can start to solve.

It isn't always easy—or comfortable—to uncover real problems. Many of us tend to avoid tough issues by ignoring them, or we blame circumstances or other people for our difficulties. But when we fail to recognize our part in causing problems, we also give away our power to find solutions. For example, if we blame our poor grades on the teacher or the school, we become powerless to raise them. By accepting responsibility for ourselves, we empower ourselves to direct our own lives.

Step Two: Gather Information

Up-to-date information is needed for solving problems and making decisions. Even well-trained experts conduct research when confronted with new problems. For example, when physicians begin working with patients who have unresolved health problems, the doctors gather as much information as possible. They observe the patient, ask questions, and run diagnostic tests. They call on their own knowledge. They may discuss their findings with other physicians and health professionals and consult reference books and recent technical articles. In summary, they gather as much information as possible from a wide variety of sources.

Gathering facts helps prevent emotional and nonproductive reactions to life's problems. If Kathy's response to receiving low grades in pharmacology class is, "I'm just dumb and I'll never get this," she will be discouraged from seeking an effective solution. If she passed the admissions requirements for her school and is receiving passing grades in her other classes, the evidence does not support her statement that she is dumb. Insisting that she is "just dumb" becomes a way to escape being responsible for seeking solutions to the problem. It is an excuse to avoid the work of going through the problem-solving process and making needed changes.

There are many sources of information for help in addressing problems:

1. Your own knowledge and observations—what you know that relates to the problem
2. The knowledge and opinions of others, such as experts and people with special knowledge
3. Books, journals, and the Internet. There are many reader-friendly books about handling personal and professional problems
4. Classes, workshops, and conferences

The number of resources you consult depends on the size, complexity, and importance of the problem. Some situations require only your current knowledge and a quick observation. Others require extensive research. (Review the section on research in Chapter 7.)

A good professional practice is to keep up-to-date in your field by reading and pursuing continuing education opportunities. This will give you the background needed for making sound decisions. It will also enable you to more effectively judge the quality of the information you gather. Not all published information or material from the Internet is based on thorough research. It can have errors or be biased by the opinions of the writer. Up-to-date knowledge of the fundamentals of your area will help you distinguish fact from opinion, an important component of critical thinking.

Here are some potential sources of information to help Kathy with her problem:
- Her math or pharmacology instructor
- Math tests that diagnose weak areas of knowledge
- Books, articles, and workshops about math anxiety
- Basic math textbooks
- Math books for health care students
- Measurement and dosage practice problems
- Online math help (the Internet)
- The resource center and library at her school

Step Three: Develop Alternative Solutions

There may be several effective solutions for a given problem. Try a technique called **brainstorming** to think of as many ideas as possible. Write them all down, even silly or impractical ideas. Don't discard anything, because even ideas that seem foolish can lead to ones that work.

Here is Kathy's list:
- Drop the class and hope to become smarter over time.
- Drop out of school. What's the use?

- Stay in the class, keep trying, and repeat the class if I don't pass.
- Drop the class and take it later. Use the extra time to work on math skills.
- Stay in the class and spend extra time developing math skills.
- Work through a basic math textbook.
- Use learning software.
- Work with a tutor.
- Form or join a study group.
- Ask the instructor to work with me after class several times a week.
- Ask a friend or relative who is good at math to help.
- Go to a hypnotist who specializes in helping people overcome anxiety problems.
- Use positive self-talk and visualizations.
- Borrow my children's math books.
- Ask my children for help.
- Go to a learning supply store and buy math games and toys.

☐ **Prescription for Success: 9-2**
More Solutions

List at least five more ideas that Kathy might consider to solve her problem of doing poorly in her pharmacology class.

Step Four: Review Possible Results and Consequences

Now is the time to use critical thinking skills to evaluate your ideas. Review each option and ask yourself, "What would happen if I took this action?" You may find that you need to ask more questions and gather more information. Look for ideas that can be combined or that suggest other workable solutions. Let's review a few of Kathy's ideas from step three. *Drop out of school. What's the use?*

This is an emotional response that's perfectly natural when someone feels frustrated or discouraged. Possible results and consequences:
- Disappointment at not reaching her goal of a career as a nurse
- Missed opportunity to help others
- Feelings of failure and depression
- Student loans to repay and no job to help her financially
- A feeling of relief. This just wasn't for her

New questions Kathy can ask:
- How can I find out if I really am capable of learning the necessary math?
- How did I do in past math classes?
- Did I learn these skills at one time and just need to review, or did I never learn them at all?
- Do I have review materials, tutors, friends, and/or family members available to help me?
- What other career possibilities are open to me? Do I really want to change direction now?
- How much has my education cost so far? What would my student loan payments be each month if I were to drop out now?

- What other jobs am I qualified to start immediately? How much would they pay?

Stay in class and spend extra time developing math skills.

Possible results and consequences:

- She masters the math skills and does well in the class.
- She understands just enough to get by and passes the class.
- She tries but just never gets it and fails the class.
- She neglects her other classes when she spends extra time working on math skills.
- She passes all her classes, including math.

New questions Kathy can ask:

- How much math review do I think I need? Have I mastered at least the most fundamental math skills (e.g., multiplication and division of whole numbers)?
- What resources are available to help me learn the necessary math skills?
- How much extra time can I devote to learning math? (Consider job, family, etc.)

Go to a hypnotist for a cure for math anxiety.

Possible results and consequences:

- It works! She now looks forward to working with numbers.
- It doesn't work. She still experiences mental paralysis when faced with a problem that involves numbers.
- She still doesn't love math, but she can get through it to accomplish what needs to be done in her classes and on the job.

New questions Kathy can ask:

- Do I think that math anxiety is the problem, or have I just forgotten or never learned the necessary skills?
- Do I believe in hypnosis?
- Would I be comfortable trying hypnosis?
- Is there a good, reputable hypnotist in the area?
- How much does it cost? Can I afford it?

Although Kathy decides not to see a hypnotist, just considering this idea helps her realize that math anxiety may be a real problem for her. She decides to seek help from her school counselor and read a book about conquering math anxiety.

Step Five: Choose a Solution and Act on It

"It is common sense to take a method and try it. If it fails, admit it frankly and try another. But above all, try something."

—Franklin Roosevelt

After weighing the various alternatives, select the one that best fits your own mission and goals. It's easy to spend a lot of time thinking and then be afraid to take action. Think positively, make a plan, and do your best to implement the solution you have chosen. You may decide to combine several alternatives and attack the problem from different directions to increase your chances of success. Kathy decides to stay in the pharmacology class. She finds a math tutor and asks her sister to watch her children two afternoons a week to give her the extra time needed for meeting with the tutor and studying. She also decides to use positive self-talk to work on eliminating her negative feelings about math.

Step Six: Evaluate the Results and Revise Your Plan as Needed

Did you achieve the desired results? Were there unknown facts or circumstances that resulted in unexpected consequences? How can you revise your plan to get the results you want?

After working with the tutor for three weeks, Kathy realized that this person, though well-meaning, was unable to explain the concepts so she understood them. She decided to work on her own and bought a math software program that her instructor recommended. She also joined a study group to share ideas and gain support from other students. The results of her revised plan were positive. She learned the skills she needed, gained self-confidence, and passed her pharmacology class.

Prescription for Success: 9-3
Try Something!

Choose a real problem you would like to solve and go through the six-step process.

1. Define the problem.
2. Gather information. List your sources, and the facts, ideas, and opinions you find.
3. Brainstorm alternative solutions.
4. Consider the possible results and consequences. Do you have questions or need information about any of these results or consequences?
5. Describe the solution you chose and the action you took.
6. Describe and evaluate the results, and describe any necessary revisions.

On the Job

Problem Solving on the Job Here are some examples of daily problems encountered by health care workers. Your occupation may present different situations. These are examples that require thinking on the job.

- A man calls Dr. Beck's office complaining of chest pain. The medical assistant takes the call and must ask appropriate questions, apply what she knows, and decide whether the man should speak with the doctor, come to the office, or call 911 for emergency assistance.
- Dr. Beck is unhappy with the poor service he is receiving from the office's current supplier of certain medical supplies. The office manager contacts suppliers, compares prices and services, and uses the information collected to choose a new supplier.
- Rhonda is a nursing assistant at an extended-care facility. She has small children at home and must make childcare arrangements at least one week in advance. Several times during the past few weeks her supervisor has changed her schedule with only a day's notice. Rhonda wants to keep her job, but cannot continually find childcare at the last minute. She must find a way to work out this problem with her supervisor.
- Carla, a medical biller, needs to learn a new billing software system as soon as possible to avoid getting behind in her work.

Its All Part of the Job

Karen enjoys her work as the receptionist and administrative dental assistant for Dr. Sims. He has been practicing dentistry for more than 35 years and has a large number of loyal patients. He recently took in a young partner, Dr. Lewis, to help him handle the patient load. And, as he admitted to Karen, he'd like to take a little more time off now that he is getting older.

Karen's job is to keep the office running smoothly. Whenever anyone asks just what it is she does, she tells them it's "different tasks every day, but mainly it means keeping things together!" She has an opportunity to demonstrate what she means by that, when the office receives a request from Amanda, a student at a local high school, to job shadow at Dr. Sims' office. Amanda is considering a career in health care, but isn't sure she knows what type of work she wants to do. She already has developed some office skills from her part-time job at a local bookkeeper's office and thinks she might be able to apply these to something more challenging.

Karen and Dr. Sims talk over the idea. He asks Karen to interview Amanda to see just how serious she is about working in health care. Then he tells her that it is really up to her. "It sounds like it's your job she's interested in knowing more about. So I'll leave it up to you—if you think you have the time to have her here and answer her questions, it's okay with me."

"I think the interview is a good idea," says Karen. "Actually, I'm glad to see a young person take an interest in their future—and take the initiative to learn more about it."

Amanda shows up a few minutes early for her appointment with Karen and demonstrates a strong interest in learning just what it is Karen does each day. The school year ends in two weeks, so it is agreed that Amanda will spend a week in the office as soon as summer vacation begins. Karen stresses to Amanda that patient confidentiality is essential and asks her to sign a confidentiality agreement.

One of Karen's responsibilities is to greet and welcome patients when they come for appointments. Although Amanda had an idea that Karen did more than this, she didn't realize the scope of Karen's work. After a couple of days of job shadowing, her mother asked how it was going.

"I'm really enjoying it. Karen is great. She explains what she's doing. She really lets me see what's 'behind the scenes' at the office."

"Do you think this is the kind of job you might want?" asks her mother.

"Well, maybe. Karen showed me her job description and it's two pages long! I had no idea she did so much," said Amanda.

"My goodness!" exclaimed her mother. "What kinds of things are on there?"

"Well, a bunch that surprised me kind of have to do with math: ordering and paying for supplies, billing patients, handling the petty cash, doing the bank statements—things like that."

"That sounds like a lot of responsibility," comments her mother.

"Actually, I think the more challenging part of the job is when problems come up. Like with patients. Some of them don't understand why what they need done costs so much. Figuring out a plan for them to pay and following up with patients who don't pay on time. Or this week there was a problem with a supplier not delivering some supplies that Dr. Sims needed. Karen had to find another company that could get them to the office the next day. It took some doing, but she managed to get it taken care of."

Questions for Thought and Reflection

1. What are some other health care jobs that require working with math?
2. What are some possible consequences for Dr. Sims if Karen does not work accurately when ordering supplies, billing insurance companies, and handling patient accounts?
3. How do you think Karen uses problem solving strategies when dealing with challenges in the office?

Creating a Personal Reference Guide

After graduation, it's possible that you'll use your textbooks, lecture notes, and completed assignments as resources. Putting together your own reference guide adds even more value to your education by storing useful information that might otherwise be lost. Collecting information, however, is not useful if you can't find it when you need it. It can make life more difficult, rather than help, if it becomes simply another pile of stuff that gets in your way. Design an organized, easy-to-access guide. Select a medium or large three-ring binder and buy a package of index dividers. Start with a few categories and add to them as you proceed through your program. Include a table of contents to help you see what you have at a glance.

You may find it helpful to incorporate building your guide as part of your study sessions. For example, making new vocabulary lists can be part of your review for a terminology quiz. You can do the same thing when learning abbreviations, the steps in procedures, and other facts. These lists can then be included as part of your references. You will be applying the art of effective time management by accomplishing two things at the same time: creating a useful reference guide at the same time as you are studying and reviewing.

The contents of your guide will vary according to your career area and personal preferences. Here are some suggestions. Which ones do you think would be useful to include?

- Names, phone numbers, and addresses of instructors and classmates with whom you want to keep in touch. Include a sentence or two about each one for recall in the future.

- Spelling words from Tables 8-8 and 8-9 in Chapter 8 and other words you are learning and want to review periodically.
- New vocabulary words and their definitions.
- Important health care abbreviations. (When you become employed, your facility will have its own set of abbreviations you can add to your guide.)
- Useful website addresses.
- Names, titles, organizations, phone numbers, and addresses of professional contacts. Make a few notes about each person to refresh your memory later.
- Titles of interesting books, journals, and apps. Also, titles of reference books that might be useful on the job. There are pocket-sized guides and apps for many occupations that contain frequently used measurements, formulas, summaries of common procedures, and so on.
- Inspiring and helpful quotations.
- Names and addresses of professional organizations (see Appendix A).
- Sources of equipment and supplies that were used in your school. (This list may be useful on the job if you are asked to make recommendations for purchases.)
- Summaries of the procedures you have learned. If check-off sheets are used in your classes, consider including them.
- Fact sheets that list measurement systems, test values, and so on. Your textbooks may include these within the body of the book or at the end as appendices.
- Potential employers you learn about from your instructors, graduates, guest speakers, job fairs, newspaper articles, and so on.
- Memberships in professional and civic organizations.

Think of your reference guide as a "living document." Add to it as you progress through your program and career. Your guide will be useful while you are in school, during the job search, and on the job.

Your Externship

Your externship, whether it is called an "internship," "fieldwork experience," "practicum," "clinical experience," or some other name, can be one of the most valuable parts of your education. It provides the final link between your education and your future career. Experienced professionals and/or clinical instructors will guide your work in a real occupational setting. This phase of your education provides you with opportunities to do the following:

- Apply the skills learned in class
- Gain confidence in performing these skills
- Learn firsthand about the expectations of employers
- Practice working with patients
- Think and problem solve in real-life situations
- Demonstrate your abilities to a potential employer (students are sometimes hired to work at their externship site after graduation)

A successful externship requires your full attention and effort. Some students make the mistake of thinking that this part of their education is less important than their academic classes, especially if the externship is graded on a pass–fail basis. But nothing could be further from the truth! The externship really counts in the sense that you now have an impact on real people and real problems. It is also during the externship that you begin to establish your professional reputation. Your performance at this time can influence your ability to get a job.

Not every externship will be ideal. Things will not always go just as you expected or hoped. At these times, it may be necessary for you to adjust your attitude. The truth is, not every work environment will be ideal, either. Act professionally and focus on doing your best to learn and achieve your learning goals. Even difficult situations offer opportunities to practice getting along with others, adapt to a work environment, and solve problems.

Setting Goals for Your Externship

What do you hope to learn from your externship? You will increase your chances of benefitting if you write out goals that express specifically what you want to learn; what skills you hope to practice and acquire and what you hope to accomplish by the end of your externship.

It is recommended that you research the facility where you will be working as much as possible before beginning your externship. This will help you anticipate, prepare good questions for your supervisor, and set appropriate goals. Once at the site, share your goals with your supervisor and discuss what is expected of you.

As you begin your externship, ask if you can meet with your supervisor regularly, such as once a week, to discuss your progress and goals. At the same time, conduct your own personal progress checks to see if you are meeting your expectations and goals.

Having a Positive Approach

Approach your externship with enthusiasm and a positive attitude. Look forward to putting your skills into practice, meeting and learning from interesting people, and securing a good recommendation from your supervisor.

We can choose our reactions to people and events. If you find a staff member at your externship site to be especially annoying, it is natural to become angry or frustrated. But how does this benefit *you*? Negative feelings drain energy and may interfere with your focus on your work. This person is now not only annoying, but has, in a sense, taken over your emotions. Don't give negative people and situations that power.

Here are some suggestions for developing a positive attitude to your work:

- Make an inventory of the good features at your externship site. Examples: Are you encouraged to learn new skills? Are your co-workers willing to help you? Are there opportunities to help others?
- Keep things in perspective. Examples: If a patient does not want to work with an extern, don't take it personally. If your supervisor becomes upset when you make a mistake,

realize that she has many responsibilities and isn't picking on you to be mean.

- Fix your sights on your goals. Don't let everyday frustrations distract you from doing your best.
- When faced with difficulties, distinguish between what you can and cannot change, and concentrate your efforts on what you can change. Examples: You may not change your supervisor's moodiness, but you can ask for information you need from a friendly co-worker. The computer program may have glitches, but you can do your best to learn to work with it.
- Find sources of help and inspiration. Look for role models and possibly a mentor who is willing to spend some time advising you.
- Challenge your negative beliefs. Examples: You may worry that you have little to contribute to the workplace. But think about it: you have recent training and are interested in working and learning. The employer has offered you a position as an extern. Focus now on making the best contribution you can.

Keeping a Journal

Consider keeping a journal during your externship in which you record your thoughts, experiences, and feelings. (Caution: Do not record any patient names or other identifying information in your journal.) Describe significant situations and what you learn from them. For example, describe incidents in which you are either involved or simply observe that cause you to think or feel strongly. Write about your reactions, how you believe the situation was handled, and how you handled—or would have handled—the situation.

Your journal is also a good place to write out your externship goals and record your progress.

Finally, you can include a task log in your journal in which you record the new skills you are acquiring to be added to your resume when you begin your job search.

Success Tips for Your Externship

- Take advantage of the assistance and advice offered by your school. The staff has experience in setting up externships so students will have the best chance to succeed.
- Strive to have excellent attendance. If you must be absent, call the site before the time you are scheduled to arrive and let them know. Your attendance may have a significant impact on the site's ability to deliver services. (Most schools require you to notify them, too.)
- Be sure you understand what you will be expected and allowed to do. Some facilities have students start with relatively easy tasks before giving them more complex assignments. Others have students jump right in with a full set of duties.
- Learn the facility's policies and procedures that apply to your duties.
- Ask questions about anything you don't understand or want to learn more about. Try to determine the answers

for yourself first, but don't hesitate if you are unsure. This is especially important in the case of procedures that have safety consequences for you or the patients.

- Ask an appropriate person to check your work if you are unsure about its accuracy.
- Follow all rules and dress codes, even if others do not seem to be doing so.
- Be courteous to everyone. These are your future professional colleagues, even if your future job is at a different facility.
- Learn as much as possible from the staff. Observe them at work and get to know them as people. Do be careful, though, not to get involved in gossip sessions.
- Become a contributing member of the health care team. Offer to help without being asked.
- Find out how you will be evaluated. Be sure you understand the performance expectations.
- Take advantage of any resources the facility has available. Is there a technical library you can use? Does the facility have reference materials about topics in which you have a special interest? Are there additional opportunities for you to observe and talk with people about their work?
- Apply what you learn in Chapter 16, "Success on the Job." The concepts discussed there apply to externships as well as to paying jobs.

The Simulated Externship

Most health care externships take place off campus at a site such as a doctor's office, clinic, or hospital. For some programs, such as medical coding and medical transcription that do not require interaction with patients and limited interaction with coworkers, externships may be conducted as simulations. Students complete real-world work activities under the supervision of an instructor who acts as the workplace supervisor. Because of the nature of some occupations, students are able to get more hands-on practice in a simulated externship than they would if they were in a medical facility.

Just as with an on-site externship, students are expected to complete all projects accurately and submit them on time. They must apply what they learned in the classroom and are evaluated just as they would be by a workplace supervisor. Working on their own, they are likely to be required to work a certain number of hours, just as they would be at a facility—and later on the job. Students may be asked to keep track of their hours worked on a timesheet.

Success Tips for Simulated Externships

- Treat the work for an externship simulation as seriously as you would if you were on site.
- Plan your work time carefully to complete all projects on time.
- If you work on projects at home, set up a quiet space and let everyone know you are "at work."

1234 Vista Place
Caliente Springs, CA 92000
March 3, 2015

Sarah Gonzalez, Office Manager
Warm Springs Health Clinic
1234 Henderson Road
Happy Rock, CA 92001

Dear Ms. Gonzalez:

I want to thank you for the time you spent helping me to benefit from my externship at Warm Springs Health Clinic. You have a busy schedule, and I very much appreciate the time you took to teach and direct me in my duties. You were patient when I had questions and I learned a great deal from my experience.

Working directly with patients has given me the confidence to seek employment as a medical assistant. Thank you for the letter of recommendation you wrote for me. I'm sure it will be helpful as I pursue my job search. I would welcome any suggestions you might have about people in the field I could contact.

I look forward to keeping in touch with you and the Warm Springs staff.

Sincerely,

Emily Hanson

Emily Hanson

FIGURE 9-6 Example of a thank-you letter to an externship supervisor. Be sure to show your appreciation after completing your externship. *In addition to courtesy, what might be some positive consequences of writing a thank-you letter?*

After Your Externship

In addition to thanking your supervisor verbally and anyone else who helped you, write a thank-you letter to your supervisor and/or employer after completing your externship. Include a statement about what you learned and how he or she helped you to achieve your goals. See Figure 9-6 for a sample thank-you letter.

Be sure to ask your supervisor if he or she will write you a letter of recommendation. This is important, especially if this is your only work experience in the health care field. Keep this in mind as you do your externship: the skills and professionalism you exhibit here can influence your future employment prospects.

Some students are hired by their externship employer, although you should not expect to be offered a job—nor should you ask for one. Some sites prefer to continue offering opportunities to students from local schools and therefore cannot hire every good student who works with them.

Evaluating and Documenting Your Experience

Use your journal and task log to write a summary of what you learned. Marianne Ehrlich Green, author of *Internship Success*[1], suggests that students consider the following questions:

1. Did you meet your learning objectives [goals]? Explain how.

2. What was your most important contribution?
3. What new skills did you develop?
4. What were the highlights of your externship?

When asking yourself these questions, consider the areas that need improvement and how you can do better in your future employment.

Include your externship experience on your resume in either the Education or Work History section. Be sure to make it clear that this was an unpaid position completed before you graduated from your program. You can write a brief description of what you learned, the skills you practiced, or anything else that supports your job objective. Make copies of your letter of recommendation from your externship supervisor to include with your resume or to put in your professional portfolio.

Personal Reflection

1. Which of your personal characteristics do you believe will most help you have a successful externship?
2. Which personal characteristics do you need to work on to increase the benefits you will receive from your experience (e.g., shyness, impatience, or difficulty being on time)?

Paul worked in construction for many years before deciding it was time to hang up the hammer. The climbing, bending, and reaching were starting to get to him and he wanted to be able to enjoy his later years without the injuries he witnessed in older workers.

Paul wasn't ready—or financially able—to retire, so he spent some time thinking about what he wanted to do next. As a teen, he had considered the medical field, but his family didn't have the money for college so he followed his hobby of building things and went into construction with his Uncle Frank. Now in his 50s, Paul thought it might be interesting to check out a health-related career. He ended up enrolling in a medical assisting course and discovered that he really enjoyed the technical aspects of the program.

Being the oldest student in his class bothered him a bit. His study skills were pretty rusty and concentrating on reading took some effort. But he made it through his program and was happy to be assigned to a large orthopedic clinic near his home for his externship.

As the only clinic in the area specializing in orthopedics, the clinic was a busy one. Paul's supervisor, Ms. Adams, only had time to greet him and give him a very brief description of his duties. Paul spent the first couple of days trying to orient himself. As in school, it seemed like everyone was younger than him. This made him self-conscious and hesitant to ask questions about his duties and how he was to perform them. He believed that at his age, he should be able to figure things out for himself.

He tried observing the employees and thinking about what he had learned in school. The confusing thing was that much of what went on at the clinic was either unfamiliar to him or done in ways he had not been taught. Still too embarrassed to ask for help, he did what he believed were his assigned tasks as best he could, keeping to himself much of the time.

Paul believed that his work had been satisfactory, but a couple of weeks into his externship his supervisor called him into her office and informed him that some of his work was unsatisfactory—that he was not following the protocols of the clinic. At this point, Paul became upset, raising his voice and telling Ms. Adams, "I can't believe you're telling me this! I've tried hard to figure out what I'm supposed to do here—and how. I really believe I've done my best."

Ms. Adams replied, "That may be—that you've tried. But if you were having trouble, why didn't you ask for help? You never said anything, so we just assumed you were doing okay. Unfortunately, that's not the case."

Questions for Thought and Reflection

1. Whose responsibility was it to explain Paul's duties when he started his externship?
2. Whose responsibility was it after the first week?
3. What could Paul have done to make his experience at the clinic more positive?
4. What do you think he should do now?

Math Skills

Math is necessary for performing many health care tasks. Examples include measuring a child's height, calculating the correct amount of medication to give a patient, conducting tests, and determining how much to bill an insurance company. It is not necessary to be a math genius, but there are a few basics you must understand to accurately and safely carry out the responsibilities of your job. See Figure 9-7 for an example.

You may have trouble with math. The truth is, with practice, almost everyone can master the fundamentals. Some common reasons why students have trouble with math are itemized in the following list. Do any of them apply to you?

1. They either didn't learn or have forgotten how to perform basic operations, especially those involving fractions, decimals, percentages, ratios, proportions, and simple equations.
2. They don't understand the metric system, which is extensively used in health care as well as the sciences. Many Americans don't know what metric measurements refer to—how big, how much, or how long—because they don't typically use them in daily life.
3. They don't know the meaning of the many strange-looking signs and symbols called *notations*.

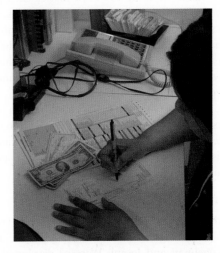

FIGURE 9-7 Math skills are required for many jobs in health care. They may involve only basic operations, but accuracy is essential. *What kinds of math skills might you need for your future career?* (From Bonewit-West K, Hunt S, Applegate E: *Today's medical assistant: Clinical and administrative procedures,* ed 2, St Louis, 2013, Saunders.)

4. They have trouble visualizing math operations in their minds.
5. They memorize formulas without really understanding them or knowing how to apply them to solve problems.
6. They avoid taking math classes. When this is impossible, they may skip class and/or not do all the homework.

Personal Reflection

1. Describe your previous experiences with math classes. Were they positive or negative?
2. Think how you use math (or could use it) in your everyday life. For example, do you understand how interest on loans and credit card balances is calculated? Do you balance your checkbook each month? Can you double a recipe or calculate how much paint to buy for a home-improvement project?

Some Truths About Math

Knowing the truth about something can be helpful. For example, if you are told that "math is really easy" and you find it difficult, you might worry that you are not smart enough to understand it. It would be better to hear that although it may not always be easy, it can be mastered with persistence and practice. So, let's talk about some truths about math.

The first is that although it can be mastered, math is not always easy or fun. The strange symbols and unfamiliar language make it seem difficult, but once you learn to use it, it helps you perform many tasks quickly and efficiently.

Another truth you can use to your advantage is that math knowledge builds on itself. You must master each principle and skill before moving on to the next. Walter Pauk,[2] a noted expert on study skills, believes that the most common reason students have difficulty with math is that they didn't understand an earlier principle or process. This means that getting behind in class can really trip you up. A failure to understand one concept can lead to failure in the next.

Finally, math is a subject in which memorization is helpful, but understanding is essential. In order for math to be useful on the job, you must be able to apply it to new situations. You can do this only if you understand how concepts, operations, and formulas work.

Relieving Math Anxiety

Some students feel helpless and even stupid when faced with math. These feelings have been labeled **math anxiety**. Stanley Kogelman and Joseph Warren[3] developed a series of workshops to help people of all ages approach math with confidence. They firmly believe that math problems are more emotional than intellectual. The material in this section was adapted from their book *Mind over Math*.

Kogelman and Warren suggest that you start by accepting your feelings of anxiety and realizing that many students experience the same feelings. By being aware of and experiencing your emotional reactions, you are in a better position to handle them. The next step is to develop a positive attitude about learning and using math. Having confidence in yourself is one of the most important factors in developing math ability. As an adult student, for example, you have more life experience than you had in grade school. Research has shown that most adults can learn arithmetic in a relatively short time.

Avoid saying, "I can't do math." Negative self-talk defeats you before you even start! It is difficult to concentrate and focus, which is necessary when learning math, when you are anxious and nervous. In other words, math anxiety itself, not your lack of ability, can be a major cause of your problems with math. Relax and take your time. Read and work through math books and problems slowly and carefully. Don't worry if you have to go over a concept many times before you get it. That's okay! If you do feel really stuck, take a short break. The unconscious part of your mind will continue to work, and you may find that the "impossible" problem you left is not so difficult after all.

Finally, don't make the situation worse by avoiding math. Attend all classes, do the studying, and complete all the assignments. Ask questions in class. Stay with it. Work all the examples in your book and do lots of practice problems. Explanations often don't make sense until you've actually worked with the problems yourself.

Q&A with a Health Care Professional

Debbie Sholter

Debbie is a medical assistant in a single-physician office. Debbie describes the use of math in her everyday duties.

Q Can you tell me how you use math and numbers in your work?

A Sometimes we have to convert kilograms and pounds from one to the other. This happens when we get medical records and the patient's weight has been recorded in kilograms. These are usually out of country records. We use the English measurement system—pounds—so I have to change them. I need to make them uniform so we can track things like weight gain and loss. This is important because weight changes can provide clues to a patient's condition. An unexplained weight gain, for example, might mean that a cardiac patient is retaining water.

Q Are there other kinds of conversions you have to make?

A Yes, with medications. Lots of them come in doses for adults, so I have to cut them down for children. You have to calculate by the patient's weight, so you may have to divide or multiply carefully—you can't make any mistakes here! Too much medication can do real harm to the patient.

Another thing with medications is taking health history information. If a patient is taking medications, we have to find out what these are and accurately record the dosages. So we have to understand metric measurements and units and know abbreviations like mcg and mg. Thyroid replacement, for example, comes in micrograms. It's important to understand how diagnostic test numbers relate to medication doses.

Q How about business uses of math?

A I keep a price sheet and collect money from patients. Everything has to add up correctly. For certain insurance companies, we have to calculate percentages to know what the patient should pay—their co-payment, that is.

Then we have to track payments and make change. Many people use credit cards, but some do use cash. So we have to make change accurately.

Some offices do their own billing. The staff has to prepare statements for insurance, calculate write-offs, add the daily intake of money, prepare deposit slips, and take the money to the bank.

Q Do you help with any purchasing?

A Yes, I buy supplies for the office, both front and back. I try to get the best deals by comparing prices. I do this by calculating the price per unit, per test, etc. This also helps the physician determine how much to charge patients. I go through prices at least annually because they change and new suppliers become available. Some employees are paid bonuses, so saving money affects everyone.

Success Tips for Mastering Math

Choose from among the following study techniques the ones that best fit your preferred learning styles:

- Make flash cards for learning "math facts," such as the multiplication tables, formulas, and common conversions.
- Draw pictures of concepts to help you understand them.
- Use paper plates, clay, blocks, and other materials to make shapes and help you see how the parts relate to the whole in fractions and decimals.
- Look for examples of math applications in everyday life: shopping, bills, bank statements, recipes, weights, measurements, taxes, and interest on loans.
- Read math explanations out loud. Be sure you understand each word or idea before moving on.
- Try to translate math concepts into words you are familiar with.
- Mark your book with questions or your own explanations.
- If you don't understand the explanations in your own books or materials, look for others in the library or bookstore, or ask your instructor for resources. Sometimes a different approach helps.
- Buy or borrow a book with exercises and answers. Look for online resources.
- Be proactive. Ask questions about anything you don't understand.
- Write down any calculations the instructor does in class. Be sure to include each step so you can review it later.
- Join or form a math study group.
- Learn how to check your work for correctness. For example, use multiplication to check division problems.

- Try explaining important concepts to someone else. By having to talk about it, you may clarify and understand it better.
- Explain concepts and processes in writing. Pretend you are writing a letter to a friend in which you describe what you are learning in class.
- When studying math, plan to concentrate fully. Remove as many distractions as possible, and try to spend at least 20 minutes of focused time before taking a break.

Math Review

"Most of the fundamental ideas of science are essentially simple, and may be, as a rule, expressed in a language comprehensible to everyone."

—Albert Einstein

Math has its own special language. For example, when referring to a fraction, it is awkward to say "the bottom half" or "the number underneath." Its proper name is "denominator," and knowing this makes talking about it easier. See Table 9-1 for the definitions of common math terms.

The figures in the section "Math Operations Review" contain more math vocabulary along with a brief review of some of the operations commonly used in health care—and commonly forgotten by students! The purpose of the figures is to help you recall math skills you have already learned, not to teach new material. As you are reading the explanations and looking at the examples, keep bear in mind that there are different "right ways" to work out a problem. For example, division problem calculations are not set up the same way in every country—or even in every part of the United States. As you go through the material in the figures, try working the examples. Sometimes explanations don't make much sense until you work with the numbers yourself.

The Multiplication Chart

Knowing the products of all the possible combinations of the numbers 1 through 12 is a great time saver. This is not a substitute for learning how to multiply, but a way to increase your efficiency. It is also a good study aid for learning the multiplication tables. To use the chart in Box 9-2, find the intersection of the two numbers you wish to multiply, one from the row across the top and the other from the far left column. For example, to multiply 3 times 4, find the 3 in the top row and the 4 in the first column. Move down the column from the 3 and across the row from the 4 until the lines meet at 12. This is the answer. Study the chart in Box 9-2, or make flash cards for any combinations you need to memorize. You can also use graph paper to set up blank tables to fill in to review and quiz yourself.

The multiplication chart can also be used as a tool to reduce fractions if the numerator and denominator appear in the same column. For example, for $^{12}/_{96}$, follow both 12 and 96 straight across to the far left column: 12 becomes 1 and 96 becomes 8; $^{12}/_{96} = ^{1}/_{8}$. The fraction may need to be reduced further. For example, $^{24}/_{48} = ^{2}/_{4}$; $^{2}/_{4}$ can be further reduced to $^{1}/_{2}$.

TABLE 9-1

The Language of Math

Word or Phrase	What It Means	Examples
Digit	Any of the numerals 0 to 9	The number 834 has three digits: 8, 3, and 4
Whole number	A number that has no fraction or decimal	5, 67, and 1893 are whole numbers
Mixed number	A number that has two parts: a whole number and a fraction	$1\frac{1}{3}$, $4\frac{1}{2}$, $17\frac{2}{5}$ are mixed numbers
Factors	The numbers being multiplied in a multiplication problem	$8 \times 10 = 80$ 8 and 10 are the factors
Product	The answer to a multiplication problem	$8 \times 10 = 80$ 80 is the product
Dividend	In a division problem, the number to be divided	$72 \div 8 = 9$ 72 is the dividend
Divisor	The number by which the dividend is divided in a division problem	$72 \div 8 = 9$ 8 is the divisor
Quotient	The answer to a division problem	$72 \div 8 = 9$ 9 is the quotient
Cubic measurement	Measure of volume, or the amount of space that something takes up. Medications are sometimes measured in cubic centimeters. (See Table 9-2 for an explanation of the centimeter)	To calculate the volume of a box, multiply the height by the width by the length A box that is 3 feet long, 2 feet high, and 5 feet wide = $3 \times 2 \times 5 = 30$ cubic feet
Place value chart	A chart that shows the unit values of the places that follow the decimal point	Tenths 0.1 Hundredths 0.01 Thousandths 0.001 Ten thousandths 0.0001 Hundred thousandths 0.00001

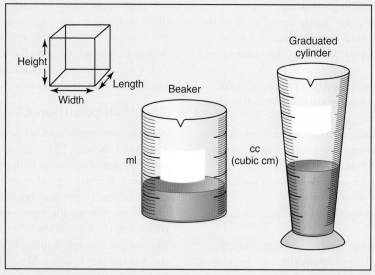

Volume is a measurement of space, such as in a box or containers of various shapes.

Making Sense of the Metric System

The **metric system** is an obstacle for many students. It is actually a very logical system of measurement based on multiples of 10. Used in most countries other than the United States, it also serves as the measuring system for science and health care. People who come to the United States find it difficult to learn our units of measurement. Our units have names that don't follow any pattern: "inch," "foot," "yard," "pound," "mile," and so on.

To make things even more confusing, some of these words—"foot," "yard," and "pound"—have other meanings as well!

Here are some facts to help you better understand the metric system:

1. It works on a base of 10. This means that the units of measurement are created by multiplying to make larger units and dividing to make smaller units by powers of 10 (10, 100, 1000, 10,000, etc.).

BOX 9-2 **Multiplication Chart**

1	1	2	3	4	5	6	7	8	9	10	11	12
2	2	4	6	8	10	12	14	16	18	20	22	24
3	3	6	9	12	15	18	21	24	27	30	33	36
4	4	8	12	16	20	24	28	32	36	40	44	48
5	5	10	15	20	25	30	35	40	45	50	55	60
6	6	12	18	24	30	36	42	48	54	60	66	72
7	7	14	21	28	35	42	49	56	63	70	77	84
8	8	16	24	32	40	48	56	64	72	80	88	96
9	9	18	27	36	45	54	63	72	81	90	99	108
10	10	20	30	40	50	60	70	80	90	100	110	120
11	11	22	33	44	55	66	77	88	99	110	121	132
12	12	24	36	48	60	72	84	96	108	120	132	144

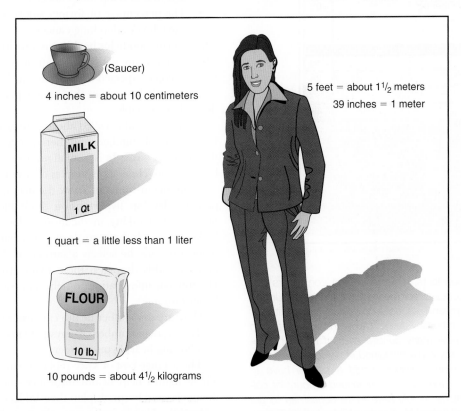

FIGURE 9-8 The metric system as it applies to measurements is easier to understand if you think in terms of how each unit compares to our more familiar U.S. units of measure. *Label a few things around your house or apartment in metric units.*

2. Prefixes that designate multiples of 10 are added to the basic units of measurement to make them larger or smaller. The same prefixes are used for all the basic units, so you have to remember only one set. (Examples: *milli*meter, *milli*liter, and *milli*gram are all one thousandth of a unit of measurement.)

micro-	0.00001
milli-	0.001
centi-	0.01
deci-	0.1
deka-, deca	10
hecto-	100
kilo-	1000

3. A knowledge of decimals is important for understanding metric units of measurement. (See the "Math Operations Review" section for a review of decimals.)

Americans who don't often use the metric system find it difficult. We know about how far a mile is, but we may be lost if someone asks us if we'd like go on a 5-kilometer walk. The easiest way to begin understanding the metric system is to learn the names of the various weights and measures and then get a feel for what each one represents. Then you can start doing conversions between the two systems, and this requires some math. Figure 9-8 illustrates some examples of metric equivalents. Figure 9-9 shows a common application of the metric system found on every grocery store shelf.

Nutrition Facts

Serving Size 1 cup (228g)
Servings Per Container about 2

Amount Per Serving

Calories 250   Calories from Fat 110

	% Daily Value*
Total Fat 12g	18%
Saturated Fat 3g	15%
Trans Fat 3g	
Cholesterol 30mg	10%
Sodium 470mg	20%
Total Carbohydrate 31g	10%
Dietary Fiber 0g	0%
Sugars 5g	
Proteins 5g	
Vitamin A	4%
Vitamin C	2%
Calcium	20%
Iron	4%

* Percent Daily Values are based on a 2,000 calorie diet.
Your Daily Values may be higher or lower depending on
your calorie needs:

	Calories:	2,000	2,500
Total Fat	Less than	65g	80g
Saturated Fat	Less than	20g	25g
Cholesterol	Less than	300mg	300mg
Sodium	Less than	2,400mg	2,400mg
Total Carbohydrate		300g	375g
Dietary Fiber		25g	30g

For educational purposes only. This label does not meet the labeling
requirements described in 21 CFR 101.9.

FIGURE 9-9 Nutrition facts, required so that consumers can see what their food contains, are reported in metric units. Understanding what these mean is especially important today, with our increased emphasis on healthy eating. *Using the information in Table 9-2, calculate how many ounces each of total fat, cholesterol, and carbohydrates are contained in the food described on this label. How many servings would a person have to eat to obtain 100% of the daily recommended amount of calcium? How many calories would have to be consumed to get 100% of the calcium?* (From U.S. Food and Drug Administration, Labeling & Nutrition, http://www.fda.gov/Food/IngredientsPackagingLabeling/LabelingNutrition/ucm114155.htm)

Table 9-2 contains explanations of common metric units and compares them to the U.S. measuring system.

Statistics

Statistics is the science of collecting and analyzing large quantities of numerical data. The data can be expressed in a number of ways. Two common ways are **percentages** and **averages**. The following examples of percentages would be of interest to health care providers:

- The percentage of Americans who are overweight or obese
- The percentage of current or former smokers who develop lung cancer
  - The percentage of former smokers who quit 20 years ago who develop lung cancer
  - The percentage of former smokers who quit 10 years ago who develop lung cancer

This information helps health care providers prepare to treat and care for future patients. A statistic such as the number of elderly people expected to enter nursing homes in the next 20 years is needed to ensure that an adequate number of facilities will be available.

An average (also called the mean) is calculated by adding a group of numbers and then dividing by the number in the group. A **sample** is a small number taken to represent a larger group. Here are examples of average and sample:

A physician wants to know the average age at which his patients develop hypertension (high blood pressure) and need to start taking medication to lower it. Rather than looking through the records of every patient who has high blood pressure, he selects a sample of 25. He lists the age of each, adds the ages, then divides that number by 25. He now has information to help him watch his patients for hypertension.

Here are some other health care examples using averages:

- The average number of days patients stay in the hospital following heart bypass surgery
- The average cost of knee replacement surgery

These figures help health insurance companies determine their costs and hospitals plan their budgets.

Statistics play an important role in medical research. Drug companies, for example, perform clinical trials to determine the effectiveness of new drugs. They need to determine the percentage of people participating in the trials who responded positively to the drug being tested to determine its overall effectiveness.

TABLE 9-2

Units of Measure

Type of Measurement	Units of Measurement	How It Compares with the U.S. System
Length or distance	*meter* (m) = basic unit	A little more than 1 yard (1 yard = 36 inches and 1 meter = 39.37 inches)
	millimeter (mm) = 0.001 meter	About the size of the width of a pinhead. There are just over 25 millimeters in 1 inch
	centimeter (cm) = 0.01 meter	About ⅖ (or 0.4) of an inch, the width of a child's little finger. There are about 2½ centimeters in an inch
	decimeter (dm) = 0.1 meter	About 4 inches
	dekameter (dam) = 10 meters	A little more than 10 yards
	hectometer (hm) = 100 meters	A little more than 100 yards
	kilometer (km) = 1000 meters	About ⅗ (or 0.62) of a mile
Liquids or volume	liter (L) = basic unit	Approximately 1 quart (2 liters is now a popular size for soft drink bottles; that's about ½ gallon because there are 4 quarts in a gallon)
	*milliliter** (mL) = 0.001 liter	*Very* small drop (commonly used in medicine)
	centiliter (cL) = 0.01 liter	About 2 teaspoons
	deciliter (dL) = 0.1 liter	Between ⅓ and ½ cup
	dekaliter (daL) = 10 liters	About 10 quarts or 2½ gallons
	hectoliter (hL) = 100 liters	About 25 gallons
	kiloliter (kL) = 1000 liters	About 250 gallons
Weight or mass of solids	*gram* (gm, g) = basic unit	Approximately ¹⁄₂₈ of an ounce. About the weight of a paperclip.
	microgram (mcg) = 0.000001 gram	An incredibly small amount (1 millionth of ¹⁄₄₀₀ of a pound!!) Don't be fooled, however. This can be a significant amount in health care. The body depends on *very* small quantities of certain substances to function properly. It can also be harmed by *very* small amounts of the wrong substances.
	milligram (mg) = 0.001 gram	Also very small amounts, although they are many times heavier than a microgram.
	centigram (cg) = 0.01 gram	
	decigram (dg) = 0.1 gram	
	dekagram (dag) = 10 grams	⁵⁄₁₄ of an ounce
	hectogram (hg) = 100 grams	About 3½ ounces
	kilogram (kg) = 1000 grams	2.2 pounds
Temperature	*Celsius* (commonly called centigrade)	Fahrenheit is the system commonly used in the United States. In this system, 32° F is freezing and 95° F is a sunny day at the beach
	0° C = freezing point of water	
	100° C = boiling point of water	
	Celsius thermometers are marked in one-tenth intervals	1° C = 1.8 times 1° F
	Water freezes: 0° C	32° F
	Normal body temperature: 37°C	98.6° F
	Water boils: 100° C	212° F
	Sterilization occurs: 121° C	250° F
	To convert between the two systems:	
	Fahrenheit to Celsius:	98.6° F
	1. Subtract 32 from the F temperature	98.6−32 = 66.6
	2. Multiply by ⁵⁄₉	⁵⁄₉ × 66.6 = ⁵⁄₉ × 66.6/1 = 37
		Another way to solve for approximate answer:
		66.6 ÷ 1.8 = 36.7
	Celsius to Fahrenheit:	
	1. Multiply the C temperature by ⁹⁄₅ (or 1.8)	37 × ⁹⁄₅ = ³⁷⁄₁ × ⁹⁄₅ = ³³³⁄₅ = 66.6
	2. Add 32	66.6 + 32 = 98.6
		Another way to solve:
		37 × 1.8 + 32 = 98.6

Note: Units in italics are the most common units of measurement in health care.

*A milliliter is the same amount as a cubic centimeter (cc). This is important to know in health care because these terms are sometimes used interchangeably.

Using Math on the Job Reading numbers correctly and performing math calculations accurately are critical to patient safety.

Here are some examples of how health care professionals use math:

- They calculate the correct amount of medication to administer. This is one of the most important applications of math in health care occupations. Medication is one of our most effective treatments today. At the same time, medication errors are responsible for thousands of deaths and more than one million patient injuries each year. Medications are sometimes ordered by physicians using a different system or dosage (amount) than that which is used by the suppliers. It is sometimes necessary to convert from one system to another and then calculate the proper quantity to administer. These calculations require an understanding of the various systems of measurement, as well as how to use proportions and solve equations.

- They take and record vital signs. The metric system is sometimes used when a patient's weight, height, and temperature are recorded. Blood pressure is expressed in millimeters, a metric measurement. Body temperature may be measured using either the Fahrenheit or Celsius system. Figure 9-10 contrasts the readings for normal body temperature.
- They calculate the body mass index by dividing the weight in pounds by the height in inches squared and multiplying by a conversion factor of 703.
  - Example: Weight = 150 lbs, Height = 5′5″ (65″)
  - Calculation: $[150 \div (65)^2] \times 703 = 24.96$
- They bill for services. Patient bills must be calculated accurately and recorded properly to ensure the proper payment is received from insurance companies. Adjustments must be calculated when insurance payments are posted. Some patients pay in cash, so the ability to calculate the correct change and track amounts of cash for bank deposits is essential.

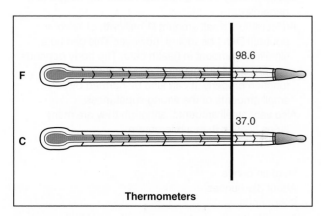

Thermometers

FIGURE 9-10 You may use both Fahrenheit and Celsius systems when working in health care. Notice how much more heat is represented in a one-degree rise in temperature measured in Celsius than in Fahrenheit. *What would a temperature of 38.4 Celsius be in Fahrenheit?*

□ **Prescription for Success: 9-4 Learn with Practice**

Practice learning the metric system by using it at home. If you don't have a measuring stick or ruler that is marked in centimeters and millimeters, buy an inexpensive one. Measure and make labels for common items. For example, the height of a doorknob is about 1 meter from the floor. As you see them over and over, you will start to incorporate metric equivalents into your thinking.

Math Operations Review

	FRACTIONS	
	The Language of Fractions	
Word or Phrase	**What It Means**	**Examples**
Fraction	A part of a whole. Always written as two numbers, one on top of the other.	½ represents 1 of the 2 equal parts into which a whole of something has been divided. ⁵⁄₁₂ represents 5 of the 12 equal parts into which a whole has been divided.
Numerator	The top number in a fraction. It tells you how many pieces of the whole you have.	In the fraction ½, 1 is the numerator. In ⁵⁄₁₂, 5 is the numerator.
Denominator	The bottom number in a fraction. It tells you into how many equal pieces a whole has been divided. The larger the number, the smaller the pieces.	In ½, 2 is the denominator. In ⁵⁄₁₂, 12 is the denominator.
Proper fraction	A fraction in which the numerator is smaller than the denominator.	¾ 3 is smaller than 4.
Improper fraction	A fraction in which the numerator is larger than the denominator.	⁴⁄₃ 4 is larger than 3. This represents a whole number and a fraction: 1⅓. (There are 3 thirds in a whole, which equals 1. ⅓ represents the additional—or fourth—third.)
Lowest common denominator	The smallest number that can be evenly divided (leaving no remainder) by all the denominators in a series of fractions. It is necessary to find this number when you want to add or subtract fractions.	The lowest common denominator for ⅙, ¾, and ⅝ is 24.
Simplest form	A fraction in which the numerator and denominator cannot be any smaller. (They cannot be evenly divided by the same number.)	½ is the simplest form of the following fractions: ²⁄₄, ³⁄₆, ⁴⁄₈, ⁵⁄₁₀, ²⁵⁄₅₀.

Continued

Operation:	Reduce fractions to their simplest form.

What to Do:	**Problem:**	Reduce ¹⁸⁄₃₀ to its simplest form.
	Step 1:	Find a number that divides evenly into both the numerator and the denominator. Both 18 and 30 can be divided evenly by 2, resulting in ⁹⁄₁₅.
	Step 2:	Ask yourself if the fraction can be reduced further. Is there another number that divides evenly into both the numerator and denominator? If not, you're finished! If so, identify that number. In our example, both 9 and 15 can be divided evenly by 3, resulting in ³⁄₅.
	Answer:	³⁄₅ is the simplest form of ¹⁸⁄₃₀. **Note:** This could also have been done in one step by dividing 18 and 30 by 6.

Operation:	Change fractions so they share the lowest common denominator. You need to do this before adding or subtracting fractions that have different denominators.

What to Do:	**Problem:**	Find the lowest common denominator for ⅙, ¾, and ⅝.
	Step 1:	Test various numbers to find the smallest number that can be evenly divided by all the denominators in a series of fractions. **Hint:** Multiply the denominators by one another to find at least one common denominator. This may not be the smallest common denominator, but it gives you a starting point. In this problem, we need a number that can be divided by 6, 4, and 8 leaving no remainder. By trying several possibilities, we find that 24 is the lowest common denominator for ⅙, ¾, and ⅝.
	Step 2:	For each fraction, divide the new denominator by the original denominator. For ⅙: 24 ÷ 6 = 4 For ¾: 24 ÷ 4 = 6 For ⅝: 24 ÷ 8 = 3
	Step 3:	Multiply each quotient (answer) from step 2 by the numerator of the corresponding fraction. This number is the new numerator. For ⅙: 4 × 1 = 4–New fraction is ⁴⁄₂₄ For ¾: 6 × 3 = 18–New fraction is ¹⁸⁄₂₄ For ⅝: 3 × 5 = 15–New fraction is ¹⁵⁄₂₄ You can now add and subtract these "new fractions" because they all have the same denominator: 24.

Operation:	Converting improper fractions to mixed numbers. You will sometimes get an improper fraction after performing a calculation, such as adding two fractions. Improper fractions must be changed because it isn't correct usage to record them.

What to Do:	**Problem:**	Convert ¹⁰⁄₄ to a mixed number.
	Step 1:	Divide the numerator by the denominator. 10 ÷ 4 = 2 with a remainder of 2
	Step 2:	If there is a remainder (R), it becomes the numerator of a fraction. The denominator is the same as in the original improper fraction. 2²⁄₄
	Step 3:	Reduce the fraction, if necessary. 2²⁄₄ = 2½
	Answer:	2½

Operation:	Add fractions.
What to Do:	**Problem:** $\frac{1}{6} + \frac{3}{4} + \frac{5}{8} = ?$
	Step 1: If the fractions do not have the same denominator, find the lowest common denominator. 24 is the lowest common denominator for these fractions.
	Convert the fraction(s): $\frac{1}{6} = \frac{4}{24}$
	$\frac{3}{4} = \frac{18}{24}$
	$\frac{5}{8} = \frac{15}{24}$
	Step 2: Add the numerators. (Keep the same common denominator.) $\frac{4}{24} + \frac{18}{24} + \frac{15}{24} = \frac{37}{24}$
	Step 3: Simplify the result if it is an improper fraction. $37 \div 24 = 1$ R 13
	Answer: $1\frac{13}{24}$

Operation:	Subtract fractions.
What to Do:	**Problem:** $\frac{5}{8} - \frac{1}{4} = ?$
	Step 1: If the fractions do not have the same denominator, find the lowest common denominator. 8 is the lowest common denominator (recall that this is the number into which both denominators can be divided evenly). Convert the fraction(s): $\frac{1}{4} = \frac{2}{8}$ (**Note:** In this case, one of the fractions contains the lowest common denominator.)
	Step 2: Perform the calculation by subtracting the second numerator from the first. $\frac{5}{8} - \frac{2}{8} = \frac{3}{8}$
	Answer: $\frac{3}{8}$
	Step 3: Reduce the fractions, if necessary. (Not necessary with 3/8.) **Note:** When subtracting mixed numbers, change them to improper fractions before subtracting the numerators.
	Here's how: Let's start with $1\frac{5}{8}$.
	Step 1: Multiply the whole number by the denominator. $8 \times 1 = 8$ Add the product (answer to the multiplication operation) to the numerator of the fraction, and use the result as the new numerator. $8 + 5 = 13$ Use the same denominator as in the original fraction.
	Answer: $\frac{13}{8}$

Continued

Operation:	Multiply fractions.	
What to Do:	**Problem:**	½ × ¾ = ?
	Step 1:	Multiply the numerators by each other and then the denominators by each other. Numerators: 1 × 3 = 3 Denominators: 2 × 4 = 8 Create a new fraction with the products: ⅜
	Answer:	⅜
	Step 2:	Reduce the fraction, if necessary.

Operation:	Divide fractions (everyone's big fear!). What you are figuring out: how many fractions will fit into another fraction.	
What to Do:	**Problem:**	¾ ÷ ½ = ?
	Step 1:	Invert (switch) the numerator and the denominator of the divisor (the number "doing the dividing"). ½ inverted becomes ²⁄₁. Use this fraction in the following steps.
	Step 2:	Multiply the numerators by each other and the denominators by each other. (That's right—you don't actually divide as we know it. This is what makes an otherwise simple operation seem confusing and hard to remember!) Numerators: 3 × 2 = 6 Denominators: 4 × 1 = 4 Create a new fraction with the products: ⁶⁄₄
	Answer:	⁶⁄₄
	Step 3:	Simplify and/or reduce the fraction, if necessary. ⁶⁄₄ is an improper fraction. Simplify by dividing 6 by 4. 6 ÷ 4 = 1 R 2 The proper fraction is 1²⁄₄. (**Note:** The remainder becomes the numerator of the fraction. The denominator is the same as in the improper fraction.) Reduce the fraction by dividing 2 and 4 by 2.
	Answer:	1½

Examples of Fractions in Health Care

Fluid intake and output

1. Janice drinks 1½ cups of juice, ⅓ cup of water, and ⅝ glass of soda. What is her total fluid input?

Changes in weight and height

2. Al weighed 175¼ pounds. After following a recommended diet, he weighs 162½ pounds. How much weight did he lose?
3. During the first month of life an infant grew ½ inch, ⅝ inch during the second, and ¾ inch during the third. How much did the infant grow in 3 months?

Units of time

4. Cassie worked in the front office for 2½ hours, in the back for 3¾, and in the lab for 1⅓. How many hours did she work?
5. If Cassie earns $16.00 an hour, how much did she earn for the work in the previous problem?

Quantities

6. A patient takes ¾ ounce of a liquid antacid twice a day. How long will a 24-ounce bottle last?

DECIMALS
The Language of Decimals

Word or Phrase	What It Means	Examples
Decimal	Like fractions, decimals represent parts of a whole. Decimals are written using a point, the same symbol as a period. When decimals are expressed as fractions, they always have denominators written in units of 10 (10, 100, 1000, 10,000, etc.).	0.3 = ³/₁₀. Both represent 3 of the 10 equal parts of a whole.

Placement Value Chart

Hundred thousands	Ten thousands	Thousands		Hundreds	Tens	Ones		Tenths	Hundredths	Thousandths	Ten thousandths	Hundred thousandths
6	5	4	,	3	2	1	.	2	3	4	5	6

Place values of the number 654,321.23456

Continued

Note: The examples for operations with decimals are worked out manually. If you use a calculator, you don't need to align the decimal points. Simply include them in the numbers you enter in the calculator. The decimal points will then appear in the right locations in your answers.

Operation: Add decimals.

What to Do: **Problem:** Add 3.96 + 4.229 + 6.1 = ?

Step 1: Line up the numbers so the decimal points are aligned.

3.96
4.229
6.1

Step 2: Use zeros to fill in the spaces to the right of the decimal point so that all the numbers have the same number of digits. (**Note:** Zero is a digit.)

3.960
4.229
6.100

Step 3: Add as you would whole numbers.

3.960
4.229
6.100
14289

Step 4: Place the decimal point in the answer directly under the points in the numbers you added.

3.960
4.229
6.100
14.289

Answer: 14.289

Operation: Subtract decimals.

What to Do: **Problem:** 72.5 − 18.453 = ?

Step 1: Line up the numbers so the decimal points are aligned.

72.5
18.453

Step 2: Use zeros to fill in the spaces to the right of the decimal point so that both numbers have the same number of digits.

72.500
18.453

Step 3: Subtract as you would whole numbers.

72.500
−18.453
54047

Step 4: Place the decimal point in the answer directly under the points in the numbers you subtracted.

72.500
−18.453
54.047

Answer: 54.047

Operation:	Multiply decimals.	

What to Do:	**Problem:**	$16.953 \times 3.52 = ?$

Step 1: Multiply as you would whole numbers. (**Note:** You do not fill in with zeros as you did in the addition and subtraction problems.)

```
   16.953
×   3.52
   33906 (2 × 16953)
 84765 (5 × 16953)
50859 (3 × 16953)
5967456
```

(**Note:** If you are using a calculator, you will not have 3 products to add together.)

Step 2: Count the number of decimal places in the two factors. To do this, start at the far right of each factor and count left until you reach the decimal point. Next, starting at the far right of the answer, count this number of places to the left. This is where you place the decimal point in the answer.

16.953–3 places

3.52–2 places

Total = 5 places

Count 5 places to the left: 59.67456

Answer: 59.67456

Operation:	Divide decimals.	

What to Do:	**Problem:**	$9 \div 2.5 = ?$

Step 1: Set up the problem as you would if you were dividing whole numbers.

$2.5\overline{)9}$

Step 2: If the divisor is a decimal, move the decimal point to the right, placing it immediately after the last digit in the number. Then move the decimal point in the dividend to the right the same number of places, adding zeros if necessary.

$25.\overline{)90.0}$

Step 3: Divide as you would with whole numbers.

```
      36
25)90.0
   75
   150
```

Step 4: Place the decimal point in the answer directly above the decimal point in the dividend.

```
      3.6
25)90.0
   75
   150
```

Answer: 3.6

Continued

Operation: Change decimals to fractions.

What to Do: **Problem:** 0.25 = ?

Step 1: Write the numbers in the decimal as the numerator (drop the decimal point). Numerator is 25

Step 2: Write the unit of the decimal as the denominator. (tenths, hundredths, thousandths, etc. See Placement Value Chart).

0.25 has 2 places (digits) to the right of the decimal point. Therefore the denominator is 100. The fraction is $^{25}/_{100}$

Step 3: Reduce the fraction, if necessary.

Both 25 and 100 can be divided evenly by 25:

25 ÷ 25 = 1

100 ÷ 25 = 4

The reduced fraction is ¼.

Answer: 0.25 = ¼

Operation: Change fractions to decimals.

What to Do: **Problem:** ¾ = ?

Step 1: Set up a division problem in which the numerator is divided by the denominator. $4\overline{)3}$

Step 2: If the dividend is smaller than the divisor, write a decimal point and add one or more zeros to the dividend, as needed. If there is already a decimal point, add the necessary zeros. $4\overline{)3.00}$

Step 3: Divide as you would with whole numbers.

$$
\begin{array}{r}
75 \\
4\overline{)3.00} \\
\underline{28} \\
20 \\
\underline{20} \\
0
\end{array}
$$

Step 4: Place the decimal point in the answer directly above the decimal point in the dividend.

$$
\begin{array}{r}
.75 \\
4\overline{)3.00}
\end{array}
$$

Answer: ¾ = 0.75

Examples of Decimals in Health Care

Temperatures

1. At 8:15 AM, a patient's temperature measures 104.5° F. At 2:30 PM, it is 101.2° F. What is the decrease in his temperature?

Quantities

2. You are to administer 5.25 milligrams of medication to a patient daily. In the morning, he received 2.5 milligrams. What is the remaining dose for today?

3. If a patient is to take 4.5 milligrams of a drug and it is available in 1.5-milligram tablets, how many tablets must she take?

Costs and expenses

4. A box of 100 disposable gloves costs $6.50 and a case containing 1000 gloves costs $49.46. Which quantity is the better deal for a large clinic that uses at least 1500 gloves per month?

Statistical data

5. In 1 year, the following costs were incurred because of injuries: motor-vehicle crashes, $199.6 billion; work injuries, $132.1 billion; home injuries, $118.1 billion; and public injuries, $82.1 billion. What was the total cost incurred for injuries that year?

PERCENTS
The Language of Percents

Word or Phrase	What It Means	Examples
Percent	A fraction with a denominator of 100 that is expressed as a whole number with a percent sign.	37% represents 37 of the 100 parts of a whole. It is the same as $^{37}/_{100}$ and 0.37.

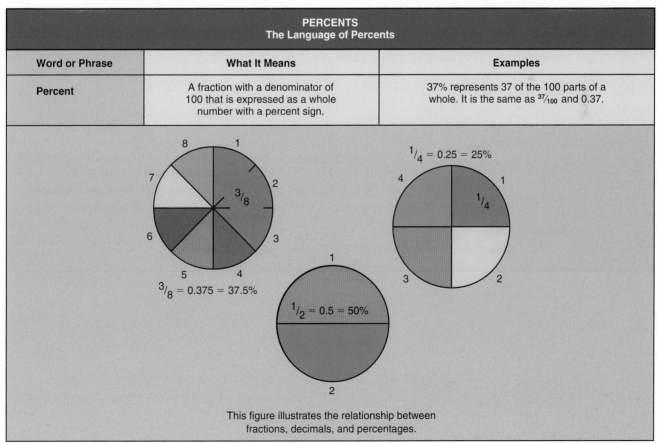

This figure illustrates the relationship between fractions, decimals, and percentages.

Continued

Operation: Change percentages to decimals.

What to Do: **Problem:** Change 41% to a decimal.

Step 1: Start counting from the decimal point and move it 2 places to the left. Fill in with zeros as needed. If the whole number does not have a decimal point written in, it is understood to be located at the far right side of the number. In this problem, the decimal point is understood to be directly to the right of the 1.

41.0

.41

Now drop the percent sign.

Answer: 0.41

(**Note:** A zero is usually added to the left of the decimal point when there is no whole number. This is done to prevent confusion if the point symbol cannot be seen.)

Problem: Change 8.5% to a decimal.

Step 1: Start counting from the decimal point and move it 2 places to the left. Add zeros if necessary.

08.5

0.085

Now drop the percent sign.

Answer: 0.085

Operation: Calculate amounts represented by percentages. This requires first converting the percentages to decimals.

What to Do: **Problem:** Find 65% of 730.

Step 1: Change the percent to a decimal.
65% = 0.65

Step 2: Multiply the number for which you want the percent by the decimal.

$$\begin{array}{r} 730 \\ \times\ 0.65 \\ \hline 3650 \\ 4380 \\ \hline 47450 \end{array}$$

Step 3: Count the number of decimal places in the two factors. Starting at the far right of the answer, count this number of places to the left. This is where you place the decimal point in the answer. **Note:** In the first factor–730–the decimal point is understood to be immediately following the zero.

Answer: 474.5

Note: Extra zeros to the far right of the decimal point can be dropped in the answer.

Examples of Percents in Health Care

Solution concentrations

1. If a physician orders a 12% solution of medication to be infused (allowed to flow into a patient) over 1 hour, how many parts of medication should be added to 100 parts of solution?

Comparisons and changes

2. In 1 year, General Hospital admitted 5343 patients. Just over 27% were patients with heart attacks. How many patients were admitted because of heart attacks?

3. The following year, the hospital initiated a heart wellness program for the community. That year, 1283 patients were admitted because of heart attacks. What was the percentage decrease in heart attack patients? (**Hint:** First calculate the difference between last year's and this year's heart attack patients.)

4. Mr. Jaspers lowers his cholesterol number from 243 to 213. By what percent does he lower his cholesterol? (**Hint:** First calculate the difference between the 2 cholesterol numbers.)

Purchasing

5. If a medical office agrees to buy all its computer and printing supplies from the Good Byte Company, it will receive a 20% discount. The office manager just ordered $7314 in goods from Good Byte. How much will the office pay after the discount?

Continued

EQUATIONS

The Language of Equations

Word or Phrase	What It Means	Examples
Equation	An equation is a statement that 2 quantities are equal. This equality is represented by an equals sign. Equations help you find values for unknown quantities by using the information you do know. The unknown quantities are commonly represented by letters, such as "x."	$x \div 12 = 18$ $6x - 4 = 30 + 26$

Working with Equations

Operation: Solve simple equations.

What to Do:

Problem: Solve for the value of x:

$5 + x = 12$

Reorganize the equation so that the unknown (x) is by itself on one side of the equals sign. Do this by adding, subtracting, multiplying, or dividing *both* sides of the equation by the same number. In this equation, subtracting 5 from each side will leave x by itself on the left side:

$5 + x - 5 = 12 - 5$

Answer: $x = 7$

Problem: Solve for the value of x:

$6x - 3 = 15$

Eliminate 3 by adding it to each side of the equation:

$6x - 3 + 3 = 15 + 3$

$6x = 18$

To get x by itself (in other words, to get 1 x), divide each side by 6:

$6x \div 6 = 18 \div 6$

Answer: $x = 3$

Note: As you see in the second problem, you may have to do more than one calculation to isolate x completely. Also, it is understood that x represents 1 x.

PROPORTIONS
The Language of Proportions

Word or Phrase	What it Means	Examples
Ratio	Expresses the relationship between 2 numbers. Ratios can be written several ways.	Most common way to write a ratio: 1:2 Other ways to write ratios: 1 to 2 ½
Proportion	Statement that 2 ratios or fractions are equal (show the same relationship between their numbers).	1:2::5:10 ½ = $^5/_{10}$ "1 is to 2 as 5 is to 10" (Why? Because 1 is half of 2 and 5 is half of 10. The two sets of numbers—the ratios—have the same relationship to each other.)

Working with Proportions

Operation: Find an unknown quantity in a proportion.

What to Do: **Problem:** Find the value of X in 1:2::10:X.

Step 1: Write each ratio as a fraction.

½ = $^{10}/_X$

Step 2: Multiply the denominators by the opposite numerators.

½ × $^{10}/_X$

$1 \times X = 2 \times 10$

$1 \times X = X$

$2 \times 10 = 20$

$X = 20$

Step 3: Solve for X, if necessary. (Not necessary in this problem.)

Step 4: Write out the completed proportion.

Answer: 1:2::10:20

(Say: 1 is to 2 as 10 is to 20)

Problem: Find the value of X in X:12::3:9.

Step 1: Write each ratio as a fraction.

$^X/_{12}$ = $^3/_9$

Step 2: Multiply the denominators by the opposite numerators.

$^X/_{12}$ × $^3/_9$

$X \times 9 = 9X$

$12 \times 3 = 36$

Therefore $9X = 36$

Step 3: Solve for X.

$9X \div 9 = 36 \div 9$

$X = 4$

Step 4: Write out the completed proportion.

Answer: 4:12::3:9

(Say: 4 is to 12 as 3 is to 9)

Continued

Examples of Proportions in Health Care

Medications

1. If 200 milliliters of solution contains 25 grams of pure drug, how many grams are contained in 75 milliliters?
2. If there are 600 milligrams in three tablets of a drug, how many milligrams are there in five tablets?

Quantities

3. If a cup of canned soup contains 650 grams of sodium, how many grams are there in ¾ cup?

Measurement conversions

4. If 2.2 kilograms (kg) equals 1 pound and a patient weighs 65 kg, what is his weight in pounds?
5. A patient is directed to take 2 teaspoons of medication per dose. The bottle of medication is labeled in milliliters. If a teaspoon equals 4.93 milliliters, how many milliliters should the patient take per dose?

Prescription for Success: 9-5 What's Your Math Status?

1. Based on your review of the figures in the "Math Operations Review" section, how would you rate your knowledge of math? Is it excellent, very good, good, fair, or poor?
2. What math skills are required in your future profession?
3. If you don't know what math skills you will need, where can you find out?
4. If you rated yourself as "fair" or "poor," what plans do you have for improving?
   - Take classes at school
   - Use special services at school, such as computer lab or tutoring
   - Study on my own
   - Use workbooks with math problems
   - Use math software
   - View videos
   - Other

Summary of Key Ideas

- Practicing hands-on procedures forms a bridge between school and the world of work.
- Online classes must be approached differently from on-campus classes.
- Learning to think critically and solve problems effectively can improve your personal and professional life.
- Creating a personal reference guide can add to the value of your education.

- An externship is your opportunity to experience the real world of health care.
- The ability to learn math is based as much on our emotions as on our intelligence.
- Math anxiety can be overcome if we accept our feelings and are willing to find out what we need to learn.

Positive Self-Talk for This Chapter

- I am perfecting my skills by the work I do in lab sessions.
- I use problem solving techniques to make sound decisions.
- I am presenting myself competently and professionally on my externship.
- I am overcoming my math anxiety and learning what I need to know for health care applications.

Internet Activities

For active links to the websites needed to complete these activities, visit http://evolve.elsevier.com/Haroun/career/

1. The Centers for Disease Control and Prevention have developed guidelines for health care workers who come into contact with blood and other body fluids. Explore this site for information about diseases transmitted by blood, and write a short report about practices you can apply in school lab sessions.
2. Math.com contains links to explanations of math operations, sample problems, games, and quizzes for a whole range of math topics. Use the information on the website to learn more about a function you find difficult, and report on what you learned.

3. St Louis University maintains a site called Success in Mathematics that contains good information for students. Using the information you find, explain the difference between active and passive learning; explain how studying math is different from studying other subjects; and list two helpful hints you think might help you with math.

4. The Study Guides and Strategies website has published an excellent explanation of problem solving. Write a brief report summarizing what new information you learn about problem solving from this study guide.

Building Your Resume

1. Think about any lab classes you have taken or practical exercises you have completed for your classes. Are there examples of skills you can list on Resume Building Block 3: Professional Skills and Knowledge?

To Learn More

Benjamin-Chung M.: Math principles and practice: preparing for health career success, Upper Saddle River, NJ, 1998, Prentice-Hall

Kogelman S., Warren J.: Mind over math, New York, 1978, McGraw-Hill

Although published more than 30 years ago, this book is still in print. It is a classic on the subject of overcoming fear of math.

Lane Community College (Eugene, Ore)

https://www.lanecc.edu/math/math-review-sheets
The college has prepared review worksheets, including the correct answers, for dozens of math concepts.

MindTools

www.mindtools.com.
This website offers help for developing problem solving and practical creativity (using creativity to succeed on the job).

Palau S.M., Meltzer M.: Learning strategies for allied health students, Philadelphia, 1996, Elsevier

This book includes study techniques for various topics including math concepts used in health care occupations.

Pauk W., Owens R.J.Q.: How to study in college, ed 8, New York, 2005, Houghton Mifflin

This classic on how to study has good suggestions for mastering math in addition to reading and other skills.

Simmers L.: Practical problems in mathematics for health occupations, ed 3, Clifton Park, NY, 2013. Cengage Delmar Learning

In addition to easy-to-understand explanations, this book has many practice problems that apply to a variety of health care occupations.

Study Guides and Strategies

www.studygs.net.
This website includes excellent sections on math, problem solving, and critical thinking.

References

1. Green ME: *Internship success*, New York, 1998, McGraw-Hill.
2. Pauk W, Owens RJQ: *How to study in college*, ed 8, New York, 2005, Houghton Mifflin.
3. Kogelman S, Warren J: *Mind over math*, New York, 1978, McGraw-Hill.

CHAPTER 10

Developing Your People Skills

1. Explain the importance of having good people skills and respecting others.
2. Describe ways to better understand people whose backgrounds and beliefs are different from yours.
3. Explain the meaning of empathy and its importance in health care work.
4. Improve your effectiveness when speaking.
5. Become an active listener.
6. Use various types of questions effectively.
7. Use effective telephone techniques.
8. Become aware of how you and others communicate nonverbally.
9. Prepare and present effective oral presentations.
10. Practice good teamwork skills.
11. Understand organizational culture.
12. Identify the teaching styles of your instructors, and describe what you can learn from each.
13. Apply effective strategies when dealing with difficult people.
14. Explain the role of criticism in the learning process.

Debate Formal discussion in which two people or teams take sides on an issue, and each tries to persuade the audience to accept its point of view.

Diversity The differences that characterize people, including their native language, religious beliefs, values, and everyday customs.

Empathy Awareness and understanding of how another person feels and experiences the world.

Feedback Techniques used in spoken communication to check your understanding of what you hear another person say.

Nonverbal Communication Facial expressions, gestures, nondeliberate movements, and body positions that send messages.

Organizational Cultures The customs and practices of organizations that influence all aspects of how work is accomplished and what is considered appropriate behavior.

Stereotype An often unfair and untrue belief about people based on their ethnicity or other characteristics.

Teamwork Working with other people to accomplish a common goal. Modern patient care depends on teams of professionals working together effectively.

The Importance of People Skills

The last few chapters focused on you as an individual and the personal attitudes, habits, and skills that influence your academic and career success. In this chapter, we shift our focus to other people and how you relate to them. You can expect to work closely with many kinds of people in your career, and your ability to create and maintain mutually beneficial relationships will be an important factor in your career success.

The quality and consistency of patient care are affected by how well health care professionals communicate among themselves as well as with patients and their families. Poor communication with patients is a leading cause of malpractice lawsuits. When patients feel they are listened to and understood, trust is developed between them and their health care providers. As a result, these patients are less likely to sue, even if their treatment outcomes are negative.

At the same time, one of the most frequent complaints from employers today is that their employees lack good people skills. They don't know how to work well with others. Employees are more likely to fail on the job because of poor interpersonal skills than because they lack the necessary technical qualifications.

Good interpersonal skills are also important for academic success. Throughout your studies, you will have opportunities to learn from both your instructors and your fellow students. Your ability to communicate effectively will influence how much and how well you learn. Activities such as working on teams, practicing hands-on skills with other students, and joining study groups are ways you can start now to practice working with others. Most of life's activities take place in relation to other people, and improving the quality of these relationships can improve the overall quality of your life.

Respecting Others

"Be kind. Remember, everyone you meet is fighting a hard battle."
—Plato

By choosing a career in health care, you have accepted the responsibility to serve others. Your duties may range from performing an uncomfortable medical procedure to explaining a complicated bill for a hospital stay. You are obligated to serve all patients or clients with an equal level of care and concern, regardless of their appearance, behavior, level of education, or economic status. Not everyone will look, act, behave, or even smell as you would like them to. They will not all express appreciation for your efforts. People who feel sick may be irritable and cranky. The satisfaction you obtain from your work must be based on what you can give to others, not on what you receive from them.

Good health care practice is based on the principle that all human beings deserve to be treated with respect and dignity. The need to treat all patients equally and fairly has been recognized and endorsed by professional organizations such as the American Hospital Association (AHA). The AHA formalized this belief in "The Patient Care Partnership" mentioned in Chapter 1. Specifically, it states that patients have the right to "be treated with compassion and respect."

It is also important to demonstrate respect toward your supervisor and coworkers. The quality of work produced in any organization depends on the quality of the relationships among the people who work there, and good relationships are based on mutual respect.

Guidelines for Respectful Behavior

- **Be courteous.** Many observers today have noted that as a society we are moving away from the practice of common courtesy. Many people fail to use expressions like "please" and "thank you." These are powerful words that improve the quality of both personal and professional relationships.
- **Acknowledge the other person.** No one likes to be ignored. In school, greet others. Say "hello" to students and instructors. On the job, if you are busy working with someone else or talking on the telephone when a patient arrives, use eye contact and a quick nod to let the person know you are aware of his or her presence.
- **Don't interrupt.** Avoid breaking in when another person is speaking. Some people need extra time to compose their thoughts or express themselves. Avoid the habit of finishing sentences for others. This frustrates the speaker, and your assumption about what they planned to say may be incorrect.
- **Show interest.** Look at the other person when you are talking and listening. Show you are listening by nodding or using confirming sounds or phrases such as "uh, huh," "I understand," "okay," and so on. As you complete an encounter with a patient, don't turn your body toward the door as if to say, "Hurry up. I need to move on to something else."
- **Guard privacy.** This is good practice in your personal life. In health care, patient privacy is protected by law. It is illegal to discuss patient information with anyone who is not working directly with the patient. Make a habit of never sharing anything told to you in confidence by family members, friends, or classmates. (Patients must even give written permission before their information can be given to insurance companies, other health providers, and so on. More information about the legalities of patient confidentiality is given in Chapter 16.)
- **Avoid gossip.** Gossip can be a very serious problem in the workplace. It serves no useful purpose and can lead to hurt feelings, broken trust, and strained relationships. If it involves confidential patient matters, it can lead to a lawsuit.
- **Remain calm.** It is important to behave and speak calmly when you are dealing with situations such as emergencies or angry patients. A calm demeanor both reassures others and enables you to focus on doing what can best help the situation.

Take a look at the people in Figure 10-1. Do they appear to be showing respect for one another?

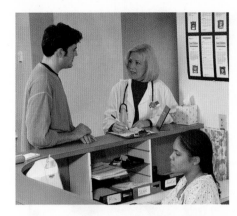

FIGURE 10-1 Respectful interaction is a necessary component of good health care, whether this is with patients, coworkers, or your supervisor. *How are the health care professionals in the photo demonstrating respect as they communicate?* (From Proctor DB, Adams AP: *Kinn's the medical assistant: an applied learning approach,* ed 12, St Louis, 2014, Saunders.)

▢ Prescription for Success: 10-1 Showing Respect

1. List three ways, in addition to those listed in the text, in which you can show respect to others.
2. Describe a situation in which someone made you feel that you were respected. How was this respect communicated to you?
3. Explain why showing respect to patients is an important part of providing good health care.

On the Job

Showing Respect on the Job The book *Health Professional and Patient Interaction* includes a conversation from a student who was finishing his clinical experience:

"This might surprise you," John said, "but do you know what I'd say is the most important thing I've learned in the last several weeks of my experiences in the clinics? I'd call it learning that little things mean a lot! Do you think that's ridiculous? For instance, I have learned the importance of pouring a glass of water for a thirsty patient, listening to the ninth inning of a baseball game between parts of a treatment, laughing at something the patient says, wiping a nose. Perhaps these things sound silly to you, but I know that I could not be getting the good results I am seeing if I had not mastered these skills along with my technical ones!" After a pause, he added with a smile, "I guess I have learned to nurture my patients a little!"

It is often the small things that show patients you care about them, and this can have a very positive effect on their health outcomes.

(From: Purtilo R, Haddad A: *Health professional and patient interaction,* ed 7, Philadelphia, 2007, Saunders.)

Appreciating Diversity

"Commandment Number One of any truly civilized society is this: Let people be different."

—David Grayson

The population of the United States is made up of people from all over the world, as illustrated in Figure 10-2. A wide variety of races, religions, lifestyles, languages, and educational and economic levels are represented in America. These variations are known as **diversity**.

Diversity also refers to differences that are not related to cultural background or race. These include age, sexual orientation, disabilities, and appearance. People who are different are sometimes ignored or treated inappropriately, sometimes even cruelly. This may not be done intentionally, so you must think about what you are doing and how it might be interpreted. For example, it is not uncommon for health care professionals to speak to younger relatives who accompany elderly patients as if the patients were not present. Other examples are using "baby talk" with the elderly or shouting at them if they are hard of hearing.

Our society can benefit from the contributions of people with different customs and ideas. By drawing from a variety of viewpoints, we increase our chances of solving the complex problems encountered in modern society. Learning from our differences can be beneficial. Many Americans, for example, find pain relief from the ancient Chinese practice of acupuncture, the insertion of very small needles into specific points on the body. Unfortunately, differences in values and beliefs about life can cause misunderstandings and even lead to violence. Learning to take advantage of the differences and to work out misunderstandings peacefully is one of the major challenges the world faces today.

Work in health care will give you opportunities to interact with people from many different backgrounds. Your personal actions and efforts to understand and serve others can contribute to a more harmonious society. The students in your school probably come from diverse backgrounds. Initiate communication with them. And if your own background is different from that of your classmates, you can serve as a source of information about your culture (Figure 10-3).

Promoting Understanding

When we learn about others, we also learn about ourselves and what it means to be human. You can enrich your life by accepting diversity and seeking opportunities to learn about different ways to view the world. Here are some suggestions to help people of all backgrounds better understand each other:

- **Put fear aside.** Many people are frightened by what they don't understand. Some are afraid that acknowledging differences among people will result in negative changes in society. In fact, the contributions of people from different backgrounds have resulted in the economic success and political stability of the United States.
- **Listen to other points of view.** Seek opportunities to interact with people whose backgrounds are different from yours. Encourage them to express their ideas and opinions. Listen carefully to what they say.

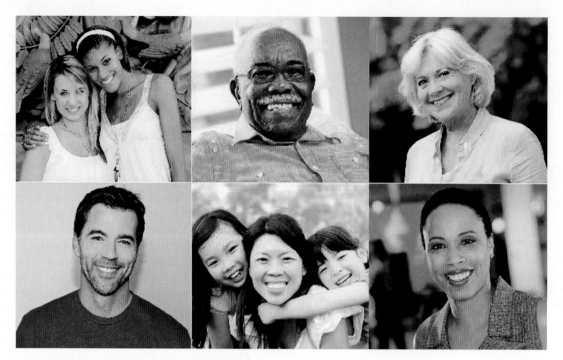

FIGURE 10-2 It is likely that you will work with people, both patients and coworkers, from a variety of cultural backgrounds. Their differences may include race, ethnicity, age, educational levels, and sexual orientation. This wide diversity can make a health care career challenging as well as rewarding. *How can you prepare to be empathetic and work effectively with people who are different from you?* (All photos © Thinkstock)

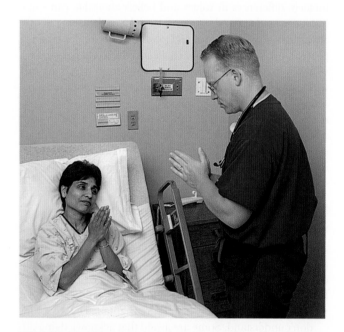

FIGURE 10-3 The nurse here is giving a traditional Hindu greeting to his patient. According to this patient's beliefs, this method of greeting honors the spirit in each of us. A simple gesture such as this helps put the patient at ease. Understanding customs that are important to your patients will promote better communication. *Are you aware of the different ethnic groups in your community? How can you learn more about their customs, especially those that relate to health care?* (From deWit S, O'Neill P: *Fundamental concepts and skills for nursing,* ed 4, St Louis, 2014, Saunders.)

- **Ask questions.** Use questions to learn more, but not to challenge the other person. For example, instead of asking, "Why do you believe that?" you could say, "That sounds interesting. Could you tell me more about that?" Your goal is to learn and understand, not to imply that the other person is wrong.
- **Avoid stereotypes.** Don't make assumptions about people because of their age, race, gender, or other characteristics. Consider each person as an individual with a unique set of characteristics.
- **Don't judge people by their appearance.** Outward appearances do not always represent who people are. To truly know people, you must talk with them and observe their actions. If you immediately dismiss them based on how they look, you may lose the opportunity to form a friendship or a beneficial working relationship. Assuming that patients "are what they look like" may detract from the care you give them.
- **Explore different cultures.** Many schools and communities sponsor activities that highlight the cultures represented in the local population. Check your local library and the Internet for other sources of information about the backgrounds of your classmates and future patients.
- **Learn about other value systems.** People are defined by their values and beliefs about how they should live. Culture is much more than typical foods and daily customs. Develop a deeper level of knowledge and understanding through conversation and by learning about the religions and important beliefs of the people in your area. See Table 10-1 for examples of cultural and personal beliefs.

TABLE 10-1

Examples of Conflicting Cultural and Personal Beliefs

Concept	Varying Beliefs
Time	It is important to always be on time for meetings and appointments. Appointment times are just estimations of when they will take place. Time is valuable and should not be wasted. Time is not a resource over which we have control. It just is. It is important to use time productively. If something is important, it will eventually get done; there is no reason to rush. The present is more important than the future. The present should be used for planning and preparing for the future.
Personal Space	The distance comfortably maintained when people are talking ranges from a few inches away (when you can feel the breath of the other person on your face) to over a foot away.
Age	Youth is valued. People should try to maintain a youthful appearance and lifestyle for as long as possible (exercise, wrinkle creams, and hair dyes). Older people are valued for their wisdom and are shown great respect. When elderly people are no longer able to care for themselves, it is appropriate to place them in a nursing or retirement home. Older people should live with and be cared for by family members until they die.
Touching	Shaking hands is okay for everyone. Only members of the same sex can shake hands with one another. Hugging is okay for everyone, even members of the same sex. Kissing is okay between women. When meeting a new person, only a slight bow is permitted, but no touching.
Gender	A woman cannot be treated by a male physician. Women and men are equal. Men are dominant. Women act as the head of most families. Women have no economic or political power.
Eye Contact	Direct eye contact is a sign of sincerity, honesty, and interest in the other person. It is a sign of disrespect. Sustained eye contact communicates hostility, aggression or sexual interest.
Personal Control	Each person is in control of his or her own life. Luck, fate, or the will of God determines how things turn out.
Spiritual Practices	There is only one God. There is more than one God. God helps those who help themselves. God punishes those who sin. God answers all prayers. There is uncertainty about the existence of God. There is no God. Witchcraft and magic can help or hurt us.
Definition of Success	Personal and professional achievement. Acquiring material possessions. Living a spiritual life. Achieving inner peace. Raising many children. Being a kind person and helping others.
Health Care Beliefs	Disease is caused by germs, environmental conditions, and personal habits such as smoking. Good health is a gift or reward from God. Illness is a punishment sent by God. Illness happens when the body's energy or humors get out of balance. Science has the best answers for preventing and curing disease. The body can heal itself naturally. Herbs are the best remedies. Only God can heal. Good health is a balance of the mind, body, and spirit. Individuals are responsible for their own health and healing.

Continued

TABLE 10-1—cont'd

Examples of Conflicting Cultural and Personal Beliefs

Concept	Varying Beliefs
Beliefs About Death and Dying	Death is a natural part of the life cycle.
	Death should be avoided at all costs.
	Dying is up to God.
	Death means the health care system has failed.
	An autopsy destroys the soul.
	Cremation frees the soul.
	Everything possible should be done to save a life.
	People who are terminally ill or suffering should be assisted to die if this is their wish.
	Families should take care of the dying.
	Hospitals or other health care facilities should take care of the dying.

- **Look for commonalities.** As human beings, we share many of the same needs, concerns, and goals for our lives. Explore what you have in common with people who seem different.
- **Offer to help others.** Expand your attitude of caring by looking for ways to help others. For example, offer to help a classmate who has trouble speaking or writing English. Or if English is your second language, offer to teach your language and customs to others.
- **Learn another language.** You may not have time now to study another language formally, but you can learn a few key phrases of any major cultural groups in your area. This will increase your effectiveness as a health care professional and your worth to an employer.

Personal Reflection

1. Which cultural groups are represented where you live?
2. How much do you know about their customs and beliefs?
3. How can you learn more?

On the Job

Diversity on the Job Everything we do is influenced by our cultural backgrounds. Being aware that differences exist can help you to better understand the people you will encounter on the job. The beliefs that many of us take for granted, such as, "It is important to always be on time," are not important to everyone. Making assumptions can result in misunderstandings. Let's look at an example. A patient has to wait 15 minutes before you can perform his lab test. In an effort to respect his time and not add to the delay, you keep conversation to a minimum and complete the procedure as quickly as possible. You believe you have been considerate. The patient, from a culture that does not consider time in the same way, is insulted. His interpretation of your behavior is that you obviously have more important things to do than work with him, so you are rushing along.

On the Job—cont'd

The "right thing" in your eyes was the "wrong thing" in his. Of course, it is impossible to know and accommodate every cultural difference that you encounter. You can, however, be aware of what types of differences exist and strive to be sensitive to them. Ask questions if you are unsure about a person's feelings or understanding of a situation. Table 10-1 lists common areas of differences among cultures.

Prescription for Success: 10-2 Getting to Know Yourself

The first step toward understanding others is knowing yourself. What are your beliefs about each of the concepts below? You may use any of those listed in Table 10-1 or you can write your own.
- Time
- Personal space
- Age
- Touching
- Gender
- Eye contact
- Personal control
- Spiritual practices
- The definition of success
- Health care beliefs
- Beliefs about death and dying

Prescription for Success: 10-3 Your Health Care Beliefs

1. What is your personal definition of "health"?
2. How much responsibility do you believe people should have for their own health?
3. What do you believe are the main causes of health problems?
4. What are the best ways to take care of health problems?
5. How do you think your own beliefs about health may influence your future work?

Experiencing Empathy

"Don't judge a man until you've walked a mile in his shoes."

Empathy means attempting to see the world through the eyes of other people in order to understand their feelings and experiences. Prescription for Success 1-6 in Chapter 1 asked you to imagine yourself as a patient with a broken arm. Mentally putting yourself in the place of someone else is necessary to experience empathy. This is not always easy to do because we are all influenced by our own beliefs, values, and previous experiences. Being empathetic requires listening carefully to others without judging what you hear. You then think about what you hear and, if necessary, ask for clarification or more information. What is the person trying to communicate or trying to hide? What clues are you getting from the person's body language? What is important to this person?

Health care professionals must have empathy with patients to understand their needs and learn how best to help them. Being empathetic sends the message, "You are important and worth my time and respect. I will make every effort to know who you are and what you need."

A key part of empathy is letting the other person know that you are trying to understand his or her experience. It is best, however, not to say that you know exactly how he or she feels. This sounds insincere because, in fact, it is impossible to know precisely how another person feels. In trying to be helpful, we may be tempted to share and compare our own stories—for example, saying, "Oh, I know just what you mean. The same thing happened to me…" and then launching into a detailed explanation about what happened to us. This shifts the focus to us and away from the person who needs the attention (Figure 10-4).

Learning to experience empathy improves all interpersonal relationships, including those with friends, family members, classmates, instructors, coworkers, and supervisors. Your relationships can be more harmonious when you make an effort to see the views of others. Here are some ways to increase your practice of empathy at home and in school:

- When you talk with your classmates, listen carefully. How are their views different from yours? What experiences have they had that explain these differences?
- Are there students who exhibit poor behavior? Why do you think they behave in this way? What are some clues that might explain their actions?
- Why do family members sometimes "act out"?
- What kinds of experiences have shaped the opinions of your friends?

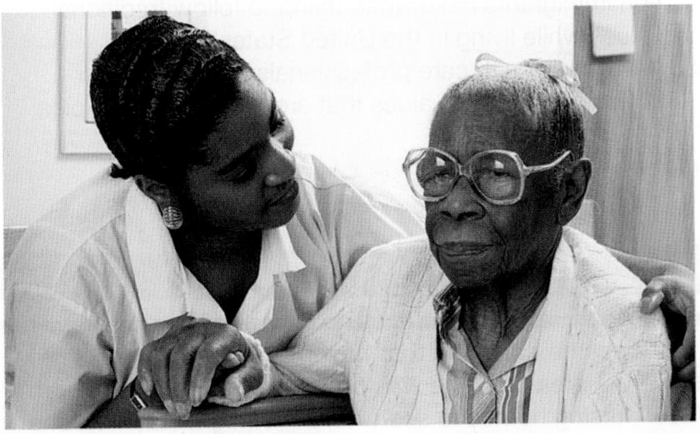

Prescription for Success: 10-4 What Would It Be Like to Be . . . ?

Answer the questions that follow for patients in the following conditions:

- Paralyzed
- In pain
- Unable to work
- Blind
- Mentally ill
- Poor and without health insurance
- Elderly and living alone
- Unable to speak English
- Having a terminal illness
  1. What emotions could they be experiencing?
  2. What could be their concerns and fears?
  3. What are their major needs likely to be, both physical and emotional?
  4. How is their condition likely to affect their quality of life?
  5. How could you learn more about each person?

FIGURE 10-4 Empathy is the first step toward helping your patients. It means focusing on the other person and attempting to understand how he or she feels. *What do you think this elderly patient may be feeling? In addition to touching her, what else could the health care professional do to help her?* (From Sorrentino S, Remmert L: *Mosby's textbook for nursing assistants,* ed 8, St Louis, 2012, Mosby.)

On the Job

Empathy on the Job A medical office manager shared the following story: The receptionist, Grace, was a very efficient woman who treated all patients courteously. One of the patients, William, was a gay man with AIDS. Grace was courteous but stiffened visibly whenever he came for appointments. She had trouble accepting his lifestyle. One day William learned that Grace's son had been a missionary in Africa. On his next visit, William brought in a scrapbook that showed his experience working with missionaries in Africa. After that, Grace was warm and friendly to William. When asked why seeing the scrapbook had changed her behavior, she said that now she was able to see William as a person and not simply as a gay man with AIDS.

Whitney has worked in nursing homes as a CNA for several years. Most of the patients she works with are elderly and she enjoys spending time with them. She is able to see beyond the wrinkles and confused behaviors of the older patients who are suffering from dementia as well as various physical ailments. But Whitney is committed to her work and believes that all patients, regardless of their condition, deserve her best efforts.

A new patient, Mr. Hirayama, has become the talk of the break room. The caregivers in his wing are full of complaints. Although many patients in nursing homes are unhappy, Mr. Hirayama has proven himself to be particularly difficult. Nothing seems to please him, he's unappreciative of the staff's efforts to be pleasant—the list goes on and on. Whitney has not met Mr. Hirayama and tries not to get involved in the complaint sessions that sometimes take place with stressed caregivers. She does understand their frustration. Working in a nursing home requires caring and sensitivity and it's not always easy. It can be hectic and the chances of burnout and employee turnover are high.

A couple of weeks later, Mr. Hirayama is moved to a private room in the wing where Whitney is assigned. She takes a deep breath before entering his room and tells herself she will simply do her best. But the truth is that her patience—and spirit—are tested.

She smiles and asks, "I'm Whitney. How are you doing today, Mr. Hirayama?"

He scowls and grumbles, "Pretty awful. This place is terrible."

Whitney sighs. "I'm sorry you feel that way. Is there anything I can do to help make things better for you?"

"I doubt it. My son has stuck me here to die. He doesn't care about me. Why should you?"

Whitney really doesn't know how to respond to this, so she gives him a sympathetic look and goes about her duties, taking his vital signs and tidying up the room.

As she leaves she says, "It was nice meeting you, Mr. Hirayama. I hope you have a good night. I'll see you tomorrow."

"Hmmmph!" he grumbles.

At home, Whitney shares her day with her husband, Rich.

"Boy," says Rich. "It sounds like you have your work cut out for you with this new guy."

"Yeah," responds Whitney. "I don't know if this is one I can reach. He may be beyond help at this point."

"What did you say his name was?" asks Rich.

"Hirayama—Mr. Hirayama."

"Is he Japanese?" asks Rich.

"I think so."

"You know, there's a fellow at work—he's a Japanese American. One day we were talking and I told him where you worked—and how many older folks were there in the nursing home. And he said that this was something hard for his family to understand—putting older family members in an institution instead of taking care of them at home."

"Rich, you've given me an idea," says Whitney. "After dinner I'm going to check some things out on the Internet."

That evening, instead of watching TV with Rich, Whitney did some web searches about Japanese culture and health care beliefs. She was surprised by what she read. And a lot of it might explain Mr. Hirayama's negative attitude and unhappiness. It also gave her a clue about his remark about his son. She learned that an important component of Japanese culture is respect for the elderly and the duty children have to care for their parents. Placing a father in a care facility could bring shame on a family. And the traditional view on illness and death is that they are impure—spiritually impure—and that poor health can be a shameful experience.

Questions for Thought and Reflection

1. Based on what Whitney learned, what are some reasons why Mr. Hirayama is unhappy and unpleasant to the staff in the nursing home?
2. Do you think Whitney's research will help her deal with Mr. Hirayama more effectively?
3. What are some possible reasons why Mr. Hirayama's son has placed him in a nursing home instead of having a family member take care of him?
4. What are other problems that first and second generation immigrants have when trying to follow traditional values while living in the United States?
5. What can health care professionals do to help their patients who have values that are different from typical American values?

Ninety-year-old Joanna had spent a lovely Christmas with her son, Dan, and daughter-in-law, Leslie, but was looking forward to returning to her home, 150 miles away. She had lived in her town for 75 years and had many friends she looked forward to seeing and activities she wanted to resume. But on January 4, just two days before she was to leave her children's house, she became very ill. Leslie called an ambulance and Joanna was transported to the local hospital where she remained for several days. She had become dehydrated and this led to delusions, confusion, and fear.

It became apparent that Joanna would not be able to leave the area until she was better, so her children visited local nursing homes to see where she might stay until she recovered enough to return home. They chose the one that seemed most home-like, had a private room, and where the director of nursing seemed friendliest.

When it came time for Joanna to leave the hospital, she became frightened and disoriented. She refused to dress and would not leave in the wheelchair van that had been arranged to take her to the nursing home. The hospital called Dan and Leslie to come and take her to the nursing home themselves.

Once Joanna and her children arrived at the nursing home, the director came out the door and approached them. Dan and Leslie expected a friendly greeting. Instead, the director simply looked into their van, asked the two nursing assistants who accompanied her if "they could handle this," and went back into the building. Leslie was unpleasantly surprised, even apprehensive. This was the very nurse who had seemed so friendly and welcoming on her first visit to review the facility! "Boy," Leslie said. "I sure didn't expect this." Dan was worried. "But," he said, "that other place we looked at really looked dreary. And they didn't have any private rooms." There were only the two nursing homes in their small city, so Dan and Leslie really didn't feel they had any choice.

Things didn't get any better. The nursing assistants entered the van. They were unsmiling, almost dour. They loaded Joanna into a wheelchair, took her to her room, walking in silence, and instructed her to "get undressed and get into bed."

Dan and Leslie were not totally comfortable leaving his mother that evening, but at least, they told themselves, she would receive nursing care. They still couldn't get over the lack of warmth, concern, or even a polite welcome to the facility. This was especially worrisome when they were told that the staff *knew* that Joanna had been scared and uncomfortable about leaving the hospital. And there was no one there to give them any information: no papers to sign, no information about the policies, visiting hours, how Joanna would be cared for—nothing. It was two days later before they met with the facility's social worker who was responsible for sharing this information.

Questions for Thought and Reflection

1. Why do you think Joanna was confused and afraid to leave the hospital with the van driver?
2. How do you think Joanna felt about having to stay in a nursing home? (Consider what she thought she would be doing at this time.)
3. How did the behavior of the nurse and nursing assistants likely influence the rest of her stay in the nursing home?
4. How would you greet Dan, Leslie, and Joanna if you were the nursing director? A nursing assistant? What would you say?
5. What would you say or do as you wheeled Joanna to her room?
6. What would you say to Dan and Leslie before they left the facility?

Oral Communication: Creating the People Connection

"Communication—the human connection—is the key to personal and career success."

—Paul J. Meyer

Many people believe they are good communicators because they are friendly and like to talk. But the ability to speak is only one part of effective communication. There are four other essential components of effective communication: listening, thinking, requesting feedback, and using and interpreting **nonverbal communication** (body language, expressions, and gestures). Successful oral communication takes place when the receiver (listener) receives and understands the intended message of the speaker. We all know this is not always the case! Let's look at how you can increase the effectiveness of your communication.

Speaking

Speaking consists of creating and sending messages. The first step in creating a clear message is to determine your purpose. In Chapter 8, we discussed the importance of determining your purpose when writing. It is the same with speaking: you need to know your communication goal. Table 10-2 contains examples of reasons for sending a message.

TABLE 10-2

Examples of Spoken Messages

Purpose	School	Job Search	Career
Provide information	Help a classmate who missed an important lecture	Describe your training to a potential employer	Give instructions to a coworker
Demonstrate knowledge	Give a presentation in class	Describe your qualifications, using examples, to a potential employer	Report to your supervisor about a workshop you attended
Persuade	Convince a friend not to cheat on a test	Present yourself successfully at a job interview	Inspire a patient to follow her exercise program
Gather information	Ask questions in class	Ask a professional contact for career information	Conduct a patient interview
Acknowledge others	Greet classmates and instructors	Thank interviewers for their time	Express an interest in your patients

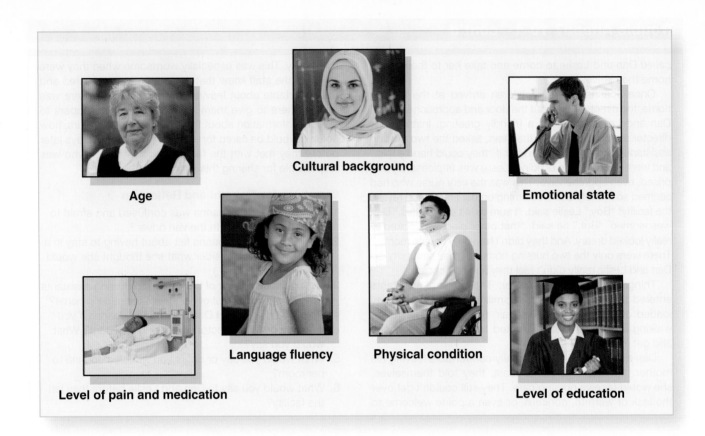

Age

Cultural background

Emotional state

Language fluency

Physical condition

Level of pain and medication

Level of education

FIGURE 10-5 It is important for patients to understand you, especially if your communication involves giving instructions about their care. Always consider who your listener is when creating your spoken message. *Think about how you would alter the same message for each person in the figure.* (All photos © Thinkstock)

Effective messages match the purpose of the speaker with the needs of the receiver. These needs are determined, in part, by the characteristics of the receiver. Figure 10-5 contains examples of characteristics you should consider in order to create appropriate messages.

Success Tips for Sending Effective Messages

- Speak from a base of sincerity, caring, and respect for others.
- Choose a level of language that is appropriate for the receiver. If a person is heavily medicated, for example, use simple words and short sentences.
- Choose appropriate vocabulary. Using medical terminology is an effective way to be precise when speaking with coworkers, but it can be confusing for patients. They may hesitate to tell you they don't understand because they don't want to seem dumb. However, ensuring that patients understand your questions and explanations is critical for their health outcomes. The inability

to understand health care providers is a major patient complaint.

- Avoid slang and nonstandard speech. These are often characteristic of certain age and social groups and can cause misunderstandings with people outside those groups. Speech that is appropriate among friends and at social gatherings may not be correct for school and work. For example, the use of the word "goes" to mean "says" is understood by many young people, but may be confusing to others.
- Speak clearly and at a moderate speed—not so quickly that you are difficult to understand or so slowly that the receiver's mind wanders. (We hear and comprehend many times faster than we speak.)
- Avoid speaking in a monotone. Speak naturally, but with expression in your voice. Make sure it is appropriate for your message. For example, speak with respect when asking questions in class, friendliness when greeting a new student, reassurance when calming fears, and firmness when giving instructions that affect patient safety.

Active Listening

"To listen well is as powerful a means of communication as to talk well."

—U.S. Supreme Court Chief Justice John Marshall

Active listening, as discussed in Chapter 7, should not be confused with hearing. Listening requires effort, whereas hearing is more passive. To listen well, you must pay attention, focus on the speaker's words, and reflect on what you hear. Active listening demonstrates respect for the speaker. It is an essential skill for the health care professional because all patients want to work with someone who listens to them and makes every effort to understand their needs. In fact, patient satisfaction surveys show that patients highly value providers who are excellent listeners and take what they say seriously.[1] The health care professional in Figure 10-6 is demonstrating active listening skills.

Think for a moment about your own listening skills. Do you sometimes catch your mind wandering and thinking about other things? Do you think about what you are going to say next? Do you argue mentally when you disagree? These habits can interfere with your attention and prevent you from hearing the speaker's message. Look over the following checklist of techniques designed to improve listening skills. Are there any you'd like to try?

- Prepare yourself mentally to listen by clearing your mind of other thoughts.
- Control the noise level of your environment as much as possible. Turn off the radio or television, look for a quiet place to talk, or move out of a busy area.
- Focus on the other person and concentrate on following what he or she is saying. Sometimes when we think we are listening, looking at the speaker, and perhaps even nodding in agreement, we are actually thinking about something else. Practice being aware of where your attention is directed.
- If you disagree with what you are hearing, try not to engage in mental arguments. Internal self-talk interferes with your ability to listen. It is usually easy to understand people we agree with. It takes more effort to hear people we disagree with, but only by listening carefully can we begin to understand another's point of view.
- Practice making quick mental notes about points you need to clarify. Work on being able to do this without losing track of what the person is saying.
- Focus on what is being said rather than how it is said. Move beyond the speaker's appearance, manners, language level, or even odor. Try not to let unpleasant factors about the person interfere with your ability to concentrate on what he or she has to say.
- Acknowledge the person even if you are taking notes or performing a test or procedure while he or she is talking. Look at the person from time to time and make eye contact.

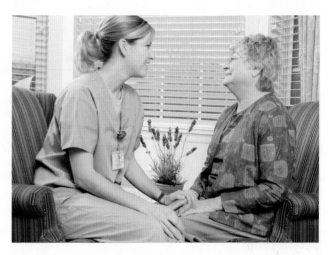

FIGURE 10-6 Listening well is as important—sometimes more so—than speaking well. *In what ways is this health care professional's body language demonstrating that she is actively listening?* (From Sorrentino S, Remmert L: *Mosby's textbook for nursing assistants,* ed 8, St Louis, 2012, Mosby.)

Listening effectively is one of the most valuable skills you can develop for both personal and professional success. It can increase your learning, your effectiveness in helping others, and even your popularity. At the same time, it is a skill many people neglect because they assume they know how to listen. Working to improve your listening skills is one of the most important actions you can take to work well with others.

Feedback

Feedback is a communication technique used to check your understanding of what a speaker says. Even when you listen carefully, there may be times when what you hear is not what the speaker intended. We have all experienced the misunderstandings that occur when we assume we understand the speaker's message—and then learn that the intended message was quite different!

There are several methods for giving and requesting feedback. Here are three of the most common kinds of feedback:

1. **Paraphrasing.** This means saying what you heard in your own words so that the speaker can confirm or correct your statement.
2. **Reflecting.** This is similar to paraphrasing but you repeat what the other person says using words as close as possible to his or her own words. This gives the person the opportunity to confirm or add additional information.
3. **Clarifying.** This means asking the speaker to explain what he or she means.

See Table 10-3 for examples of each kind of feedback.

TABLE 10-3

Examples of Feedback

	What the Speaker Says	Feedback
Paraphrasing		
School	This week's assignment is on page 83 of your workbook. Complete exercises 3 through 8.	Let me make sure that I have it right. We're to do exercises 3 through 8 on page 83 in the workbook and hand them in on Friday.
Job search	We really need employees we can rely on to be here on time every day. It's also essential for them to get along with their coworkers.	It sounds as if two of the most important characteristics you are looking for are punctuality and the ability to work well with others.
Career	It really hurts most when I get up in the mornings. I feel a little better as the day goes by.	It sounds as if the pain is much worse when you first wake up in the morning but decreases during the day.
Reflecting		
School	Well, I don't have any time for a study group because of my work schedule.	You said that you don't have time to join our study group because of your work schedule? (You suspect there may be another reason, and if it is known, arrangements could be made for the person to join the group.)
Job search	Here is a copy of the job description. It contains most of the duties required for this position, although there are some others.	The job description contains most of the duties required but there are a few others? (The interviewer has given the impression that more may be expected than just what is listed on the job description.)
Career	I haven't lost any weight because the diet the doctor gave me isn't working.	You haven't lost any weight because the diet isn't working? (There may be other reasons, such as not following the diet exactly, lack of exercise, and so on.)
Clarifying		
School	The tests in this class are really tough. You'll see!	You said the tests in medical terminology are really hard. Can you give me an example of a question?
Job search	It's easy to find. We're really close to the Cross Town Shopping Center.	You said you are close to the Cross Town Shopping Center. Can you tell me about how many blocks away that is?
Career	I give him the medication on schedule but ever since he's been taking it his behavior has been kind of strange.	Can you explain what you mean when you say your son has been acting "strangely" since he started taking the medication?

Trouble Ahead? 10-2

Until today, Christie had been pleased with herself and her life. Just six months ago she completed her nurses training and passed the state licensing exam. Now, at age 22, she is a registered nurse and has a job at a nursing home.

While in school, she studied hard and took pride in the grades she received in most of her courses. She especially enjoyed anatomy and physiology and classes on nursing procedures. But as she told her friend, Nadine, one day on the phone, "I just don't understand why all the emphasis on communication skills. It seems like the instructors are always going on about it. Good grief, I'm great at communicating."

"That's true," said Nadine. "You always have something interesting to say—the latest news and gossip."

"Right! In fact, I've got something good to tell you about right now. Remember Gerry, the girl I told you about in class—I thought she was carrying on with Jim? Well, I heard she's pregnant."

"Get out!" exclaimed Nadine.

"No kidding! But listen, I've got to go. My next class starts in 15 minutes."

Once on the job at the nursing home, Christie applied what she believed to be her good communication skills by befriending other staff members, chatting with the patients, and sharing juicy stories to keep everyone entertained. She noticed that not everyone seemed interested in spending much time visiting with her, but she figured these people were simply too busy working or not the friendly type.

Christie thought things were going just fine until today when Sarah Caldwell, the nursing director, called Christie into her office. "Christie," she said. "I've got to talk with you about how you are communicating with the other staff and patients."

"You must be kidding," exclaimed Christie. "I'm one of the best communicators around here. Some of the staff don't even talk—"

"Christie!" interrupted Sarah. "I'd like to know how you're defining 'communicate' because what I'm hearing about you certainly does not fit my definition. Especially for a professional."

"I like people. I like to talk. I like to share the news," Christie explained.

"Well, the 'news' as you call it that you are sharing consists mainly of gossip, according to what I'm hearing. And gossip really has no place here."

"That kind of takes the fun out of things," responded Christie.

"Here in the nursing home—or any health care facility where you might work—the goal of communication is not to have fun. It's to listen to what other people are saying—learn about them and their needs. Talking just to be entertaining is not helpful."

For once, Christie didn't know what to say. She wasn't sure she agreed with Sarah. After all, what kind of an impersonal place was this? She told Sarah she would think about what she had said.

"I certainly hope so," said Sarah. "In other ways, you are a good nurse. But if this doesn't stop, it is grounds for dismissal. I won't have a choice."

Questions for Thought and Reflection

1. What is wrong with Christie's idea of "good communication"?
2. What essential parts of good communication does Christie seem to be missing?
3. What do you think Sarah Caldwell's definition of communication might be?
4. How does Christie's situation demonstrate how "soft skills" such as communication can be as important as technical skills?

Asking Questions

"No man really becomes a fool until he stops asking questions."
—Charles P. Steinmetz

Scientific discoveries and technological advances are the result of people asking questions. What causes…? What would happen if…? How can we…? Asking questions is a powerful learning tool. You can increase your knowledge and understanding in school by asking questions. Yet many students sit through hours of classes and never ask a single question. Take advantage of your opportunities to learn and get ready to ask good questions in class. Here are some tips to get started:

- **Prepare ahead for class.** If you haven't read the assignment or completed the other homework, you won't have the background information on which to base a question.
- **Write questions down.** Suppose you did the reading and remember that there were several points you didn't understand, but you didn't write them down, and now you can't remember what they were! Don't let this happen to

you. When you are studying and during lectures, write down questions as you think of them so you can ask them at the appropriate time.

- **Don't be embarrassed.** No one wants to ask what they think is a dumb question. But if you already knew everything, you wouldn't be in school, right? Instructors welcome questions in class and are usually pleased when students take an interest in the subject. (Exception: You don't pay attention in class and/or don't read the assigned material and then ask lots of questions that force the instructor to repeat what he or she has just finished saying.)
- **Ask the questions later.** If all the class time is taken up with the lecture or the instructor never gets around to your lab group, arrange a time to ask your questions later. Be willing to make the extra effort to get the information you need.
- **Be brave.** Have you ever found yourself so confused in class you can't even phrase a question? This is exactly when you should ask a question. Try something like, "I'm lost here. Could we go back to…?" Avoid waiting until you're so far behind that you don't have a chance of catching up.

Staff at Bend Family Dentistry

The staff at Bend Family Dentistry discusses the importance of communication in the workplace.

Q What can you tell me about communication in this office?
A Simply put, communication is everything. It's even more important than what we actually *do.*

Q Can you explain what you mean by that?
A We've found that the most common reason patients transfer here from other dentists is miscommunication. It wasn't the quality of the dental work. They just didn't understand what was going on or didn't feel that the staff really cared about them. We know we need to explain things to patients—what we're doing and

Continued

why. Why they need seven fillings. Why a crown costs $1200. And we have to do this in a nice way. We can't tell them it's their fault that they don't brush well and never floss. We can't lecture them. But we can treat them kindly and explain what we've found and what we believe needs to be done.

Q What part does inter-staff communication play?

A A big one. Patients pick up on poor inter-staff communication, and it makes them uncomfortable. You never want them to feel there is any friction or that their information didn't get passed along to the person who needed it.

You should speak to your coworkers as you would like to be spoken to. You really have to value them and consider their input and their feelings. And remember that there is always more than one way to do something, so be accepting of differences among staff. When you're talking with the dentist, you have to think about what you're saying. Identify the important points, summarize, and communicate clearly. Share any information about patients you think will help the next person who is going to work with them.

Q Besides good communication, what else is important?

A Doing your share of the work—and maybe a little extra. Knowing your job and what your responsibilities are.

Help others, clean up, answer the phone if necessary. Look for things to do—sometimes it's not obvious, but learn to observe and see what needs to be done.

Think to yourself, "What could I do to fill in and help the situation?"

Dr. Hester always says that he wants the work environment here to be "like a waltz where everything is smooth, cool, and okay." This means that our goal is to make everyone's job easier. We want the dentists to be able to focus on clinical work and the patients. The dental assistants learn to know what the dentists want and need.

Q People don't usually enjoy going to the dentist. How do you handle this as dental professionals?

A We start with ourselves. One of our sayings here is "leave your stress at the door." We can't expect patients to feel okay about being here if we aren't. So we try to be calm and reassuring. We listen to patients. They may be nervous and talkative—they may express views we don't agree with. When this happens, we are respectful and keep our personal views to a minimum. Patients who are really afraid may be angry, arrogant, or just grumpy. Again, we listen and try to be attuned to their needs. Maybe they need more explanations. They may need to know exactly what's going to happen and what they will feel. If they have had trouble in the past, we ask them what went wrong, how they felt, and what we can do to help the situation. Our goal is to establish confidence and trust so they can be more comfortable.

Types of Questions

There are four basic types of questions:

1. **Closed-ended.** Can be answered with a "yes" or "no" or in one or two words. They are used for getting specific facts.
2. **Open-ended.** Require a longer answer and request explanations, descriptions, examples, and other details.
3. **Probing.** Based on what the other person has already told you. The purpose is to acquire additional information.
4. **Leading.** The question is worded to provide a possible answer. Leading questions can be helpful with people who find it difficult to communicate because of injury, language barriers, shyness, or other problems that make communicating difficult. However, these questions should be used with great care because they may encourage the other person to simply agree because he or she doesn't really understand the question or thinks you have provided the correct answer.

See Table 10-4 for examples of each kind of question.

Prescription for Success: 10-5 And the Question Is . . . ?

Write two examples of each of the four types of questions.
1. Closed-ended
2. Open-ended
3. Probing
4. Leading

Success Tips for Asking Effective Questions

- **Choose the right place.** Some important questions are personal, embarrassing, or potentially difficult to answer. A question for the instructor about a low grade you believe to be unfair is best asked in private, not during class. An interview with a patient with acquired immunodeficiency syndrome (AIDS) must be conducted out of the hearing of others.

TABLE 10-4
Examples of Questions

Type of Question	Examples
Closed-ended	What is the date of the math test? Can we use our calculators? Have you ever had surgery?
Open-ended	How would you recommend that we study for the math test? What is your understanding of why you need surgery?
Probing	Could you give us an example of the kind of question that will be on the test? Can you describe how you found it easier to walk after you had the surgery?
Leading	Did you decide not to do the exercises at home because you didn't understand the instructions?

- **Choose the right time.** Asking your supervisor a question about your performance when he or she is ready to leave the office isn't fair to either of you.
- **Avoid challenging or judgmental questions.** Your choice of words and tone of voice can communicate the negative message, "You are wrong, and I demand an explanation." For example, questions like, "Why did you do that?" or "What were you thinking?" may draw a defensive reaction or no response at all. A major goal of communication should be to encourage discussion so that issues can be resolved.
- **Know what not to ask.** There is a difference between showing interest in others and asking questions that are too personal and may offend. To show concern without prying, you can say something like, "You seem really upset. Is there some way I can help?" This allows the person to reveal as much information as is comfortable. If you must ask potentially embarrassing questions, explain why you are asking them and how the information will be used. Assure patients that anything they say will remain confidential, as required by law.
- **Know what's legal.** Some questions, especially when asked in hiring situations, are illegal. These include asking about age, marital status, number of children, and other matters that are not related to job performance. (See Chapter 14 for more information.)
- **Allow silence.** Some people need more time than others to think and prepare a response. Unless it is obvious they don't understand the question, don't feel that you must speak to fill the silence.

On the Job

Asking Questions on the Job On the job it will be important to know how and when to ask questions. For example, never proceed with a task if you are unsure about any part of it. It is smarter to ask than to take safety risks, waste supplies, or make it necessary for someone else to redo your work. Questions are also a good way to show interest in your job and gain a better understanding of your duties.

Gathering information from patients is an important part of most health care occupations. In order for physicians and others to make diagnoses, they need information about family history, symptoms, lifestyle habits, and anything else that affects health.

Effective Telephone Technique

The telephone provides an important link between patients and health care providers. The voice that patients hear on the phone may be their first contact with a facility. Not only does it give the first impression, it also may provide important communication the patient needs to make decisions about his or her health care. According to one health care marketing consultant, the person who answers the phone in a facility, whether it be a hospital or a single-physician office, serves as a front-line public relations representative. He goes on to say that perhaps only 10% of the callers to physicians' offices are made to feel "comfortable, welcome, and cared about."[2] Your goal should be to inspire confidence in the care your organization can provide. Keep in mind that the caller may be ill, anxious, confused, or worried.

You can see how important good phone skills are. Many are based on common sense: speak at a moderate speed in a clear, pleasant voice; be polite, saying "please" and "thank-you;" focus on the caller and listen actively; and carefully document the call in writing.

Other components of good telephone technique include:
- Identifying yourself. Your employer may have a standard greeting.
- Quickly assessing the level of understanding of the caller and speaking appropriately.
- Using nontechnical words.
- Addressing the caller by name.
- Ending the conversation on a positive note, as appropriate: "Thank you for calling." "We look forward to seeing you at your appointment next week." "I'm glad you're feeling better." "I hope you have a good day."

Nonverbal Communication

More than half of the content and meaning of our messages is communicated nonverbally through our movements, posture, gestures, and facial expressions. In fact, nonverbal communication is often more revealing than verbal communication because we are usually not aware we are doing it—it is not completely under our control. For example, telling a friend that you are "fine" when you have a worried expression on your face sends a mixed message. The friend is more likely to believe your face than your words. Nonverbal communication can either emphasize or distort the content of verbal messages. See Figure 10-7 for an example of nonverbal language.

Use the following questions as a starting point to become more aware of your own nonverbal language.
1. Do you have nervous habits, such as jiggling your leg or playing with your hair, that distract from or distort your messages? These habits can give the impression that you would rather be somewhere else.
2. Is your general posture upright or slouching? Do you face the person you're talking with or partially turn away, as if looking for escape? Leaning slightly toward the other person communicates interest.
3. Do you assume an open and accepting body position? Crossing the arms, for example, can be a sign of being closed to what the other person is saying.
4. Do you use gestures to emphasize or add meaning to your words? Or are they routine habits that add nothing to your message? Gestures are especially helpful when used for demonstrations and to communicate with people who have limited ability to understand spoken language, such as very young children, non-English speakers, and the hearing impaired.

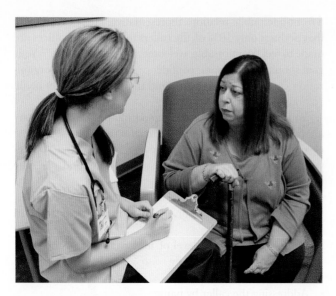

FIGURE 10-7 Take care to notice the body language of your patients, coworkers, and supervisor. *What can you tell about how this patient is feeling from her facial expression and body language?* (From Yoder-Wise PS: *Leading and managing in nursing,* ed 6, St Louis, 2015, Mosby.)

Prescription for Success: 10-6 What Does It Mean?

Choose a time and place to observe people (politely!) as they are communicating. The exercise works best if you cannot hear what they are saying.
1. Give at least three examples of nonverbal behaviors you observe.
2. What do you think they mean?
3. How can you become more aware of your own nonverbal communication?
4. Are there any gestures you often use when speaking? If so, describe what they are and what they mean.

Prescription for Success: 10-7 Rate Your Communication Skills

1. Do any of the areas listed below need improvement?
   a. Sending clear messages
   b. Listening actively
   c. Requesting feedback
   d. Asking good questions
   e. Understanding nonverbal communication
   f. Demonstrating the appropriate nonverbal communication
2. If so, what can you do to improve them?
3. What resources, including people, could help you improve your communication skills?

5. Does your face express interest or boredom? In class, do you usually face the instructor or look out the window? When an activity is announced, do you roll your eyes and exchange pained looks with other students? Poor attitudes are easy to read and can negatively affect the quality of the class by annoying the instructor or putting him or her on the defensive. Learning to control your facial expressions is important because as a health care professional you will need to maintain expressions that convey caring and reassurance even in difficult situations.

6. Do you smile when it is appropriate? Does your face send the message "I'm glad to be here talking with you"?

7. Do you maintain appropriate eye contact? Failing to look at the other person while you are speaking tends to communicate a lack of sincerity, interest, or respect. (Exception: people from some cultures may be offended or distraught by direct eye contact.)

In addition to monitoring your own nonverbal communication, practice observing it in others. This will be important when working with patients who may be unable or unwilling to fully communicate with you verbally. Learn to "listen between the lines." Do the speaker's words and actions match one another? Are there any nonverbal signs of confusion, fear, or anger that you should take into account? Does your instructor give any of the nonverbal messages, discussed in Chapter 7, that communicate what is most important for you to learn?

Ask for clarification if verbal and nonverbal messages seem to conflict. Use the feedback and question techniques discussed previously. Be willing to take the time and make the effort to get the true message. You can improve the interpersonal relationships in all areas of your life by combining an understanding of nonverbal communication with active listening and feedback.

Giving Presentations with Confidence

Many students find speaking in front of a group to be a frightening experience. This is a fear worth conquering, because the ability to speak with confidence can increase your opportunities to grow professionally and advance in your career. Proper preparation and a lot of practice can take the terror out of public speaking. See Figure 10-8 for examples of self-talk that affect confidence.

Preparing an oral presentation requires some of the same skills you use when writing, such as conducting research and organizing your material. It is said that an excellent way to learn something is to explain it to someone else. Try making oral presentations positive experiences by focusing on how you can learn from them.

Preparation

The six steps for preparing a presentation listed here are similar to the suggestions given in Chapter 8 for writing a paper.

Step One: Choose your topic early. It should be something you want to know more about or something you have strong feelings about. (Note: If you must speak on a topic you disagree with, as sometimes happens in a **debate** on a controversial subject, this is a chance to practice seeing other points of view and experiencing empathy.)

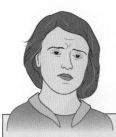

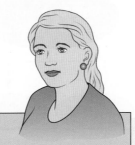

Negative Self-talk
I can't speak in front of others.
No one is interested in what I have to say.
I'll never remember my speech.
I'll shake and lose my place.
This is a nightmare!

Positive Self-talk
With practice, I can speak well.
I have something of value to share with others.
I can effectively use notes to guide my speech.
I can research until I feel comfortable with my material.
This is an opportunity to build my self-confidence!

FIGURE 10-8 You can use a good attitude and positive thinking to turn public speaking monsters into friends. Preparation and practice can give you the confidence you need to make successful presentations. *How do you feel about giving presentations to groups?*

Step Two: Be clear about your purpose: inform, persuade, demonstrate, encourage people to take action, entertain.

Step Three: Find out about your audience. What is their background? How much do they know about the topic? What are their beliefs? What is their interest level?

Step Four: Identify what you need to find out, and then do your research. Make sure you have accurate, up-to-date facts. Health care is constantly advancing and changing. Start now to develop the habit of verifying all information you use or distribute to others. In this sense, preparing for a presentation is like preparing for a test: master your material so you'll "know that you know."

Step Five: Organize your information using one of the techniques suggested in Chapter 8 to use when writing. These include idea sheets, note cards, questions, and mind maps.

Step Six: Divide your presentation into the following three parts:

1. **Part One: Introduction:** "Tell the audience what you're going to tell them."
   - Engage your listeners with an interesting story or fact. Give them a reason to pay attention. Why is this topic important to them? What should they know about it? How does it relate to their lives? Approach your audience with the positive attitude that you have something to offer them.
2. **Part Two: Body:** "Tell them."
   - This part takes up the most time. In it you explain and develop your ideas; give supporting facts, details, and examples; narrate events; and tell stories. This is the "meat" of your presentation.
   - Put the body of your speech together so it flows smoothly. For example, you might number your major points. Tell your audience how many points there will be and then announce each one as you come to it, for example:
     - "The kidneys have five important functions. The first is the regulation of fluid and electrolytes." (You then explain how they do this.)
     - "The second function is regulation of blood pressure." (More explanation.)
     - "The third is…" (etc.)
3. **Part Three: Conclusion:** "Tell them what you've told them."
   - Briefly review your major points, show how they tie together, and summarize why they are important. Tell the audience what action you want them to take or how they can use what you have told them.

It is especially important for oral presentations to be put together in a logical, organized way so that your audience can follow you.

Memory Joggers

It is usually a bad idea to read directly from your paper when giving an oral presentation. You may be tempted to look only at your paper instead of at the audience. Presentations that are read lack the warmth of human interaction and are less interesting for the audience. It is better to become familiar with your material and then use one of the following prompts to help you remember what you plan to say:

1. **Note cards** with key points.
   A. Advantages: Small and easy to handle. Prevent you from reading directly from your paper. Encourage you to practice beforehand and become familiar with the material.
   B. Watch out for: Having too many cards and getting them confused. Failing to number the cards and getting

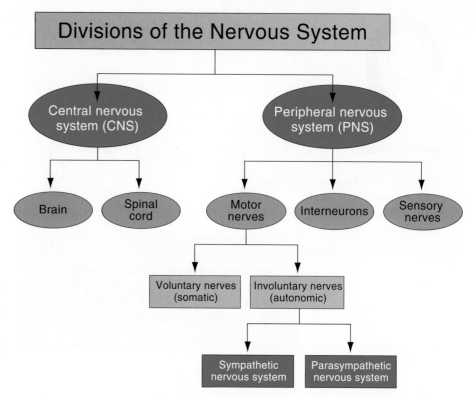

FIGURE 10-9 An example of an effective visual for an oral presentation. Keep your visuals clear and simple to highlight and illustrate your major points. *How would this diagram help your audience better understand the structure of the nervous system?* (From Gerdin J: *Health careers today,* ed 5, St Louis, 2012, Mosby.)

them out of order. Fiddling with them, which can distract the audience. Not including enough information on them and forgetting what you meant to say about each point.

2. **Outline** on full sheets of paper.
   A. Advantages: Includes more information than note cards and may increase your confidence in remembering what you plan to say.
   B. Watch out for: Rattling the paper while you speak. Looking at the paper instead of the audience. Holding the paper with both hands and failing to use natural gestures while you speak.
3. **Mind map** with major topics and supporting points in graphic form.
   A. Advantages: Easy to see major points at a glance. Especially helpful if you don't need a lot of notes to remember what you plan to say.
   B. Watch out for: There may be less room on the page to include detail, so be sure you know your material. Sometimes mind maps have words written at angles which are difficult to read quickly. Make sure you set it up in an easy-to-read format so that you don't get lost.
4. **Key points** written on PowerPoint slides, charts, or listed on the board. Figure 10-9 contains an example. Slides can serve both as visual aids for the audience and as a guide for you. See Box 10-1 for tips on creating effective PowerPoint presentations.
   A. Advantages: You and the audience are working together and sharing the experience of looking at the same materials. Listeners may become more involved if they are listening as well as seeing. This technique also helps

---

BOX 10-1 Tips for PowerPoint Presentations

- Keep it simple.
  - Don't use too many slides.
  - Use only a few words and images on each slide.
  - Don't write chunks of text, such as paragraphs.
- Avoid fancy transitions between slides.
- Use good quality images, not "cheesy" clipart.
- Use a large, simple font.
- Illustrate, don't repeat what you have just said.

---

the audience follow your presentation. Take care, however, to explain each point, rather than simply reading the list. The audience can do this for themselves!
   B. Watch out for: Poorly prepared visual aids that have too much information on them or lettering that is difficult for the audience to see. Equipment failures such as a balky computer or not having an extension cord (or discovering at the last minute that the equipment you need is being used by another class!). Prior planning and consulting with the instructor are critical to prevent being tripped up during your presentation.

Practice

"The audience is not the enemy. Lack of preparation and practice is."

Give yourself the best chance possible to give a smooth presentation by practicing it a few times in advance. Run through your presentation in front of a mirror, and then try it on friends and family members. Use the materials that will serve as your prompts to make sure they are clear and easy to follow. Time yourself to find out if you need to lengthen or shorten your presentation.

Should you memorize what you plan to say? Unless you are entering a formal speech contest or it is part of the assignment, this is usually not necessary or even a good idea. First, it is time consuming. Second, it can make you sound stiff and unnatural. Finally, and perhaps most important, if you forget a line or lose your place, it can be hard to get back on track. The resulting long pause is uncomfortable for both you and your audience.

Whenever possible, check the room where you'll be giving your presentation for details like the following:

- Is there a place to put down your cards or outline, or will you have to hold them as you speak? If you are short (like me), can you see over the podium?
- Do you know how to operate the computer or other device? Can the people in the back row read the material?
- Is there chalk or a pen available for the blackboard or white board? Will you have time to write out what you need? Is there an eraser?
- Is there a place to hang your charts, graphs, and other illustrations? Will you need tape, tacks, and so on?
- If you have models, samples, or any other objects to show, is there a place to put them down? Will the audience be able to see them? Will you pass them around?

Success Tips for Making an Oral Presentation

- Before you start to speak, take a deep breath, smile, and look at your audience. Even if you don't feel glad to be there, act as if you are. Try putting yourself and everyone else at ease.
- Look at the audience while you are speaking. Make eye contact with them. Look around the audience, not just in one direction. Catch the eyes of people who appear to be listening attentively and are "with you" to increase your feelings of support.
- Pause briefly if necessary. Some speakers even use pauses for dramatic effect. If you need a moment to gather your thoughts, stay calm. It is better to pause than to nervously ramble on or repeat filler words ("uh") that, if overused, are distracting. Pauses also give the audience time to reflect on what you have said.
- If you do lose your place or blank out a whole portion of your talk, stop and take a breath. Try not to panic. Acknowledge the audience with a smile or a nod (they may be as nervous as you are), and then concentrate on getting reorganized.
- Shift your focus from yourself to the audience. Remember that you have prepared well and have something of value to share. The audience needs this information, and you are being of service by sharing it with them.
- An old trick used by speakers is to imagine the audience in a funny situation: dressed in silly costumes, wearing big fake noses, standing on their heads—anything to change your perception of them as a threat.
- Consider organizing a buddy system. If you are already in a study group with classmates, that might do the trick. Practice your speeches with each other and offer constructive suggestions. Ask them to "cheer you on" by making

eye contact when you are speaking, signaling when your time is almost up, or letting you know if you should speak louder. Ask them to help you with handouts or visual aids. You will feel less alone.

On the Job

Giving Presentations on the Job Health care professionals who belong to professional organizations may be asked—or may volunteer—to give presentations at meetings and conferences. They may share information about innovative practices at the organization where they work, new products their employer is exploring, or something they have learned in a workshop or through their own research.

Providing patient education is becoming more important, and sometimes this takes place in groups. Shorter stays in hospital and larger numbers of outpatient surgeries mean more patients need to learn self-care techniques they will use at home. Some facilities offer group classes presented by nurses and other professionals. For example, all prospective knee-replacement candidates may be required to attend a class about the surgery, what to expect, how to prepare for it, and their postoperative recovery.

Developing Your Teamwork Skills

Modern health care delivery relies on specialized professionals who work together. Look through the descriptions for health care jobs and you will see "team player" and "teamwork" mentioned in many of them. **Teamwork** refers to the efforts of individuals to coordinate their work to achieve common goals. High-quality patient care depends on how well people communicate and function as members of a team.

People do not always work together easily and naturally. Competition, rather than cooperation, is built into many aspects of our educational system. As a student, for example, you may be competing for grades, especially on tests that are scored on a curve. On the job, there may be competition for pay raises, bonuses, and recognition by the supervisor, but competition can get in the way of providing good care. The focus in the workplace must be on serving patients, not on competing with coworkers. Teamwork is so important in health care that the National Healthcare Foundation Standard # 8 is devoted entirely to teamwork criteria.[3] See Box 10-2 and Figure 10-10.

You can begin practicing teamwork in school. Group activities assigned by instructors and lab sessions provide excellent opportunities to prepare for real work situations. You can practice cooperating in study groups. Many students report disliking group activities, saying they far prefer being responsible for their own work. If you feel this way, be aware that learning to work together and knowing how to encourage group members who fail to do their part are essential job skills. Welcoming opportunities to work with others while you are still in school is a good strategy for future career success.

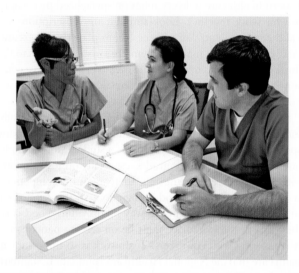

FIGURE 10-10 A group of health care professionals working together—teamwork in action. *What does the body language of the team members tell you about this meeting? Do you think it is a productive meeting? Why or why not? Do you think the team members are benefitting from the meeting? Why or why not?* (From Yoder-Wise PS: *Leading and managing in nursing,* ed 6, St Louis, 2015, Mosby.)

Differences Among Team Members

When team members support one another, work can become a more pleasant experience. On the other hand, teams in which members don't get along can slow down the work process and make life difficult for everyone. People have differences that can interfere with communication, cause hurt feelings, and disrupt the workflow. Understanding and taking advantage of these differences can help teams flourish rather than fight.

We all have different work styles and preferences. Identifying and taking advantage of the differences between team members helps prevent misunderstandings and allows each one to make a useful contribution. There are no right or wrong work styles. Ignoring differences, however, can decrease the effectiveness of the team and reduce the satisfaction of the people on it.

Here are some common work styles and preferences. As you read the list, check the ones that apply to you.
* Working methodically and completing one task or part of a task before moving on to the next.
* Working on several projects at the same time.
* Working alone and being responsible for your own work.
* Working with others in situations in which cooperation determines the success of the project.
* Working with details. Enjoying striving for accuracy and neatness.
* Thinking of ideas, but preferring to let someone else carry them out.
* Receiving assignments with clear deadlines.
* Knowing exactly what is expected.
* Receiving general instructions and a final due date. Figuring out by yourself how to get it done.
* Generating new ideas, products, and ways to work. Enjoying being creative.
* Receiving a lot of guidance. Having someone check and approve your work as it progresses.
* Working with little supervision. Asking questions when you need help.
* Preferring quiet and order.
* Finding noise and activity stimulating.

After reading this list, you can see how work styles are not only different but even contradictory! It is not surprising that people sometimes find it difficult to work together. Attempting to understand the views and needs of your coworkers and supervisors is part of empathy, discussed earlier in this chapter. Applied in the workplace, empathy contributes to establishing good relations among staff members and creating a positive work environment.

Success Tips for Being an Effective Team Member

* **Understand the ground rules and agreements.** These may not be formally stated or written down, but they are important for keeping the lines of communication open and preventing misunderstandings.
* **Be clear about the purpose and goals of the group.** Everyone should know what is to be accomplished. Have you

been assigned a specific project? Or is the goal an ongoing effort related to your role as a student or an employee?

- **Do your part—and then some.** Follow through and complete any work you have been assigned or have volunteered to do. Let the group know if you run into problems. Ask for help. Someone may be willing to pick up the slack. Letting things go can result in serious consequences, such as affecting the group's grade, endangering patient safety, or costing the facility money.
- **Listen to what others have to say.** What can you learn from them? What are their ideas on how to get the work done? What are their needs? What can they contribute?
- **Speak up.** Share your ideas and opinions.
- **Take advantage of differences.** If you are the leader, maximize group efficiency by assigning tasks that are appropriate for each member.

Case Study 10-2

Teamwork—it was a word Jim had heard a lot in his health care classes. So much, in fact, that he had gotten tired of hearing the word. In addition to lectures about teamwork, many of the assignments in his classes involved working with others. Sometimes it had worked out okay. Everyone did their part and the group completed the project. But often—too often, in fact—there were problems. The students disagreed, one or two members didn't make any contribution and the others had to pick up the slack. Jim had begun to wonder if teamwork was overrated.

"Geez," he told his friend, Mike. "This group stuff in class is frustrating. I wish the instructors would just let us work on our own. That way, I'd know I could get the assignment done."

"Yeah," Mike responded. "In my mechanics class, the guy wants us to work together in little groups to diagnose car problems. I don't get it. I thought I'd be working on my own when I got a job."

Jim was fairly quiet by nature—not really shy but he just preferred to work on his own. One of his reasons for wanting to become an ultrasound technician was the independent nature of the work: the one-on-one with the patients, the interpretation of the images taken. But Jim realized that if working in groups—practicing teamwork—was a part of his education he would just have to accept it. He did his best to contribute to the group efforts.

When Jim began his job search after completing his education, he learned that most technicians work in hospitals. He had done well in school and received a job offer from St. Mary's Hospital. As part of his orientation, he learned that he would be expected to attend a weekly staff meeting. And as it turned out, the imaging department was seeking input from its employees—even new ones, like Jim—to participate in setting goals for the department to increase their efficiency as well as patient satisfaction with scheduling, communication, and follow-through. Jim was assigned to work with two other technicians and a physician to research health care provider–patient communication and suggest ways in which hospital staff could improve their communication skills.

Questions for Thought and Reflection

1. Do you think Jim will succeed as a team member at his new job? Why or why not?
2. Do you think the team approach will be more successful in making positive changes at the hospital than the employer making all the decisions? Why or why not?
3. What part do you think teamwork will play in your chosen profession?

Prescription for Success: 10-8 Go, Team!

1. Describe at least three teams to which you belong or have belonged at work, school, church, etc.
2. Describe your role on each team.
3. How is or was the work assigned?
4. How are or were group decisions made?
5. How could each team be or have been more effective?

Understanding Organizations

Organizations, such as schools and dental offices, have a personality, just as individual people do. These personalities are known as **organizational cultures**, and they include the goals, rules, expectations, and customs of the organization as a whole. Schools have cultures, too. For example, some are very formal and emphasize respect for authority. Students are required to address their instructors by their titles and last name. Uniforms must be worn, and the rules are strictly enforced. At other schools, the atmosphere is more casual, with students and instructors on a first-name basis. At some health care facilities, people eat lunch together, celebrate birthdays and holidays, and meet after work. At others, there is a clear distinction between work and social life. Some organizations stress orderliness, engage in detailed planning, and have clear work assignments. Others move at a fast pace, with informal job descriptions and planning done "on the run."

It is important to be aware of the culture you are part of—or plan to join—to see if it matches your preferences or if you could at least adapt to it. Sometimes we can learn from a culture that has values we would like to develop in ourselves. For example, if you have poor study habits and find yourself in a strict school, this can be a great opportunity to get the encouragement you need to develop new habits.

Understanding Your Instructors

Instructors are individuals who have their own ideas about education, teaching methods, and the proper roles of teachers and students. Understanding what is important to your instructors will help you benefit fully from your classes. You will use the same skills to identify the characteristics of your future supervisors so you can work with them more effectively.

The following are some common characteristics of instructors, along with some suggestions about what you can learn from each of them:

1. **Strict.** Rules are emphasized. They are clearly explained and there are consequences if they are broken.

   You learn: Good habits for work situations in health care in which rules must be followed to ensure patient and worker safety.

2. **Value appearance.** Students must be neat, with clean, pressed uniforms, and polished shoes. Points may be deducted from grades for infractions of the dress code. Students who arrive out of uniform are sent home to change. (In a work environment, improperly dressed employees may also be asked to leave.)

   You learn: To practice the habits of excellent hygiene and an appropriate professional appearance that are critical in health care work. (Remember: Your professional career began when you started school.)

3. **Believe students should be responsible for their own learning.** Instructors with this philosophy may allow you to go all term without ever mentioning that you haven't handed in all your homework assignments. You interpret this as meaning that it's not important and are shocked to receive a final grade of D or F. Never assume that no nagging means "not important." The same can happen at work. An employee may not be told about unsatisfactory work performance until the day of a formal evaluation or the initiation of a disciplinary process.

   You learn: To take responsibility for yourself and what you must do. On the job, supervisors don't have the time to remind you constantly about your tasks. It will be up to you to get them done.

4. **Believe they must monitor students closely.** Some instructors believe it is their responsibility to prompt students to complete their work. They give constant reminders, check their students' progress frequently, call those who are absent, and generally provide "super-support." They are like those supervisors who are very organized and nurturing and are willing to tell employees what has to be done. They provide a lot of feedback.

   You learn: To work with frequent deadlines and a hands-on manager to meet deadlines and avoid falling behind in your work. Be careful, however, that you don't become dependent on continual help, because you can't always count on it being there for you.

5. **Value order.** The classroom is neat and tidy, lectures follow a clear pattern, and class activities are well planned.

   You learn: To practice orderly habits when necessary. Although your home may be comfortably chaotic, order is necessary in the health care environment. Forms must be filled out in a very specific way, tests performed in

a prescribed order, and disinfecting procedures carried out precisely. Tidying up the classroom or lab before you leave is a good habit to develop, and your instructor will certainly notice and appreciate your efforts.

6. **Value creativity over order.** Classes may seem disorganized. Lectures are mixed with interesting stories and don't follow an orderly plan. Group activities and creativity are emphasized over doing things the instructor's way.

   You learn: To be creative and think for yourself, to work with classmates, and to practice the teamwork skills discussed in this chapter.

Take advantage of different teaching styles to help you improve your weak areas. For example, if an instructor uses a lot of group activities and you prefer to work alone, you now have the opportunity to increase your ability to work with others, something you might not choose to do if it weren't required.

Working with Your Instructors

If you have difficulty with an instructor, the first step in resolving the problem should be to speak privately with him or her. If you go straight to a school administrator, neither you nor the instructor has had the chance to explore the problem and try to work out a solution together. Furthermore, the administrator doesn't have personal knowledge of the situation. The problem has been moved away from its source. However, if speaking with the instructor fails to resolve the situation, inquire about the proper procedure to follow at your school. If you have problems with your supervisor at work, you are expected to speak with that person first. How to handle interpersonal difficulties with a supervisor properly is discussed in Chapter 16.

When meeting with an instructor or supervisor to discuss a problem, it works best if you prepare for this in advance. Think about what you want to discuss and accomplish. Prepare some notes of the points you want to address. At the meeting, let the other person know that your goal is not to complain, but to resolve the issue. Learn about their views by asking questions and listening carefully and nondefensively. Express your own view of the situation and then discuss the problem in terms of possible solutions.

Most instructors decide to teach because they want to share what they have learned about their profession. They are motivated by concern for their students. This does not necessarily mean they strive to be liked by their students, because this is not the purpose of teaching. Their job is to train students to be excellent health care professionals. You may not like all your instructors, but given the chance, they all have something of value to share with you.

> ## Personal Reflection
>
> 1. How would you describe each of your instructors?
> 2. What can you learn from each of them?

Dealing with Difficult People

"One of the best ways to persuade others is with your ears—by listening to them."

—Dean Rusk

People problems cannot be avoided entirely. There will be classmates who annoy you, who don't do their share of the work on a group project, or who take up a lot of class time with questions because they never read the assignments. Family members may criticize you because they are upset about the amount of time you spend studying. Friends may be jealous of your future career opportunities. Some of your future patients, clients, coworkers, or supervisors may be a challenge, too. Learning to get along with difficult people helps make life more pleasant and productive.

In difficult situations, it is sometimes necessary to separate your role from who you are as a person. It may be your position that is a problem for someone else. For example, your family may be annoyed about your role as a student because of the time it takes you away from them. Or a patient may take his anger out on you as a representative of the clinic with which he has a problem.

Empathy, which we discussed earlier in this chapter, can help. Listen carefully to the other person. Try to see the world from his or her point of view. What could explain his/her behavior? Could there be personal problems you don't know about? Is it possible that you have done something unintentionally to hurt his or her feelings? Acknowledge the other person's feelings without agreeing to feel the same way. For example, you could begin your discussion like this: "I can see why you feel that way but…" and then state your view. Acknowledging the validity of the other person's feelings often decreases the negativity. Remain calm and courteous. Reacting negatively only makes the situation worse. (This does not mean you have to take verbal or physical abuse. If this occurs, seek the assistance of your instructor, other school personnel, or your supervisor.)

Seek solutions to interpersonal problems by being honest and "up front." Tell the other person what you see as the problem and explain how it affects you. For example, in the case of a lab partner who is never prepared to practice the assigned procedures, you could say, "I feel really frustrated when you continually come unprepared. I'm worried that I'm losing an opportunity to learn and I can't afford to do that." Simply venting your feelings or arguing won't solve the problem; it could even make it worse. Work towards a mutually acceptable agreement. Using the lab partner example, you could ask, "Can you agree to come to class prepared?" When there are serious consequences at stake, such as your grades or work performance, let the other person know what you plan to do if the situation is not resolved. Tell your lab partner, "If I can't depend on you to come to the lab prepared to work with me, I'll have to ask the instructor to allow me to change lab partners." As you attempt to find a solution, try to keep a positive attitude. From our discussion about attitude in Chapter 3, remember that it doesn't make sense to give an unpleasant person the right to ruin your day. Do what you can to seek a positive solution and then move on.

We learn and develop professionally when we engage in all types of relationships, both positive and negative. Expressing kindness toward a troublesome classmate or giving an instructor the benefit of the doubt are signs of maturity. It's easy to be professional when things are going well. True professionals can also deal effectively with challenging situations.

Dealing with Criticism

Criticism and constructive suggestions about your work present you with opportunities to learn. In school, you are paying for instruction that includes correction of your work. Your teachers would not be acting responsibly if they awarded inflated grades or withheld criticism to avoid hurting a student's feelings. It would be unfair to allow students to perform work incorrectly because this would only set them up for failure on the job, where the consequences could be more serious.

You may be criticized for your behavior or work results when you are on the job. This may come from your supervisor, a coworker, or even a patient. No one likes to be criticized and it is natural to react strongly. Dismissing the criticism as unfounded, becoming angry, taking the criticism to heart or feeling worthless are common reactions. These feelings and actions are natural but not very helpful. A more constructive response is to pay attention to the message, examine the criticism, and consider it carefully. Then decide if any or all of it actually applies to you. If it does, you can choose to benefit from it and engage in self-improvement. If it does not, consider talking over your feelings with the person who gave the criticism to see where the misunderstanding lies.

If you receive criticism that seems harsh, try to focus on the content and not on the way it is delivered. Not all instructors and supervisors are skilled at giving suggestions. If you don't understand what you did incorrectly, ask for clarification. It is your responsibility to learn as much as possible. Feelings must be put aside, if necessary, to ensure that you gain the skills necessary to be a competent health care professional.

Giving Constructive Criticism

The purpose of constructive criticism is to provide the person receiving the criticism with an opportunity to improve. This is based on the assumption that behavior can be changed for the better. It is important, when giving constructive criticism, to focus on the problem behavior rather than on the person. Suppose you have a coworker who frequently fails to return equipment to its designated storage space, causing you to waste time looking for items you need to do your work. State the problem behavior clearly: equipment is not being returned and this is affecting your efficiency. Avoid negative statements about the other person such as he/she is inconsiderate, a poor coworker, disorganized, and so on. Judgmental statements about personal characteristics tend to put people on the defensive and make them less willing to examine their behavior and make positive changes.

Here are a few more suggestions for giving criticism that helps rather than hurts:

- Choose a private location to talk, and allow enough time for the other person to respond and ask questions.
- Try to see the situation from the other person's point of view (empathy).
- Include positive statements along with the criticism.
- Be clear when explaining the problem. Give specific examples that illustrate the problem.

Neither giving nor receiving criticism is easy, but if this is done well and taken in the spirit in which it is intended, it can contribute to our learning and growth.

Summary of Key Ideas

- The ability to get along with others is necessary for career success.
- All human beings deserve to be treated with respect.
- We are all human beings, in spite of our differences.
- Empathy is essential for a caring health care professional.
- The ability to listen well is as important as the ability to speak well.
- The keys to effective oral presentations are preparation and practice.
- Understanding the work and teaching styles of others will increase your ability to work with them effectively.
- You can learn from difficult situations.

Positive Self-Talk for This Chapter

- I respect other people and try to learn something from everyone I meet.
- I value the differences between people and strive to promote understanding among people.
- I practice empathy with others.
- I have good communication skills.
- I prepare well and speak confidently in front of groups.
- I work well with others and make valuable contributions to teams.

Internet Activities

ⓔ For active links to the websites needed to complete these activities, visit http://evolve.elsevier.com/Haroun/career/.

1. The University of Washington Medical Center has developed a cultural diversity guide. Although some of the information applies specifically to this medical center, most of the material addresses cultural diversity in general. Read the online presentation and write a summary of what you learn about diversity in health care.
2. Read the Mindtools.com article, "Tolerance in the Workplace: Respecting Others' Differences." Write a summary of what you learn with ideas that can be applied to the health care workplace.
3. Use the search term "active listening." Choose one or more websites to research and write a short report explaining why listening can be difficult for many people. Then list some techniques for improving one's listening skills.
4. Use the search term "giving effective oral presentations" and look for five tips you think may help you.
5. Using the sources you find on the Internet, such as the University of Washington's Culture Clues™, research a culture and write a paper describing their medical and health care beliefs.

Building Your Resume

1. Think about how you will use your communication skills to ask questions about jobs of interest, to listen actively to find out about jobs and the needs of employers, and to explain your education, work history, and other qualifications.
2. Using Resume Building Block #4: Work History, in Chapter 2, list any transferable skills related to communication, interpersonal, or teamwork skills you acquired during previous employment. These are skills all employers look for in future hires. Are there any specific examples you can use during interviews to support your qualifications in these areas?

To Learn More

Luckmann J.: *Transcultural communication in health care*, Clifton Park. NY, 2000, Thomson Delmar Learning

From this book, you can learn about the cultural values and beliefs of a wide variety of people, including Latinos, Muslims, Native Americans, and Hasidic Jews. The author's purpose is to help students increase their self-awareness and become more sensitive to cultural differences.

Milliken M.E.: *Understanding human behavior: a guide for health care providers*, ed 8, Clifton Park. NY, 2012, Delmar Cengage

This reader-friendly book gives practical information to assist health professionals to understand and work effectively with their patients.

Purtilo R., Haddad A., Doherty R.: *Health professional and patient interaction*, 8th ed., Philadelphia, 2012, Saunders

Good discussions and examples of how to empathize and communicate with patients.

Tamparo C.D., Lindh W.Q.: *Therapeutic communications for health care*, ed 3, Clifton Park. NY, 2008, Delmar Cengage

Easy to read and full of specific details and examples.

University of Washington Medical Center, Patient and Family Education Services Culture Clues

Culture Clues™ are sheets containing tips for clinicians. They are designed to increase awareness about concepts and the preferences of patients from a number of diverse cultures including Albanian, Chinese, Latino, and Somali.
http://depts.washington.edu/pfes/CultureClues.htm.

References

1. Anderson R, Barbara A, Feldman S: What patients want: a content analysis of key qualities that influence patient satisfaction. Available at: http//www.drscore.com/press/papers/whatpatientswant.pdf.

2. Hirsch, L: Phone skills can make or break your healthcare business. Healthcare Marketing, Physician Marketing. Available at: http://www.healthcaresuccess.com/blog/healthcare-rketing/phone-skills-can-make-or-break-your-healthcare-business.html.

3. National Consortium on Health Science and Technology Education: National Healthcare Foundation Standards and Accountability Criteria. Available at: http://www.healthscienceconsortium.org/docs/Foundation_Standards__AC_October_2013.pdf.

Becoming a Professional

1. Define professionalism in health care.
2. Explain the importance of professionalism in health care.
3. Develop and maintain a professional attitude and a professional appearance.
4. Describe customer service as it applies to health care.
5. Practice therapeutic communication skills.
6. Explain how to adapt communication to special situations.
7. Develop positive relationships with your coworkers.
8. Develop strategies for effectively dealing with change in the health care workplace.
9. Develop the technical skills needed for your occupation.

Affordable Care Act A comprehensive federal law signed by President Barack Obama in March 2010 that provides for a fundamental reform of the U.S. healthcare and health insurance system.

Bedside Manner The manner that health care workers assume toward and how they interact with patients.

Coping Minimizing negative emotions arising when you experience negative events.

HIPAA Acronym that stands for the Health Insurance Portability and Accountability Act, a U.S. law designed to provide privacy standards to protect patients' medical records and other health information.

Professional Attitude How an individual views their workplace and job tasks.

Professionalism An all-encompassing concept that describes how one thinks, looks, and acts on the job.

Soft Skills Nontechnical, but important, skills such as ability to communicate, time management, and getting along with others.

What Is Professionalism?

Professionalism refers to your total package, how you think, look, and act on the job. It includes everything from your technical skills to your appearance to your work habits. When the word "professionalism" is used, it usually is understood in the positive sense. That is, it is a compliment to be told that you are acting professionally.

Soft skills are major components of professionalism. These are personality traits and personal qualities such as the following:
- Work ethic
- Attitude
- Self-confidence
- Adaptability
- Optimism

In addition to traits, soft skills include skills such as time management, problem-solving, and effective communication. It is reported that for many occupations, soft skills are as or even more important than occupational (technical) skills. For example, a medical assistant may be skilled at giving an injection, but if she cannot work effectively with a patient who is terrified of needles, there is a good chance the patient will not return to this particular clinic. Although soft skills cannot be easily measured, such as computer and math skills can, it is obvious when they are lacking.

Your level of professionalism influences your interaction with others, including patients and their family and friends; coworkers; and supervisors. It encompasses everything you do, both on the job and in your personal life. The underlying value of professionalism is a commitment to goals that meet the needs of others.[1]

That sounds like a lot—and it is! Professionalism means applying what you learn in school. In this chapter, we will pull together the skills, both technical and "soft," presented throughout this book and show how to apply them to be successful on the job (Figure 11-1).

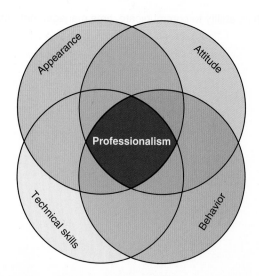

FIGURE 11-1 Professionalism includes four major categories. *How would you rate yourself in each category?*

In Chapter 1, we discussed what patients and employers want from health care workers. We will expand on these wants and needs and talk about what you can do to meet them.

See Box 11-1 for a variety of definitions of professionalism in health care.

The Importance of Professionalism in Health Care

"Identity as a health professional carries with it expectations on the part of society, as well as privileges and responsibilities."

—Ruth Purtilo and Amy Haddad

Workers in every industry who display professionalism are valued by employers and consumers. However, professionalism takes on extra importance in health care. Consider the difference between a customer buying a pair of shoes—or even a large purchase such as a car—and the same person as a patient seeking treatment for a health problem such as heart disease. In which case is the person most emotionally involved? Most vulnerable? Having the most to lose? While most people consider shopping or getting a haircut to be pleasant experiences, almost no one looks forward to a visit to the doctor, dentist, or hospital. Helping to ease the worries and fears of patients is the responsibility of everyone on the health care team.

Your professionalism can instill trust and provide competent care to the individuals who come to you for assistance. This is true whether you provide direct patient care or work behind the scenes to support the health care process.

> **Prescription for Success: 11-1 What Do You Think?**
>
> *"Healthcare professionals have a tremendous obligation. The most important thing is that healthcare professionals have higher standards than most professions because they are dealing with the dignity of patients and their ability to be healed."**
>
> —Robert J. Wolff, PhD
>
> Do you agree with Dr. Wolff? Write a short essay explaining why or why not.
>
> *From Healthcare professionalism: How important is proper bedside manner?". Available at: http://source.southuniversity.edu/healthcare-professionalism-how-important-is-proper-bedside-manner-132067.aspx.

Professional Attitude

A **professional attitude** is how you view your work. In turn, your attitude determines how you act, forming the foundation for your actions. Health care workers with professional attitudes take their work seriously. They recognize their own importance in the workplace and develop positive habits such as being on time, interacting courteously with everyone, and keeping their skills up-to-date. Your attitude drives everything you do and is a major determinant of your career success and personal happiness.

Your professional attitude affects the quality of not only your life, but the lives of others. Most jobs in health care consist of direct human contact and what you do and say influences everyone with whom you interact. Even in jobs with minimal patient contact, such as medical coding and billing and lab technology, the quality of your work, influenced by your attitude, can affect others in significant ways.

Sometimes it can be challenging to maintain a positive attitude. Not everything in every job will be to your liking. There may be frantically busy days, difficult patients, and annoying coworkers. If you choose to focus on these negatives, you are likely to adopt a bad attitude. In these situations, you need to remember that your attitude is under *your control*. As discussed in Chapter 3, how you respond to situations is more important than the circumstances themselves. You can interpret events positively, neutrally, or negatively. If you habitually choose to concentrate on the positives in your work environment, you will likely experience a more satisfying work life.

Prescription for Success: 11-2 Attitude Makes the Difference

How do you think the attitudes of the health care workers in the following examples are likely to affect their work today? And their customers and patients?

1. Julie, a pharmacy technician, is not thrilled to be at work today. Her dog is sick and she really didn't want to leave home him alone. On top of that, she almost ran out of gas on the way to work and had to stop at a station near work that is more expensive than the one she usually goes to. She imagines that this will be the day when the most demanding and difficult patients come by to get their prescriptions.
2. Carlos, a physical therapist assistant, is anticipating a good day. A recent graduate, he has been on the job for 3 weeks working alongside Amy, the supervising therapist. Today Amy is going to have him work with some of the patients on his own.
3. Dana, a dental assistant, hopes that the patients who Dr. Hopkins works with today are a better bunch than most of the people who came in yesterday. Talk about losers! Some of them hadn't been to a dentist in years! And then they complained about how much work they needed to have done.
4. Zach, a surgical tech, heard he will be working with Dr. Sims next week. This is not good news—in fact, he dreads what's coming up. He's heard about Sims' tantrums and short temper with everyone he works with.

Personal Reflection

1. Are you aware of how your attitude affects your life?
2. Do you consider yourself to have a positive attitude?
3. If not, what might you do to develop a more positive outlook?

Professional Appearance

Your appearance communicates the level of respect you have for yourself and for patients. Your appearance can influence the impression patients have about your competence. To summarize what was discussed in more detail in Chapter 2, there are several characteristics that define a professional appearance in health care:

- Conservative
  - Avoid extreme styles, revealing clothing, heavy make-up.
- Neat and clean
  - Details count! Clothes should be clean, pressed, and in good shape; shoes clean and in good repair.
- Safe
  - Avoid anything that can be caught by patients or equipment, such as long hair worn loose and dangling jewelry. Avoid fragrances and long and/or painted fingernails in which bacteria can hide.
- Good hygiene
  - Bathed, odor-free, clean teeth and hair.

If you were to be in close contact with a person, such as a medical or nursing assistant, how would *you* want them to look—and smell? Always keep in mind how your appearance affects others. See Figure 11-2 for an example of appropriate workplace appearance.

The Business of Health Care

We don't always think in terms of health care as a business, but to be able to provide services we must consider the business side: revenue, expenses, employees, legalities, and marketing. Health care is actually a huge industry. In fact, it is the largest service industry in the United States with spending in 2012 of $2.8 trillion.[2]

It is also the fastest-growing sector of the U.S. economy, employing over 18 million workers.[3]

Customer Service

Customer service, or more to the point, *excellent service*, is a phrase frequently heard these days relating to health care (Box 11-2).

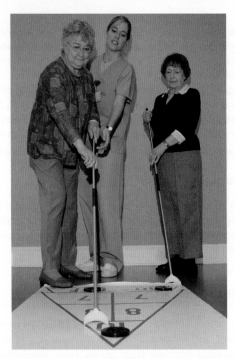

FIGURE 11-2 A professional appearance communicates competence. *Describe in detail what makes this nursing assistant's appearance appropriate.* (From Sorrentino S, Remmert L: *Mosby's textbook for nursing assistants,* ed 8, St Louis, 2012, Mosby.)

BOX 11-2 Excellent Service

The author of one study concluded that excellent service consists of four elements:
1. Deliver the promise of quality healthcare.
2. Provide a personal touch.
3. Go the extra mile.
4. Resolve problems well.

From Johnston R: Towards a better understanding of service excellence, Managing Service Quality 14: 129–133, 2004.

Patients are becoming more demanding about services, along with having more choices of providers.[4] A number of surveys and studies have been conducted to learn what patients expect from their health care encounters. In one survey of 6000 patients, the top priorities of health care consumers were friendly staff and convenience. The survey also found that patients are less forgiving of negative experiences than retail customers and more likely to depend on personal experience and recommendations from friends and family when choosing a health care provider.[4] For these reasons, patient satisfaction is taken seriously by both those who pay for services, such as medical insurance companies and Medicare, and the providers of health care. Health care providers, along with the government, are increasing their efforts to promote and measure patient satisfaction. For example, the famous Mayo Clinic has developed a training program called *PLEASE CARE* to increase the professionalism of allied health staff[5] (Figure 11-3).

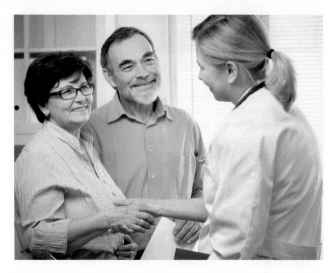

FIGURE 11-3 Friendliness is highly valued by patients as they enter the health care environment. *What is this health care professional's body language communicating to this couple?* (Copyright AlexRaths/iStock/Thinkstock.)

Your Effect on Patients

"Too often we underestimate the power of a touch, a smile, a kind word, a listening ear, an honest compliment, or the smallest act of caring, all of which have the potential to turn a life around."

—Leo Buscaglia

A major component in delivering excellent customer service in health care is how the providers of care interact with patients. The nature of patient–provider interactions, referred to as "**bedside manner**," affects patient outcomes. Poor bedside manner, characterized by an uncaring attitude, poor listening skills, and the inability to clearly convey information to patients, can have negative consequences. At the same time, patients who perceive good bedside manner are more likely to follow treatment and instructions, have more positive health outcomes, and be satisfied with the care they receive. In fact, some studies report that many patients value good bedside manner and listening skills more than clinical competence.[6]

Behaviors on the part of the health care provider, such as rudeness, a cold attitude, and poor listening skills can increase a patient's fears and anxiety. In addition, it can negatively affect potential benefits of the health care encounter.

Consider the potential consequences of the following situations:
1. When Kathy, who is obese, feels that nurse Jennifer is talking down to her, she feels humiliated and angry and soon stops focusing on the instructions that Jennifer is giving her about improving her diet.
2. Medical office receptionist Kalina is not happy to see elderly and lonely Mr. Harris who visits the immediate care clinic at least once a week with a perceived ailment. Her impatience shows when she greets him with, "And what is it *this* time, Mr. Harris?"
3. Medical assistant Mike greets teenage Greg with, "I'm here to take your medical history," then never looks up

from the laptop on which he is recording the information. Finally, Mike asks, "So what are you here for?" but doesn't really seem to listen when Greg tries to explain the symptoms he finds embarrassing to talk about.

- Do you think these patients will benefit from the interactions they are having with their health care providers?
- Will they follow the instructions given them?
- Are they likely to return to the same facility the next time they need care?

Keep in mind that respect will not always be mutual. Patients who are experiencing illness or injury may take out their frustrations and fears on those who are trying to help them. Some patients will have values and lifestyles in opposition to your own—those who have committed crimes, for example. These situations call for a high level of professionalism on the part of the health care worker to avoid being judgmental and uncaring.

What are the characteristics, then, of good bedside manner? Although each patient has different expectations and perceptions of bedside manner, the following were repeatedly reported as important in a number of studies:

- Good listener
- Caring, compassionate, and kind
- Sensitive
- Empathetic
- Respectful

Strive to be a health care professional with good bedside manner who contributes to, rather than takes away from, positive experiences and results for the patients (Figure 11-4).

Today's employers want to hire employees who can help them deliver the high quality of service that patients want—and deserve. Developing a professional attitude along with good soft skills can help you become one of those valued employees.

Personal Reflection

1. Think about health care encounters you have had, both positive and negative. How was your experience influenced by the health care providers who worked with you?

Prescription for Success: 11-3 Make It Positive for Patients

1. In the section, "Your Effect on Patients," Jennifer, Kalina, and Mike have poor interactions with patients. Describe, either in writing or role playing, how these encounters could be more positive.
2. Explain how more positive encounters might benefit these patients.

A Professional Service Model

The SullivanLualin Group in San Diego works with health care organizations to increase their patient satisfaction. They developed a service model, C.L.E.A.R., to organize and present simple behaviors that enhance customer satisfaction.

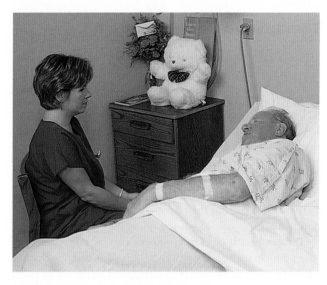

FIGURE 11-4 A comforting, caring bedside manner can positively affect patient outcomes. *What might this patient be experiencing? Why do you think the nurse is sitting instead of standing next to the bed? What is she communicating with her posture and facial expression?* (From deWit S, O'Neill P: *Fundamental concepts and skills for nursing,* ed 4, St Louis, 2014, Saunders.)

CONNECT *Make a great first impression*	• Acknowledge patients immediately, even non-verbally if necessary.
	• Use eye contact and smile.
	• Introduce yourself, and tell what your job is (if appropriate).
	• Wear your name badge so patient can see it and read it.
	• Use the patient's name.
	• Keep your voice warm and welcoming; be polite: say "please" and "thank you."
LISTEN *Make patients feel valued and listened to*	• Use eye contact and a pleasant expression.
	• Use head nods to indicate you're paying attention.
EXPLAIN *Ensure patients understand information and instructions*	• Tell patients what you're doing.
	• Use simple language (not abbreviations or acronyms).
	• Tell patients what's going to happen.
ASK *Make sure patients get their needs met*	• Ensure patient's comfort with information, surroundings.
	• Ask for other questions.
RE-CONNECT *End visit on positive note*	• Check with roomed patient every 10 minutes and say, "Thanks for your patience."
	• Acknowledge patients/others as they depart saying, "Take care."

From SullivanLuallin Group, 3760 4th Ave., San Diego, CA 92103. Used with permission.

Therapeutic Communication

"We are much more likely to respect a patient's decision or action if we understand its rationale."

—Ruth Purtilo and Amy Haddad

In health care, communication takes on special significance. Did you notice that most of the behaviors in the C.L.E.A.R. model discussed in the previous section involved communication? The communication techniques used in health care interactions are often referred to as "therapeutic communication," defined as the face-to-face process of interacting that focuses on advancing the physical and emotional well-being of a patient.[7]

Today's health care environment can be especially challenging for patients. They may be forced to change doctors whenever their insurance plan changes. The doctor or other professional they do see may have limited time to spend with them. When they are seriously ill or injured, they may have to see a specialist they've never met. And modern, complex technology can be intimidating.

Another factor has increased the need for good communication with patients: the Affordable Care Act, signed into law in 2010. The changes brought about by this law have resulted in many more Americans with health care insurance and therefore, increased access to health care. Many of these individuals have visited doctors infrequently and are confused by how insurance works and the health care system itself.

Allied health personnel are playing an increasingly important role working with patients to inform and create a bridge between patients and physicians, dentists, therapists, and other providers. You may be the critical link that makes the difference between a satisfied patient and one who seeks care elsewhere.

Listening

"When people talk, listen completely. Most people never listen."

—Ernest Hemingway

The starting point for effective communication is *listening*. Listening demonstrates respect and shows that you care. It is only through listening and *hearing* what others are saying that you can understand and assess their needs. And only by knowing their needs can you determine how to best meet those needs.

In satisfaction surveys, patients list being listened to as a major factor. One study showed that patients value good listening skills more than clinical competence. Furthermore, when patients feel listened to, they are more likely to share the information that helps the health care provider to correctly assess and treat their conditions. They are also more likely to follow the directions given for their self-care.[8]

Active listening, discussed in Chapters 7 and 10, is a skill you can learn and improve with practice. Box 11-3 includes

BOX 11-3 Listening Actively

- Remove distractions as much as possible.
- Focus on the other person and pay attention.
- Look at the other person (if using a computer, look up often).
- Maintain eye contact, if culturally appropriate.
- Empathize—try to imagine how the other person feels and understand his or her point of view.
- Don't interrupt.
- Don't think about what you are going to say next.
- Don't argue mentally with the speaker.

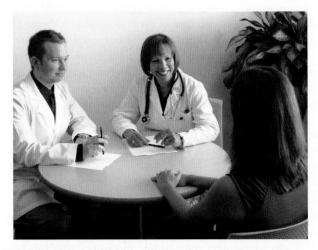

FIGURE 11-5 Being able to listen well is one of the most important skills for a successful career. *Do these health professionals appear to be listening actively? Why or why not?* (From Elsevier: *Job readiness for health professionals,* St Louis, 2013, Saunders.)

a review of its components and Figure 11-5 shows an illustration of an encounter involving active listening. In health care, active listening has even more meaning. It requires listening with a "third ear." This means noting what the patient is *not* saying, picking up on hints not directly stated, and trying to determine the real meaning of the patient's words.[9,10]

Personal Reflection

1. Pay attention to your listening skills over the next few days.
2. Do you think you really "hear" what people are saying?
3. Do your listening skills need improving?
4. What can you start doing now to improve them?

Verbal Communication

Sending effective verbal messages was discussed in Chapter 10. When speaking with patients, it is especially important

TABLE 11-1

Examples of Health Care Questions

Closed-Ended	Open-Ended	Probing	Leading
Are you feeling better?	Can you tell me about how you are feeling today?	Do you feel better since starting the medicine the doctor prescribed?	You look like you're feeling better today, right?
Are you in pain right now?	Can you describe the nature of the pain?	When do you feel the most pain?	It looks like you are in pain now, right?
Did you take all the tablets the doctor prescribed?	Can you describe how you felt after taking the medication?	Did you feel worse after taking the medication in the morning or in the evening?	Did you stop taking the medication because you felt better?
Are you doing your exercises every day?	Which of the exercises are you doing each day?	Which exercises are you finding most difficult?	You don't believe the exercises are helping your recovery, do you?

that your messages are clear and complete because how you are understood can have direct consequences on their well-being. Consider the following patient characteristics when composing your message to increase the chance that it is understood:

- Level of education
- Knowledge of his or her condition
- Native language
- Age
- Sensory impairments
- Level of pain, medication, confusion
- State of emotion, such as fear or anger

This leads us to a word about medical terminology. Students spend many hours learning these words. But they are not everyday words for most people. Limit their use when communicating with patients. They may become confused, but hesitate telling you they don't understand, not wanting to appear dumb or wasting your time. Take care to always adjust your language to your listener's level of understanding.

Once you have determined the appropriate level of communication for your listener, the next step before you begin to speak is to establish, in your own mind, the purpose of your communication. What do you hope to accomplish? Reassure? Secure information? Inform? Organize your message with your purpose in mind.

In addition to words, the tone of your voice sends a powerful message. Do you sound warm? Interested? Or is your voice a monotone, communicating boredom and lack of interest? Your voice should be pleasantly pitched—not too high. Here are other suggestions for speaking in a professional manner:

- Use proper grammar.
- Speak at a moderate speed.
- Don't mumble.
- Avoid slang, especially that which is common to one age or cultural group.

- Avoid constantly repeating words or expressions such as "like" and "you know."
- Avoid very casual language such as "cool," "he goes" (instead of "he said"), and "sucks."
- Never use swear words.

Questions

An important component of verbal communication in health care is asking questions. The four major types of questions were described in Chapter 10. Let's review and then look at the examples in Table 11-1 that apply specifically to health care:

1. Closed-ended: can be answered with one word or "yes" or "no." These questions are useful for obtaining facts.
2. Open-ended questions: require a longer answer. Good for learning about a patient's condition, needs.
3. Probing: acquire additional information. Responder supplies more information.
4. Leading: question gives clue to provide answer.

Asking good questions facilitates communication and encourages patients to share in making decisions about their health. Some commonly phrased questions aren't likely to tell you anything useful. Here are some examples, along with suggestions for improvement.

Not very helpful: "Are you okay?"
Better: "You seem upset. Do you want to tell me about it?"
Not very helpful: "Do you understand how you need to change your diet?"
Better: "Okay, can you tell me three ways you plan to change your diet?"

For the first question in each pair, the easy—but maybe not complete, or even correct—answer is "yes." The patient, out of embarrassment or concern for your time, may simply respond with a "yes" when the real answer would be, "I don't know." Or "I don't understand." Patients may also remain silent when you ask them questions. Rather than being a sign of understanding, this may indicate the opposite—a complete *lack* of understanding.

Patients should also be encouraged to ask their *own* questions. This enables them to share in making decisions about their health. They may be stressed by the health care environment, as well as feeling vulnerable. These conditions can promote "white-coat silence"—the reluctance of patients to ask questions.[11] You can encourage them to overcome this silence by asking them:

- What questions are on your mind?
- What more would you like to know about your condition/treatment options/test results/etc.?
- Do you have questions about how to contact us if you experience side effects from the medication? Do you have questions about how you are to perform your exercises at home?

Prescription for Success: 11-4 Asking Good Questions

Ask about each of the following four situations using the following types of questions in this order: (1) open-ended, (2) close-ended, and (3) leading.

Example: Inquire about how a patient is feeling.
(1) Are you feeling better today?
(2) Tell me about how you're feeling today.
(3) You're feeling better today, aren't you?

1. Ask about a patient's success following the weight-loss diet the physician prescribed.
2. Ask a patient if he feels okay to drive home.
3. Inquire about whether a patient understands why he is having an x-ray.
4. Ask a coworker about his sick child. (You've heard around the office that the child is getting better.)

Feedback

Feedback is a technique for checking both your understanding as well as that of your listener. As explained in Chapter 10, feedback can take several forms. Because it is so important for you and patients to understand each other, these are important tools in your communication toolbox. Here are examples in which the three types of feedback are used:

You work in the billing department of a large clinic. Mr. Gonzalez calls and states that he doesn't understand why he received a bill from your office.

Feedback: Mr. Gonzalez, if I understand correctly, you don't understand why you received a bill from our office. Is that right?

Reflect: You received a bill from our office and you don't know what it's for?

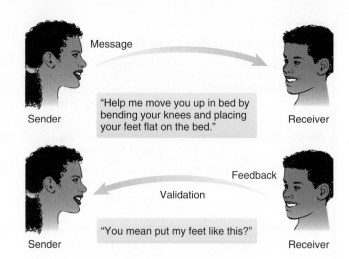

FIGURE 11-6 Feedback helps ensure that a message is received and understood. *Look for opportunities in your daily interactions to use feedback to clarify messages you aren't sure that you have understood correctly.* (From deWit S, O'Neill P: *Fundamental concepts and skills for nursing,* ed 4, St Louis, 2014, Saunders.)

Clarify: Can you tell me why you believe you shouldn't have received this bill?

Mrs. Sanborn tells you, the medical assistant, that she doesn't agree with the doctor's recommendation to have her child immunized.

Feedback: You are saying you don't agree with Dr. Shultz about having Emily immunized?

Reflect: You don't think Emily should receive the recommended vaccinations?

Clarify: What are your reasons for not wanting to have Emily immunized?

Learn to use feedback to ensure that you understand the messages that patients are trying to convey. Figure 11-6 illustrates the feedback process. Table 11-2 shows examples of a variety of therapeutic communication techniques.

Nonverbal Communication

Nonverbal communication, introduced in Chapter 10, usually communicates even more meaning than words. Recall that it includes movements, posture, gestures, and facial expressions. These are emotional responses done unconsciously which is why they may contradict what a person says. You may say you are interested in what a patient is saying, but if you are looking at your watch, your body language says something else. Here are some specific suggestions for showing respect and putting patients at ease:

- Sit at the same level.
- Face and lean toward the other person.
- Make eye contact.
- Smile warmly.
- Use a friendly, reassuring tone of voice.
- Look up frequently and make eye contact when taking notes or entering data into a computer (Figure 11-7).

TABLE 11-2
Therapeutic Communication Techniques

Technique	Examples	Rationale
General leads	"Go on." "I see." "Please continue."	Encourages patient to continue or elaborate.
Open-ended questions or statements	"Tell me more about that feeling." "I'd like to hear more about…"	Encourages patient to elaborate rather than answer in one or two words.
Offering self	"I'm here to listen." "Can I help in some way?"	Shows caring, concern, and readiness to help.
Restatement	Patient says, "I tossed and turned last night." Nurse says, "You feel like you were awake all night."	Restates in different words what the patient said; encourages further communication on that topic.
Reflection	Patient says, "I'm so scared about the surgery; anesthesia terrifies me." Nurse says, "Something scares you about anesthesia?" Patient looks scared. Nurse says, "You look scared."	Reflects received message back to patient. Also encourages further verbalization of feelings. Reflects feelings. Can also be used if patient is unable to verbalize or if nonverbal information doesn't match the verbal.
Seeking clarification	Patient says, "Having my little girl come to visit me was so hard. I'm so upset." Nurse says, "Something about your daughter's visit upset you?"	Seeks clarification about the source of the upset feeling. Helps the patient clarify thoughts or ideas.
Focusing	"Do you have any questions about your chemotherapy?	Asking a goal-directed question helps the patient focus on key concerns.
Encouraging elaboration	"Tell me what that felt like." "I need more information about that." "Tell me more about that experience."	Helps the patient describe more fully the concern or problem under discussion.
Giving information	"The test results take at least 48 hours." "You will get a preoperative injection that will make you sleepy before you are taken to the operating room."	Provides the patient with information relevant to specific health care or situation.
Looking at alternatives	"Have you thought about…?" "You might want to think about…" "Would this be an option?"	Helps patients see options and consider alternatives to make their own decisions about health care.
Silence	Patient says, "I don't know if I should have chemotherapy, radiation, or both." Nurse remains silent, sitting attentively but quietly.	Allows patient time to gather thoughts and sort them out.
Summarizing	"You've identified your alternatives pretty clearly." "You are aware of the important signs and symptoms to report to your physician; you plan to make an appointment next week."	Sums up the important points of an interaction.

From: deWit S, O'Neill P: *Fundamental concepts and skills for nursing,* 4 ed, St Louis, 2014, Elsevier.

Even if your day is hectic, try to maintain a relaxed manner so that patients don't feel rushed and as if they are just a number. If you are the first person to greet an incoming patient, give them a smile and nod of recognition, even if you are busy with someone else, on the phone, or completing a computer entry. Let patients know they are welcome and will be attended to shortly.

Learning to read the body language of others is just as important as being aware of your own. Do the patient's words match his or her body language? Most obvious are facial expressions that display worry, fear, or anger. Other signs are more subtle, as shown in Table 11-3.

A word of caution: the meanings listed in Table 11-3 are *suggested* reasons for behaviors. Always check out their meaning by asking questions. For example, a person who is cold may cross her arms and lean forward. Fidgeting or appearing distracted may be due to pain. It is important not to make assumptions.

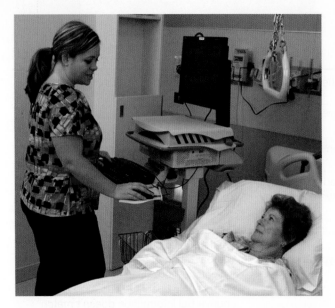

FIGURE 11-7 Although this nurse is entering data into the computer, she remains focused on the patient. *How do you think the patient would feel if the nurse didn't make eye contact with her, but simply looked at her computer as she worked?* (From deWit S, O'Neill P: *Fundamental concepts and skills for nursing,* ed 4, St Louis, 2014, Saunders.)

Prescription for Success: 11-5 Meaning through Motion

Choose a television program that has more dialogue than action. Turn off the sound for 10 or 15 minutes and watch the body language of the actors. Write a list of what appear to be the emotions of the characters based on what they do rather than say.

TABLE 11-3
Body Language Messages

Behavior	Possible Meaning
Picking at clothes	Have an idea or opinion but are unwilling to share
Slumped shoulders	Depression, discouragement
Finger-tapping	Impatience, nervousness
Shrugged shoulders	Indifference, discouragement
Rubbing the nose	Puzzlement
Whitened knuckles and clenched fists	Anger
Fidgeting	Nervousness
Open body posture, leaning forward	Responsive
Open body posture, leaning back	Considering, evaluating
Closed body language, leaning forward	Skeptical, possibly angry
Touch face, cover, mouth, pull on ears, look back and forth or up and down	Not truthful

From: Tamparo CD, Lindh WQ: *Therapeutic communications for health care,* ed 3, Clifton Park, N.Y., 2008, Delmar Cengage; Body language can tell you if your patient will commit to care: what you see is what you should hear. Chiropractic News. Available at: http://www.chiroeco.com/chiropractic/news/3358/802/body-language-can-tell-you-if-your-patient-will-commit-to-care-what-you-see-is-what-you-should-hear-/.

Trouble Ahead? 11-1

Linda and her husband, Steve, worked and raised their family in southern California. Linda was a successful office manager for a real estate agency and Steve worked in the airline industry. They both enjoyed their jobs and were able to send their two children to good universities.

But Los Angeles is a huge city and was feeling more crowded by the day. It had been exciting when they were younger, but now it seemed like more of a battle to get anything done. And the traffic kept getting worse. Commutes to work could take well over an hour—sometimes it took two hours if there was an accident or other problem.

Steve and Linda talked it over and decided to consider moving to a smaller community. They both enjoyed outdoor recreation—fishing, hiking, and camping—and getting out to areas they could enjoy was getting more difficult as the areas around Los Angeles built up. They considered how much they had saved for retirement and Steve realized that his knowledge of the airline industry might lend itself to consulting. So one spring, they sold their house, packed up, and moved to a small city in northern California.

Linda became involved in the community, volunteering at the library, helping raise money for charity, and pursuing her hobby of knitting. Steve did find jobs consulting; the only drawback was that he had to travel to where the companies were, and this sometimes meant being gone for a few weeks at a time. This was not a problem until Linda began experiencing abdominal discomfort. At first, she thought it was indigestion, or perhaps stress. She had been quite busy lately and her daughter had recently moved in—temporarily—after separating from her husband.

Linda finally decided she had better get checked out at the local clinic and made an appointment. Being relatively new in town, this meant finding a new doctor and then waiting until there was an appointment available. When she called to inquire about an appointment, she was immediately put on hold. When the receptionist finally came on the line, she was obviously in a hurry and wanted to get something scheduled and move on to the next thing. Linda, having emphasized customer service in her office management career, saw this as a red flag. But it had turned out that not every doctor in town accepted her insurance, so she didn't have many choices. Her stomach pains had increased, she was starting to lose weight, and she was becoming increasingly worried, so she went ahead and made an appointment.

Once she had seen the physician, she was sent to the clinic's lab for a blood draw. Linda was nervous—she very much disliked needles, but it was obvious with her sighing and eye-rolling that the lab tech thought it was silly for a grown woman to be afraid of such a thing. So Linda gritted her teeth and got on with it.

The first blood tests didn't reveal anything, but with continuing symptoms Linda went through a series of imaging tests that required her to drink unpleasant liquids. Steve was away at a job during this time, so it was particularly stressful. She really could have used his support. One of her worst days during the time before her condition was finally diagnosed as Crohn's disease was when the technician in charge of performing a diagnostic test commented, "Gee, we don't do many of these tests. Most people's insurance doesn't pay for them." While the test was being conducted, Linda overhead the same technician say to a coworker, "Well, I hope she doesn't have what we're testing for here. Lots of people who have that don't make it."

Questions for Thought and Reflection

1. List the instances of unprofessional behavior exhibited by the staff at the clinic.
2. How could some of the encounters with Linda been handled better? Be specific.
3. How do you think the staff affected Linda's physical condition? Her emotional condition?
4. If you were brought in as a consultant to improve the customer service at this clinic, how would you start?

Adapting Communication to Special Situations

While you must consider the needs of each person with whom you are communicating, you may encounter patients who have needs beyond the usual:

- Individuals who are terminally ill
  - Many dying patients want to express their fears and concerns. A major problem reported is being ignored or having their communication disregarded. Let them know that you are available and willing to talk about whatever concerns they may have.
- Individuals with sensory impairments
  - Hearing loss: a growing percentage of the population, due to aging, has various degrees of hearing loss. Face them directly with light showing your face, remove noise sources, and speak slowly and clearly.
  - Blindness: announce your presence and introduce yourself, explain what you are going to do in detail, and communicate verbally what would otherwise be communicated with gestures, etc.
  - Aphasia (difficulty or inability to express speech): eliminate background noise; ask yes-no questions; give choices of possible answers; use visual prompts. Enable patient to point, use hand gestures, or draw (Figure 11-8).
- Individuals who do not speak English
  - Determine the level of English the patient speaks and understands.
  - Use simple words and short sentences.
  - Use pictures and gestures.
  - Request frequent feedback.
  - Request an interpreter, if necessary.
- Individuals who are angry
  - Remain calm and polite.
  - Listen carefully.
  - Express concern.

- Answer questions.
- Address their concerns.
- Individuals who are in pain, medicated, or disoriented
  - Speak slowly and clearly.
  - Use simple language.
  - Repeat information as necessary.
  - Return when they are better able to communicate.[12]

Prescription for Success: 11-6 Creating Effective Messages

How would you design your message and method of delivery for the following situations?

1. You need to give a 4-year-old an injection. It might hurt a bit.
2. You are explaining to an angry patient on the phone that his insurance company refused to cover the entire cost of a procedure.
3. You are explaining an exercise (physical therapy) to a blind patient who has had a knee replacement.
4. A hospice (dying) patient you have grown fond of tells you she is afraid of dying because she worries about her teenage son being on his own.
5. You need to explain the purpose of a medication to a patient who has a significant hearing loss.

Consideration for Coworkers

A component of professionalism is considering the needs of others. There are times when it will be necessary to put their needs before your own. A good habit to practice is to continually ask yourself, "How does my behavior affect other people?"

For example, consider how you manage your time: arriving late to work and to meetings inconveniences coworkers and may cause patients to wait unnecessarily; failing to meet work deadlines may have negative consequences for your supervisor.

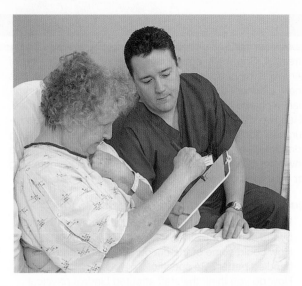

FIGURE 11-8 Sometimes special communication techniques are necessary when working with patients. In this photo, the health care professional is helping an aphasic patient to communicate her needs. *Think about the frustration experienced by patients who have sensory or physical impairments that interfere with their ability to communicate. How can health care professionals encourage and comfort them?* (From de-Wit S, O'Neill P: *Fundamental concepts and skills for nursing,* ed 4, St Louis, 2014, Saunders.)

In order for a health care facility to run efficiently, supervisors must know that employees are dependable and responsible: that they follow through and perform their work as assigned, are well organized, and are willing to adapt to the constant changes taking place in today's health care environment. Your goal should be to help your supervisor solve problems, not become another problem that he or she must deal with.

Have consideration for your coworkers, and treat them with respect. Practice good communication skills with them. Good interpersonal relations among coworkers help deliver better health care. In fact, one study showed that when doctors were more courteous to operating room staff, their patients were more likely to survive and avoid complications than the patients of doctors who were rude.[13] It is known that when people are treated poorly, they tend to treat others poorly in turn. Common courtesy spreads more good than you might think. So don't take your coworkers for granted—greet them with a smile and say "please" and "thank you."

In addition to courtesy, there are other ways to show consideration in the workplace:

- *Don't be a complainer.* Constantly complaining and whining can bring everyone down. Seek solutions: discuss problems with your supervisor and offer possible solutions. Try the problem-solving method explained in Chapter 9. If the situation cannot be changed, seek ways to adapt.
- *Avoid TMI—too much information.* It is common for coworkers to become friends, socializing during and after work. But it is best to avoid sharing too much personal detail, especially personal problems. And your personal or work problems should *never* be discussed with patients. They have come to resolve their own problems, not to hear about yours.

- *Don't be a backstabber.* Talking behind a coworker's back or taking credit for something positive that you didn't do can destroy your relationships at work.
- *Don't blame others.* Accept responsibility for your mistakes.
- *Work neatly, put things away.* Don't cause others to waste their time picking up after you or looking for supplies and equipment you didn't put back in their place.

For additional discussions of interpersonal skills, including teamwork, see Chapter 10, "Developing Your People Skills" and Chapter 16, "Success on the Job."

Adapting to Change

"Progress is impossible without change, and those who cannot change their minds cannot change anything."

—George Bernard Shaw

During the last few decades, health care has changed more rapidly than at any time in history. Being able to adapt to continual change has become an essential part of professionalism. Here are examples of changes you may encounter during your career:

- Your organization—hospital, clinic, home health agency—is purchased by another.
- There are radical changes in policies.
- New government laws and regulations go into place, such as **HIPAA**, the **Affordable Care Act**, and new Medicare guidelines.
- New technology becomes available and you must learn to use it.
- New drugs, treatments, and diagnostic tools are developed.
- Cost control measures, such as downsizing, are adopted by your organization.

Change can be upsetting, especially if its consequences are unknown or difficult to implement. It is natural to resist a change that means an increased workload, the need to learn new policies and procedures, the possibility of being moved to a different location—or of losing one's job altogether. In fact, resistance to any change is a natural human response because we are creatures of habit. We like to know what to expect when we go to work each day.

There are a number of ways of **coping** with and handling change in a professional manner. Start by accepting the fact that change is going to occur—it is a fact of life. For example, computers were not widely used in the workplace until the 1980s. People who began their careers before that had to learn a whole new way of doing their work. By acknowledging that there will be future, unknown changes, you can be better prepared to adapt.

Make a decision to approach change with a positive attitude: look for the benefits and new opportunities that may be open to you. How can you contribute to making transitions as smoothly as possible? Work to become an asset to your organization—someone who can be counted on to pitch in and get things done. Decide to be part of the team that helps accept and adjust to the change, rather than being another problem for the organization. And consider this: personal growth is the result of challenging yourself and trying new things.

To avoid being blindsided by change, be attentive. Keep up on the news of trends, discoveries, and government policies, such as the Affordable Care Act, that might affect your career. Follow the advancements in your field by reading journals, attending workshops and conferences, and researching on the Internet. Maintain communication with your coworkers and supervisor to learn about possible changes in your workplace.

Here are some additional coping strategies for dealing with change:

- Keep up with your own work focusing on what *you* can control.
- Use stress reduction techniques, such as meditation, to combat fear and anxiety (see Chapter 3).
- Do a self-evaluation to determine where you best fit into the organization.
- Consider ways to learn new skills if these are required by the changes.

Prescription for Success: 11-7 Dealing with Change

Assume the role of a supervisor in a busy, medium-sized urban clinic. Your clinic has recently been purchased by a large health care organization from out of state. Some of the anticipated changes are new policies about employee compensation, benefits, vacation time, etc.; a new computerized system for patient management and billing; and more on-site reviews from the corporate office. The clinic was previously owned by a small group of long-time physicians who, while requiring that employees provide good care to patients, managed on a friendly, almost family basis. No one knows whether the changes will be positive or negative.

Describe how you help prepare your staff for the upcoming—and largely unknown—changes that will soon occur.

Case Study 11-1

Martha grew up in conditions that surprise many Americans. Her family's house was not much better than a shack and was one of the 630,000 households in the United States without complete indoor plumbing. Her mother had several children and did her best to stretch the food so that they all had something to eat at least once a day. Martha's father was sometimes there, sometimes not. A real "charmer," he had other children around the county.

Martha later told friends that living like that "either breaks you or makes you." In her case, she became a hard worker. She knew that if she wanted anything, she'd have to get it for herself. She left home at age 16 to marry Craig, her 18-year-old boyfriend. Over the years, she cleaned houses, worked for an office-cleaning company, and took on jobs mowing lawns to contribute to the household income. Craig worked on farms and he and Martha were able to build a life that was better than either had known as children. They chose to wait before having their own children, not wanting to raise them in poverty.

Just before he turned 30, Craig was driving a tractor when it rolled over on him. In addition to broken bones, he suffered a head injury which caused him to lapse into a coma. He died three weeks later. Martha was heartbroken and it was months before she pulled herself out of grief and depression.

Martha wasn't sure what to do with her life now. A friend who had helped her during this dark, difficult period suggested that she look into going to school. Martha laughed. "Carrie, you know I never even graduated high school. What would I be doing going to school now?"

"Well, the work you've done before is tiring and it's getting you nowhere. When you and I spent those last days with Craig in the hospital and then the nursing home, I got to thinking about what it would be like to be a nurse," said Carrie. "And it seems to me that's something for you—you're kind and sweet."

"Carrie, are you nuts? Did you see what those nurses were doing—with the medicines and those things they had

Craig hooked up to. I mean those people had some skills. They had to be smart."

Carrie looked at her friend. "Martha, think about it. You've shared with me how your life was. You came from nothing. And look what you've got now because you've worked hard."

It took some convincing, but Martha did decide to take a course to become a certified nursing assistant (CNA). Maybe later she'd see about nursing, but for now, becoming a nursing assistant seemed like something she might be able to manage. And at the same time, Martha earned her GED by passing the General Educational Development tests.

Martha worked hard and received her certificate. She was hired by the same nursing home where Craig had been taken after the hospital determined there was nothing more they could do for him. That was hard at first, but then she thought of it in a new way: she could help others who had gone through what she had. Her experience had taught her that not just the patient—but also the family—needed help and comforting. So she always made an effort to be especially kind to them.

Martha sometimes found her work challenging and tried to develop habits to help her get all her tasks done efficiently. After she had been working for a few months, there was news that the nursing home had been bought by a large company that owned nursing homes and assisted living facilities all over the country. Everyone was talking about it, worried that at best, there would be lots of changes or at worst, they would lose their jobs. Martha was especially worried. She had worked hard to become proficient at her job; learning wasn't easy for her and she had become attached to the patients and didn't want to be forced to leave because she couldn't adapt to the new ways.

Martha's supervisor, Ms. Trent, sensed that Martha was concerned. She called her into her office. She started the conversation by telling Martha what a good job she was doing and how her kindness had been noted.

"Thank you, Ms. Trent. But it may be more than kindness the new owners are looking for," said Martha.

Continued

"I have met some of the people from their corporate office and I must admit they are concerned about efficiency. It seems to be happening everywhere—wanting more done while saving on expenses. But I just want you to know that I'll do my best to recommend you."

Martha thanked Ms. Trent and that night began to think about how she could do her part to survive any changes that might occur. She decided to call Erin, an instructor from her CNA training. Erin had been especially helpful in helping Martha develop the study skills she needed to complete her program. She wondered if Erin might have some advice on how she could best learn the new computer system Martha had heard was coming from the new owners. It also

occurred to her that maybe the new owners would want to keep the CNAs who knew and had cared for the patients. Maybe she had something of value to offer them.

Questions for Thought and Reflection

1. Do you think Martha's background will help her adjust to any changes brought by the new owners?
2. What do you think of Ms. Trent's conversation with Martha?
3. What is your opinion of Martha's attitude about herself being of value? Will this help or hinder her?

Mastery of Knowledge and Technical Skills

An essential component of your professionalism is knowing what you are doing. In other words, being technically competent. In order to not harm patients or disrupt the health care process, you must perform your occupational skills accurately and to the best of your ability. Performing a lab test incorrectly, administering the wrong medication, making errors when preparing insurance claims—these can have harmful consequences. Remember that the primary goals of patients are to relieve their symptoms and restore their health. Your job is to help them achieve these goals.

Attending classes, studying to learn rather than simply to pass tests, and practicing hands-on skills to develop mastery are all steps to becoming technically competent. As discussed in Chapter 3, students should think in terms of the future when studying—how their current actions while in school will influence their future careers. Keep the big picture in mind when you study: how you will someday use the knowledge and skills you are acquiring now to help others.

It is not possible to anticipate every situation you will encounter once on the job. This is why it's important for you to be able and willing to think for yourself and learn on the job. Here are some suggestions for dealing with situations when you aren't sure what to do:

• Think through the situation. What did you learn in school that you can apply?
• Ask a coworker or your supervisor. Never hesitate to ask a question for fear of appearing foolish.
• Learn from your mistakes. No one is perfect. Use mistakes as opportunities to handle difficulties as well as to learn something new.
• Seek resources to continue learning. These include the Internet; your facility's library, if available; professional journals; classes and workshops; and professional conferences.

Personal Reflection

1. Are you satisfied with the progress you are making to master the technical skills needed for your future occupation?
2. Do you need to improve your study habits?
3. Do you need to put more effort into your classes?

Prescription for Success: 11-8 Envision Your Future

Imagine yourself working in your future career. Write a detailed description of yourself, including how you look; how you will communicate with others; what values will guide your work habits.

Summary of Key Ideas

• Professionalism includes your attitude, appearance, actions, and competence.
• The professionalism of health care workers influences the success of the health care system.
• A high level of professionalism can be acquired through learning, effort, and practice.

Positive Self-Talk for This Chapter

• I am developing my professional skills and qualities.
• I have what it takes to be a successful health care professional.

Internet Activities

For active links to the websites needed to complete these activities, visit http://evolve.elsevier.com/Haroun/career/.

1. Use the search term "professionalism in health care." Select at least five articles to read and then write a short paper in which you explain how the professionalism of

health care workers helps patients achieve better health outcomes.

2. There are online tests available to measure how you cope with change and stress. Organizations with such tests include Queendom's "Coping & Stress Management Skills Test" and CERA's "Stress & Coping Self-Test".

3. Enter the search term "professional healthcare appearance images." Take a look at the results and list five characteristics that the health care workers share.

Where to Find More Information About Professionalism in This Book

TOPIC	CHAPTER
Employers: desired professional behaviors	1
Patients: what they want from health care workers	1
Appearance	2
Attitude	3
Time management	3
Personal organization	3
Demonstrating respect for others	10
Listening skills	7, 10
Speaking skills, feedback, asking questions	10
Nonverbal communication	10
Teamwork	10
Empathy	10, 16
Integrity and honesty	16
Respecting confidentiality	16
Responsibility	16
Thinking	9, 16
Solving problems	9, 16
Continuing to learn	16
Adapting to changing conditions	16
Keeping current	17
Making decisions	9, 16

Building Your Resume

1. Consider the importance of your professional and "soft" skills in your future employment. What are your own strengths that you can offer an employer?

2. Start a list of your professional skills for use in Building Blocks # 1, Introduction, and # 3, Professional Skills and Knowledge.

To Learn More

Chapman E: Life is an attitude! Staying positive when the world seems against you, Menlo Park, Calif, 1992, Crisp Publications

Davis C: Patient practitioner interaction: An experiential manual for developing the art of health care, Thorofare, NJ, 2011, Slack

Job readiness for health professionals: Soft skill strategies for success, St. Louis, 2013, Elsevier

Makely S: Professionalism in health care: A primer for career success, ed 4, Upper Saddle River, NJ, 2012, Pearson

Tamparo CD, Lindh WQ: Therapeutic communications for health care, ed 3, Clifton Park, NY, 2008, Delmar Cengage

References

1. Purtilo R, Haddad A: *Health professional and patient interaction*, ed 5, Philadelphia, 1996, W.B. Saunders.
2. National health expenditures 2012 highlights. Available at http://www.cms.gov/Research-Statistics-Data-and-Systems/Statistics-Trends-and-Reports/NationalHealthExpendData/downloads/highlights.pdf.
3. Centers for Disease Control and Prevention. Available at: http://www.cdc.gov/niosh/topics/healthcare/.
4. Fuscaldo D: What patients want, expect from health-care providers. Available at: http://www.foxbusiness.com/personal-finance/2012/08/07.
5. Locke GR 3rd, Berndt M, Woychick N, Gilles K, Schryver M, Brennan M: Professionalism among allied health staff. The PLEASE CARE program, *Minn Med* 90:47–49, 2007. Available at: http://www.ncbi.nlm.nih.gov/pubmed/17899850.
6. Adams D: Doctors urged to mind bedside manners. March 21, 2005. Available at: http://www.amednews.com/article/20050321/profession/303219970/2/.
7. Therapeutic communication and behavioral management. Available at: http://www.ncchc.org/cnp-therapeutic-communication.
8. Person A, Finch L: Bedside manner: Concept analysis and impact on advanced nursing practice, *The Internet Journal of Advanced Nursing Practice* 10, 2009. Available at http://ispub.com/IJANP/10/1/10734.
9. Tamparo CD, Lindh WQ: *Therapeutic communications for health care*, ed 3, Clifton Park, N.Y, 2008, Delmar Cengage.
10. Davis CM: *Patient practitioner interaction: An experiential manual for developing the art of health care*, ed 5, Thorofare, N.J, 2011, Slack.
11. Judson T, Detsky A, Press M: Encouraging patients to ask questions: How to overcome "white-coat silence." Available at: http://jama.jamanetwork.com/article.aspx?articleid=1696107.
12. Mitchell D, Haroun L: *Introduction to health care*, ed 3, Clifton Park, N.Y, 2012, Delmar Cengage, p347.
13. Park, A: Your doctor's bedside manner could affect your health. Available at: http://healthland.time.com/2011/07/19/your-doctors-bedside-manner-could-affect-your-health/.

CHAPTER 12

Beginning the Job Search

OBJECTIVES

1. Understand how a positive attitude, time, and effort contribute to a successful job search.
2. Organize your job search by creating a designated space for job-search activities and setting up a personal support system.
3. Understand the job market when planning your job-search strategies.
4. Use a variety of resources effectively to locate health care job leads.
5. Use the Internet as an effective job-search tool.
6. Know how to respond to job postings and ads.

KEY TERMS AND CONCEPTS

Cover Letter Letter of introduction sent with your resume to a potential employer.

Facebook An online social networking service.

Fax Machine Device that allows you to send documents over telephone lines.

Job Lead Log An organized list of the information you gather about various job leads.

LinkedIn A professional- and business-oriented social networking service.

Mailing Lists Subscription services that send messages on specific topics via e-mail. (Also called *Listservs*.)

Newsgroups Online discussion groups in which participants post information about topics of interest.

Reference Sheet A written list of your references including their titles and contact information.

Web Forums Discussion groups accessed via the World Wide Web in which interested individuals can take part. Also called *online communities* and *message boards*.

The Search Is On

"Employment is nature's physician, and is essential to human happiness."
—Galen

Congratulations! All the studying, assignments, labs, and externship experience are about to pay off. You are now ready to focus on the job search and reaching your goal of working in the health care field. Completing your education and graduating represent important personal achievements. Your attitude played a large part in your success. In the same way, attitude will play an important role in helping you get the right job.

The Big A: Attitude

"Remember that your own resolution to succeed is more important than any one thing."

—Abraham Lincoln

Attitude is the single most important factor in determining whether a student will find a job or not. In Chapter 3, we discussed how we have control over our attitudes and noted that any situation can be approached either positively or negatively. For example, some people are nervous and fearful about looking for a job. They worry about lacking the qualifications required by employers and see each interview as a chance to be rejected. A more positive approach is to look at the process from the employers' point of view. Think about it: health care facilities cannot function without good employees. Employers must fill positions with well-trained individuals who can help them serve their patients. *You* are a recently trained person ready to fill one of these positions.

In Chapter 2, we compared starting a new career with marketing a new product. You are now ready to begin marketing yourself to prospective employers. Knowing what skills and competencies you have is the first step in presenting yourself successfully as the person who fits an employer's needs. Students sometimes don't realize just how much they have learned. They tend to underestimate their abilities and the amount of practice they have had in applying their skills. Being aware of your accomplishments will build your self-confidence and help

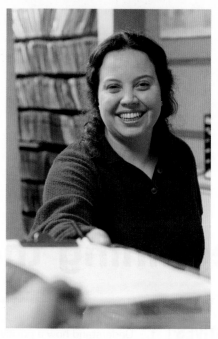

FIGURE 12-1 Your job-search goal should be to find a job that you enjoy and in which you can make a positive difference in the lives of others. Review why you chose to train for a job in health care. *How can you contribute to the success of your future employer? What are your career goals? Your attitude will influence your success. How is the young woman in the photo projecting a positive attitude?* (From Proctor DB, Adams AP: *Kinn's the medical assistant: an applied learning approach*, ed 12, St Louis, 2014, Saunders.)

you present yourself positively at interviews. Take some time now to review what you have learned, your self-assessment in Prescription for Success 1-4, and to give yourself credit for what you have to offer (Figure 12-1).

Personal Reflection

1. What do you hope to learn and gain from your first job?

Prescription for Success: 12-1 Inventory of Technical Skills

1. Refer back to Resume Building Block #3: Professional Skills and Knowledge form in Chapter 2, in which you began to list the skills you were learning in school. If necessary, gather additional sources of information to help you complete your inventory: lab checklists, course objectives, externship performance evaluations, textbooks, and class handouts.
2. Create categories, such as the following, that are appropriate for your occupational area. List your specific skills under each heading:
- Equipment I Can Use
- Lab Procedures I Can Perform
- Tests I Can Perform
- Patient Procedures I Can Perform
- Administrative Procedures
- Computer Skills and Applications

- Medical Records
- Documentation and Charting
- Medical Insurance
- Billing
- Communication Skills
  - Oral
  - Written
3. Think of examples that demonstrate your mastery of each skill, such as your performance in the laboratory or classroom, completion of special projects, or work you did during your externship experience. Are there any areas in which you demonstrated particular expertise? You can use these examples to better present your qualifications to potential employers on both your resume and at job interviews.

Focus Your Search

"To find out what one is fitted to do, and to secure an opportunity to do it, is the key to happiness."

—John Dewey

Knowing where to market yourself is the next step in carrying out a successful job search. This means identifying the type of joband facility in which you would prefer to work. In Prescription for Success 1-8 you began to identify your job preferences. As you worked through your educational program, you may have changed your work preferences.

Prescription for Success: 12-2 **What Do I Want? An Update**

Review Prescription for Success 1-8, and record any changes you have made.

1. **Type of facility:** large, small, urban, suburban, rural, inpatient, outpatient
2. **Type of population served:** economic status, age range, gender, ethnic groups
3. **Work schedule:** steady employment, per diem, flexible hours, fixed hours, overtime, days only, evenings and weekends
4. **Specialty area**
5. **Type of supervision**
6. **Work pace:** fast, moderate
7. **Amount of interaction with others** (All health care professionals are part of a team, although some work more independently than others.)
8. **Range of duties:** wide variety, concentrate on a few

As we discussed in Chapters 1 and 3, it is sometimes necessary to set short-term goals to achieve long-term career success. When seeking an entry-level position, you'll do better if you are open to a variety of possibilities. School career services personnel report seeing students lose good opportunities by setting limits that are too restrictive. For example, some students don't want to have long commutes. But passing up a good position at an excellent facility by refusing to consider jobs just outside your immediate area may not be a good career move. In the long run, driving an extra 10 minutes may be worth the inconvenience.

Making a Commitment to the Job Search

"You can't try to do things; you simply must do them."

—Ray Bradbury

Obtaining a job has been compared to actually working at a job. It can take a lot of time and effort. You'll be most successful if you dedicate a portion of each day to your search and be on call to follow up quickly on leads. Employment professionals recommend that job seekers spend between 20 and 40 hours per week on job-search efforts. In this and the following chapters, you will learn about the many activities necessary to conduct a successful search, such as the following:

- Preparing inventories of skills and examples
- Networking
- Finding leads
- Conducting searches on the Internet
- Writing and revising your resume
- Assembling your portfolio
- Writing letters
- Contacting references
- Creating a **reference sheet**
- Preparing for and attending interviews
- Writing thank-you notes

Failure to spend adequate time on these activities is one of the major reasons why people fail to get hired. You can apply many of the time-management tools and techniques suggested in Chapter 3 to your job search (Figure 12-2).

Personal Reflection

1. How strong is my commitment to finding a job?
2. How much effort am I willing to make?

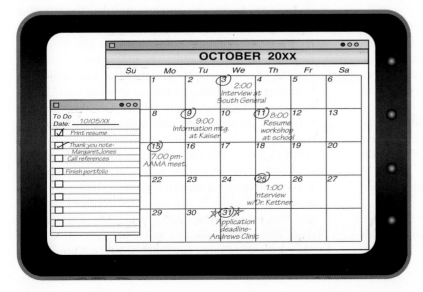

FIGURE 12-2 Being organized and using time wisely are just as important when you are looking for a job as they were when you were in school. *Create a schedule and to-do list for each week to ensure that you are ready to pursue all opportunities. Use a paper or electronic calendar to keep yourself on track.*

Time Management Tips for Your Job Search

- **Prioritize.** The job search should be your main focus, apart from your family and personal health. Dedicate sufficient time and attention to achieving this goal. Looking for a job *is* your job. Determine which search activities are the most productive, and spend the majority of your time on them.
- **Keep a calendar.** Missing—or even being late for—an interview is a sure way to lose a job even before you are hired. Take care to note all appointments and follow-up activities accurately, and check your calendar daily. If you haven't developed a calendar system yet, now is the time to start.
- **Plan a weekly schedule.** Decide what needs to be done each week, and create a to-do list to keep you on track. It's easy to reach the end of the week and discover you've accomplished only half of what needed to be done.
- **Plan ahead.** This is very important. Suppose that one morning you are notified that a hospital where you want to work is scheduling interviews for later the same day. You don't want to miss out because you haven't completed your resume or don't have a clean shirt to wear. Being prepared leads to being hired. Make sure your car is in good running order or that you have other reliable transportation.
- **Plan for the unplanned.** The unexpected tends to strike at the worst possible moment. Keep an extra printer cartridge on hand. Have extra copies of your resume printed. Leave early for interviews in case you get lost. (Better yet, take a dry run a day or two in advance to learn the route. Check out alternative routes in case of traffic.)

Setting Up a Job-Search Central

Create a personalized employment headquarters by designating a space for job-search activities. Save time and prevent losing important information by gathering your resources and supplies in one location. Check the list in Box 12-1 to see if you have what you need.

Your Job-Search Records

Each person's job search is unique. Creating personalized job-search records will help you focus your efforts, keep track of phone numbers and website addresses, and the name of the office manager at the clinic where you last interviewed. A three-ring binder gives you the flexibility to add pages and keep everything organized. If you prefer, create computerized folders and files. Choose the content that will best support your efforts. The purpose of this resource is to save you time and effort. Here are some suggestions for information to start with:

- A list of professional contacts (from your Personal Reference Guide, discussed in Chapter 9)
- A list of professional organizations (also from your Personal Reference Guide; see Appendix A for a list of health care organizations)

BOX 12-1 Job Central Checklist

- Telephone
- Telephone directories, including Yellow Pages
- Computer, printer, and supplies
- Dictionary (may be online)
- Good-quality paper for your resume and **cover letters**
- Matching envelopes
- Extra copies of your resume
- Note paper or thank-you cards
- Calendar, planner, or electronic planner
- Job-search notebook

- Copies of Prescriptions for Success 12-1 and 12-2
- Resume Building Block forms from Chapter 2

Job Lead Log

A **job lead log** consists of forms, either paper or computerized, on which you record all your job leads and contacts. See Figure 12-3 for an example.

If you have more than one version of your resume (for example, different objectives to match specific jobs), indicate on your lead log which version you sent, place a copy of the resume on the next page in your binder, or refer to the computer file name. This way you'll know how to respond if you get a call for an interview and ensure that you take the correct resume to the interview. (Chapter 14 contains more information about interviews and what to take with you.)

Students who prefer to use a computer for tracking can set up an Excel spreadsheet or another form, such as a table in Word, to record their job-search activities. Regardless of the method you choose, design something that is easy for you to use, and be sure to keep it up-to-date.

Dialing for Jobs

The telephone provides a vital link with potential employers and job lead sources. The telephone can be one of the job seeker's best friends. It can also be a barrier if not used properly. Employers form an impression of you based on your telephone manners, so be sure they hear you at your best. The following suggestions for making calls will apply to your telephone habits on the job as well as during the search to get a job:

1. Be prepared, with pen and paper, to take notes.
2. Prepare what you plan to say ahead of time and be as brief as possible without rushing or speaking too quickly.
3. Be courteous, never pushy. If the receptionist cannot connect you to the person you wish to speak with, leave a clear message and ask for a good time to call back.
4. Speak clearly and distinctly. Don't mumble or use slang or nonstandard speech that the listener may not understand.
5. When making appointments or gathering important information, listen carefully and repeat (use feedback) to make sure that you have the correct name, date and time, address, suite or office number, and so on.
6. Always thank the other party and end the call graciously.

JOB LEAD LOG

Source of Lead

☐ Personal contact   ☐ Printed ad   ☐ Referral from school   ☐ Internet

☐ Other

Facility Name: _____

Contact Person: _____

Address: _____

Telephone Number: _____

Fax Number: _____

Website Address: _____

Contacts and Follow-up Action

Date	Action (Called, sent resume, sent thank-you note, etc.)
_____	_____
_____	_____
_____	_____
_____	_____
_____	_____
_____	_____
_____	_____
_____	_____
_____	_____
_____	_____
_____	_____
_____	_____

FIGURE 12-3 Use a job lead log to help keep yourself organized. *Make a few copies or create a version on your computer now so you'll be ready to record leads as you find them.*

It is *critical* that your school, potential employers, and other contacts be able to reach you in a timely way. Be sure the telephone number you distribute is accurate and includes your area code. If you have an answering machine and/or voicemail, call your number to make sure it is working properly. The outgoing message should be simple and professional. Avoid the use of music, jokes, or clever remarks, such as "You know what this is and you know what to do." (This also applies to your e-mail address. If it's too cute or strange, it may send the wrong message to any potential employer who sees it.) Instruct everyone who might answer the telephone about proper telephone manners and how to write down a message. Every contact represents you and employers don't have time to deal with rude adults or untrained children. If you are away from the telephone during office hours and don't have a cell phone or an answering machine, give an alternative number where someone reliable can take messages for you. Consider getting an inexpensive cell phone with prepaid minutes. Don't lose out on jobs because you can't be contacted.

Communicating by Fax

Some employers want you to fax your resume. If you don't own a **fax machine** or a computer that has a fax capability, find a print, postal, or business supply store that provides this service. Some schools will fax student resumes to potential employers. When sending documents by fax, the print on the original must be clear and dark for maximum-quality transmission. Be sure there is at least a 1-inch margin on all sides so nothing gets cut off.

When faxed resumes are requested, it is best to follow the employer's instructions. Mailed resumes may arrive too late to be considered. Demonstrate that you are resourceful and can follow instructions. If you don't hear from the employer in a couple of days, call to make sure your resume was received.

Setting Up a Support System

Your job search will be easier and more pleasant if you have people available who care about your success and are willing to help you. They can provide technical support or offer friendly encouragement. Could you use some help with any of the following tasks?

- Proofreading your resume and other written materials (more than one person should proofread).
- Role-playing with you to practice interviewing.
- Discussing postinterview evaluations. (Postinterview evaluations are covered in Chapter 15.)
- Acting as a cheerleader.
- Helping you to keep things in perspective and not to get discouraged.

You may want to work with just one other person who is qualified to help you in many areas. Or you could enlist the help of several "specialists." Be sure the people you choose are qualified to spot spelling and grammatical errors and are comfortable about giving you constructive feedback. They should know when you need a push and when you need a hug. Consider asking for support from friends, family members, classmates, school personnel, and health care professionals. If you have a mentor, this person may be an excellent choice.

Most people will be happy to support your efforts to secure employment. Take care to keep your support system intact. Be considerate of everyone's time, be prepared when you have meetings with them, and show appreciation for their help.

The career services department at your school provides specific help and support to students as they conduct their job search. Find out what services are provided. In addition, some schools and communities have job clubs or support groups for people seeking employment. Consider using these resources to supplement your support system. They can offer additional viewpoints, encouragement, and helpful suggestions.

Prescription for Success: 12-3 My Support System

Think about the people in your life who are qualified to help you in your job-search efforts. Who can you ask to help you with each of the following?
1. Proofreading your resume and other written materials
2. Interview practice
3. Postinterview evaluations
4. Encouragement

Understanding the Job Market

Employment conditions vary from one geographic location to the next. And economic conditions change over time. Think about the following factors when planning your job-search strategies:

- Local employment customs
- Current economic conditions
- Current employment rate
- Trends in health care delivery
- Medical advances
- Changing government regulations

Local customs vary on what is considered acceptable dress for the workplace. In some parts of the country, health care providers dress casually, with men sporting long hair and even wearing an earring. In other areas, anyone who showed up for work looking like this would be sent home to change—or worse, sent home for good!

Local and national economic conditions affect the job seeker. When the economy is strong and unemployment is low, job seekers have the advantage. When the economy slows down, competition heats up and it becomes more difficult to find a position. At the same time, some health care occupations are experiencing shortages of applicants, and this makes finding a job easier for qualified candidates.

Health care occupations are also affected by state and federal laws. The demand for certain occupations is influenced by the reimbursement (payment for services) policies of both government and private insurance companies. Knowing what's happening in your local area as well as being aware of the national trends is important when planning both your initial job search and your long-term career strategy. Your local newspaper is a good source of information. Look in the business section for articles about the economy and local employment trends. Health care trends and major facilities are often featured. For example, a state law that increased the required nurse-to-patient ratios in California hospitals was reported in the newspaper. The predicted result was (and will be for the next few years, at least) a shortage of registered nurses to meet employer needs. This information is valuable for the recent nurse graduate or a student who is considering nursing as a career. Articles about major health care employers can give you an edge when choosing where you want to work. Knowing something about the facility to which you are applying enables you to present yourself at interviews as a candidate who has taken the time to learn about the employer.

Many newspapers publish a special weekly or monthly section dedicated to employment. These are good sources of information. They contain articles about resume writing, lists of local agencies that assist job seekers, and announcements of job fairs. News magazines such as *Newsweek, Time, U.S. News and World Report,* and *Business Week* contain many articles about health care topics. The Internet provides access to a wide variety of topics from literally millions of sources. For example, the Bureau of Labor Statistics maintains a website (www.bls.gov/ooh) with reports on employment trends and the national labor market for specific occupations. Apply the research techniques discussed in Chapter 7 when conducting your job search.

> **Prescription for Success: 12-4**
> **What's Going On?**
>
> Use your research skills to find answers to the following questions:
> 1. What is the unemployment rate in your area?
> 2. Who are the major health care employers?
> 3. What are the current hiring trends in health care?
> 4. How may these conditions affect your occupation?
> 5. How may they influence your job-search strategies?

Locating Job Leads

There are many ways to find job leads, ranging from talking with people you know to searching the Internet. You can increase your chances of finding the job you really want by using a variety of lead sources. Don't limit yourself to the one or two methods you find easiest or most comfortable to use. People who work in sales know that it usually takes many calls to make a sale. In the same way, the more sources you use in your job search, the greater your chances of finding the right job for yourself. Employment experts recommend that no more than 25% of your time be spent on any one job-search method. See Figure 12-4 for a look at the wide variety of sources available.

When the economy is slow and there are few job openings, networking and developing personal contacts can be the most effective methods for finding a job. You may not find the "perfect job" under these economic conditions. Looking for an opportunity to gain experience may be the best strategy. When the economy is booming or there is a shortage of qualified workers in your field, you are likely to have a larger selection of opportunities. Under these conditions, you may find that responding to job postings and directly contacting potential employers are very effective methods. It is a sure thing that you will experience all types of job markets during your career. The economy and employment levels run in cycles, and you must be prepared to deal with changing conditions.

Career Services at Your School

The staff at your school wants you to succeed. The goal of health care educators is to train future workers, and a sign of *their* professional success is when a graduate becomes satisfactorily employed. Schools have personnel who are trained to help students find jobs. These people work to develop relationships with local employers. Your school may be contacted about job openings before they are even advertised. It is time-consuming for employers to review resumes, set up appointments, and interview large numbers of applicants. The success of a health care facility depends on the quality of its employees, so it is important for them to find and hire the right people. Considerable time, expense, and doubt can be avoided if employers know they can count on local schools to provide qualified candidates. So how can you be among those who are recommended by your school?

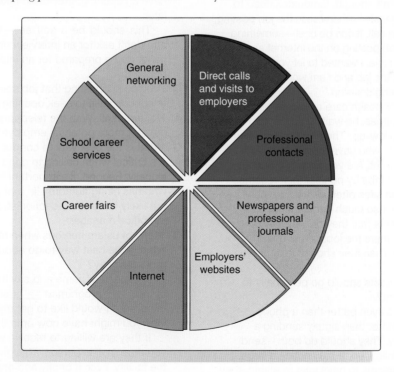

FIGURE 12-4 Use a variety of sources to increase your chances of finding the right job for yourself. *List the ones you think will be most helpful to you. Ask your instructor and/or career services personnel for their advice on which sources have been the most successful for students at your school.*

- Get to know the career services staff. Introduce yourself early in your program. Don't wait until you are beginning the job search. Seek their advice about how you can best prepare in advance for successful employment.
- Treat school staff with the same courtesy and respect you would an employer. They cannot risk the school's reputation with employers by recommending students who are rude or uncooperative.
- Maintain an excellent attendance record. Schools report that this is the question asked by nearly every employer about students. It ranks above inquiries about grades. (Even great skills are no help to anyone if you aren't there to use them!)
- Participate fully in any career development classes or workshops that are offered. Attend every session and complete all the assignments. Conduct yourself in practice interviews as if they were the real thing.

- Follow up on any leads you are given, even if you don't think the job is for you. Attend all the interviews scheduled for you. A failure to show up embarrasses the school and may result in the employer refusing to consider candidates from your school in the future. Take advantage of all opportunities to meet potential employers. You will gain valuable confidence-building interview practice. Even if the job isn't the one for you, the employer may know about one that is.
- Keep the school informed about how to contact you. If you move and career services can't find you, they can't help you.
- Let the school know when you are hired. Many agencies that regulate and accredit schools require annual reports to monitor graduation and job placement rates. These act as school report cards and are important for schools to stay in good standing. If the staff has taken the time to help you, return the favor by giving them the information they need to complete their reports (Figure 12-5).

Q&A with a Career Services Professional

Melva Duran

Melva is the former director of Career Services at Kaplan College in San Diego, California.

Q With so many job seekers out there, how can graduates increase their chances of being noticed by employers?

A I think many graduates make the mistake of simply submitting a resume or application. When using the Internet, they may believe that once they've pushed the send button, it is up to the employer. But I have found that this just isn't enough. Graduates need to follow up. Unless requested otherwise in the job posting, this could be a phone call. It can be brief—something like, "I noticed your job posting on the Internet and I've sent an application online. I wanted to let you know I'm very interested in the job and I am wondering when you'll be making a hiring decision."

I even had a major health care employer tell me that after he receives resumes, he waits a day or two to see if he receives any follow-up. Then he only reviews the resumes of applicants who have followed up!

Q You mention the Internet. Are you finding that many graduates are getting jobs by posting their resumes?

A Actually, the large job sites often attract too many resumes—there is just so much competition. So I recommend to students that they browse the job postings to identify where the jobs are and find potential employers. Then they should go in person with their resumes.

Q So you believe applicants should go personally to places of employment?

A Oh, yes, I think that's even better than a phone call—and certainly better than simply sending a resume electronically. They should do both—send a resume and then follow up. If they notice a large, local employer that seems to have jobs available, they should go to the facility. When talking to a contact person, they should state their interest in employment, ask about current hiring and other jobs that might be available, and if there is anything else they should do to apply for jobs.

Q How about cold calling—do you recommend it?

A Absolutely! In fact, I've had good success with this method when graduates have trouble getting hired. I advise them to dress professionally and go to buildings that have potential employers. This is a better and faster approach than calling on the phone. Employers may be looking to hire, and this saves them time and money spent on posting the job. Even if they don't have an opening, they often take the resume and call later.

This should be a soft sell—that is, don't be pushy and don't ask for an interview on the spot. On the other hand, do be prepared for an interview because that can happen!

Q Are you suggesting that job seekers should not make telephone calls to seek openings?

A No, not at all. With the telephone, you can obviously contact more potential employers.

Q What is the best way to conduct a phone search?

A It's critical when calling to conduct yourself professionally. Second, it's important to speak with someone who has hiring authority. In a physician's office, this is not likely to be the receptionist, so you need to ask for the office manager.

Q Many of us are nervous when making these calls. What is the best way to go about it—what should graduates say?

A First state your name and say that you are a graduate of the _____ program at _____ school. Then say something like, "I would like to get my resume to you for any jobs you might have now or in the future."

If they are willing to receive your resume, it is best if you drop it off in person. This gives you a chance to see the facility, even if briefly and only the front office, and it gives someone there the chance to see you. (Be sure to dress professionally!) So before hanging up, ask for the address and any special directions.

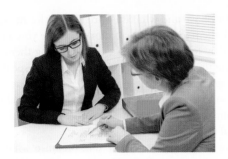

FIGURE 12-5 Take advantage of the career services department at your school. While their job is not to "place" you in a job, they have valuable expertise and contacts with local employers. *Be at your professional best when working with all the school personnel so they can recommend you with confidence.* (Copyright AlexRaths/iStock/Thinkstock.)

Networking

Many people learn about job openings and become employed through personal contacts. In fact, some career experts believe that networking is the most effective job-search tool. It was recommended in Chapter 2 that you start early to meet people in the health care field. Professional organizations were suggested as an excellent source of contacts. In addition to providing you with useful information about your occupational area, they can be a source of job leads and referrals. If you have already met people through professional networking, let them know that you are launching your job search. Give them your business card. Don't be shy about asking for their advice about where you could apply, as well as about the job search in general. People who are successful in their careers are generally happy to help newcomers. Do show consideration for their time, and send a thank-you note when they make an effort on your behalf. It is critical for you to follow up on any leads given to you by professional contacts. Failure to do so is not only rude; it may result in the withdrawal of their support.

In addition to professional contacts, general networking can be an effective way to get the word out about your search efforts. I once learned about a job opening for a school director—a position I got and enjoyed for a number of years—from a friend who had seen the ad in the newspaper. Let the people in your life know you are seeking employment. By telling 10 people who each know 10 other people, you create a network of 110 people who know you are looking for a job. Of these 110, it is likely that a few work in health care. And most people use health care services. There is a chance that someone will know someone or something that can help you. Keep in touch with your classmates. Once they have jobs, they may be willing to pass on your name to their employers. When speaking with others about your career goals, present yourself positively and express enthusiasm about your field. People want to feel confident about passing your name along. Create a directory of your network contacts that includes their name and title, contact information, where you met, and the dates when you communicate with them.

Government-Sponsored Resource Centers

The government has established a program of "one-stop" resources for job seekers. These may be called One-Stop Resource Centers, County Career Centers, or possibly another name in your area. Sponsored by the U.S. Department of Labor, their purpose is to provide a wide variety of information and services for the public. Staff members are well informed about employment conditions, as well as specific employers, in their local areas. Ask your school about these resources or go to www.careeronestop.org for the location of your nearest center.

Direct Employer Contacts

Calling or visiting employers to inquire about job openings can be a successful strategy. These actions demonstrate motivation and self-confidence, the very qualities that can help win you a job. They are also a way to discover the estimated 80% of jobs that are never advertised—the "hidden job market." There are two ways to make contact: in writing and by telephone. If you are sending a cover letter and resume, it is necessary to find the name of the person who makes the hiring decisions for his or her department. If you are calling a small medical office, this may simply mean getting the name—and correct spelling!—of the physician. In the case of a large facility, you may have to do more inquiring by phone to find the right person. When calling, use your best telephone manners.

Craft a letter that explains why you would be a good employee for this particular employer. The letter should demonstrate enthusiasm, interest, and a desire to help the employer. Of course, this means that you know something about the employer: the specialty or services offered, typical patients, etc. Include your resume with the letter, which is directed to a specific person. Follow up in a few days with a phone call.

Calling employers by phone to inquire about job openings can be helpful if you are relocating. Phone calls provide an efficient way to contact a large number of employers. Explain that you will be moving and are unfamiliar with the area. If the facility contacted has no openings, ask if they can refer you to anyone else in the area.

Dropping in on employers gets the word out that you are looking for a job. Visiting all the offices in a large medical facility can be a productive way to spend a day. It gives you a chance to introduce yourself to at least one staff member and personally distribute your resume. If the person who greets you has time, ask for information about the facility. If this is not possible, ask who does the hiring, leave your resume, and express your appreciation. Although you should be dressed as if you were attending an interview, *do not ask* for one at this time if you don't have an appointment.

Large medical facilities, such as hospitals, often coordinate hiring through their human resources office. All resumes and applications must be submitted to this office. It can be worthwhile also to contact or visit the department where you wish to work. Ask for the supervisor and, if he or she is available, let him or her know that you have applied for work through Human Resources and are very interested in working in that department. Explain why you want to work there and ask for your application to be given consideration. If the supervisor is not available, ask to make an appointment. Don't be discouraged, however, if you are unable to make direct contact. Health care professionals today are extremely busy and simply may not have the time. If they don't, send a letter or e-mail that expresses your interest.

Your Externship Site

Students who perform well during their externship are sometimes offered jobs at the facility. Some employers even create new positions for graduates who impress them with their attitude and skills. Although it is *not* appropriate to ask your externship site for employment before completing your training there, you should work as if this were your goal. Even if the site is unable to offer you a position, your externship supervisor can serve as a valuable reference and may recommend you to another employer.

Career and Job Fairs

Some schools, community agencies, and large health care facilities organize activities to connect job recruiters with job seekers. In a single day, you may meet dozens of potential employers. You can gather information, ask questions, and submit your resume. Check your local newspaper for events in your area. Inquire if large health care organizations in your area hold career fairs or open houses.

Here are some suggestions for taking full advantage of job fairs:

- Dress as you would for an interview. If the event takes place at school and you will go directly from class in your uniform, make sure it is clean and pressed.
- Prepare a list of questions in advance. It's easier to think of them beforehand than to remember them all in a noisy room. Good questions to ask include the following:
  1. What types of jobs does your facility offer?
  2. How can I get more information?
  3. What are the most important qualifications you look for when hiring employees?
  4. Can you give me a written job description?
  5. What is the application procedure?
  6. Who do I contact to set up an interview?
- Take copies of your resume. Carry them in a large envelope or folder to keep them clean and neat.
- Smile, make eye contact, and introduce yourself to recruiters. Your goal is to get information about the types of

jobs they have and what they are looking for in applicants. Thank them for any information they give you. Leave graciously by telling them it was nice meeting them, you appreciate their help, and you look forward to speaking with them again.
- Take something in which you can collect brochures, job announcements, and business cards. A small notebook is helpful for taking notes.
- As soon as possible after the fair, organize what you collected and use your job lead log pages to record information about the people you met and what you learned. Prepare a list of follow-up activities, such as people to call and resumes to send.

Employer Meetings and Websites

Some large facilities that do a lot of hiring have public meetings during which they explain their employment needs and their application process—an in-house job fair. Contact personnel departments, watch the local newspaper, and visit employer Internet sites to find announcements. You may not have a chance to meet personally with the hiring staff, but it is still important for you to make a professional impression by dressing and acting appropriately. Be prepared to take notes and ask questions.

Many employers, especially large organizations, list jobs on their websites. They also accept applications electronically. Read more about this in Chapter 13.

Employment Ads

The "Help Wanted" section of the newspaper is one of the oldest and most traditional methods of locating job openings. Although used less as a way to advertise job openings, some newspapers still include employment ads that can be a good source of job leads. Writing a cover letter and mailing or faxing a resume is worth the time and expense it takes. Every action you take increases your chance of finding the right job.

In addition to the newspaper, many professional journals contain employment ads. These can be especially useful if you are willing to move to another area.

Using the Internet

The Internet is the newest job-search tool. It greatly expands your job-search possibilities by being available 24 hours a day. It offers a wide range of how-to information, facts about specific occupations and employers, and job postings. In fact, so much information is available it's easy to get lost in cyberspace. You may suddenly realize that you've spent three hours moving from one interesting site to another without actually adding much to your job-search efforts!

Getting Started

An excellent place to start learning about how to use the Internet for a job search is the *Riley Guide* (www.rileyguide.com). Developed by a librarian and available both in print and online, it has provided free, updated career and employment information since 1994. The website serves as a gateway to hundreds of other websites for all phases of the job search. Other good sources that have been in business for some time are Quintessential Careers (www.quintcareers.com) and CareerBuilder (www.careerbuilder.com).

General Research

Studies have shown that only a small percentage of applicants are actually hired as the result of posting a resume on one of the large employment websites; there is simply too much competition. There are literally millions of resumes online at any one time. However, the Internet is still a valuable job-search tool. It provides a vast and easily accessed source of information. You can read about health care trends, the general economy, and advances in medicine. You can scan job postings to see what characteristics employers mention most, get information about major facilities, and see samples of good resumes. To access general information, use the search engines discussed in Chapter 7 with key phrases such as "health care trends," "future of health care," "health care providers," and "health care employment." Government agencies such as the Department of Labor (www.dol.gov) and the Bureau of Labor Statistics (www.bls.gov) have information about the national job market, the laws that affect employees, and resources for job seekers.

Other effective ways to take advantage of "the net" are discussed in the following sections.

Health Care Facility Websites

Many health care facilities have websites that include photos, maps, information about the services they offer patients, and statements of their goals and overall mission. If you don't know the address, use a search engine such as Google (www.google.com) and enter the name of the company or facility. Many organizations now list their current job openings along with online applications. In fact, some facilities accept *only* electronic applications. (Chapter 13 contains information about submitting electronic resumes and completing online applications.)

Job-Posting Websites

Job openings are listed on hundreds, perhaps thousands, of websites. Although some websites are easier to use than others, most organize jobs by occupational fields, such as health care, and geographic location. The following are six general employment websites that have been operating for several years and are well-rated by users:
1. www.indeed.com
2. www.careerbuilder.com
3. www.jobbankinfo.org
4. www.monster.com
5. www.usajobs.gov
6. www.simplyhired.com
You can view the job listings on these sites without registering. If you wish to post your resume, however, you must register by supplying information such as your name, address, and telephone number. You then select a username and password to access your account each time you visit the website.

The general websites listed previously include health care categories and job postings. At the same time, there are employment websites that are specific to health care. Links are available at www.quintcareers.com/healthcare_jobs.html. If you are interested in exploring civil service (government) jobs available in veterans' hospitals (Veterans' Administration), federal prisons, or public health agencies, information about positions and the exams required for certain positions is available at:
1. www.federaljobs.net/healthcarejobsva.htm
2. http://www.careerbuilder.com/jobs/industry/government-civil-service/
3. www.federaljobs.net/exams.htm
Most professional organizations maintain websites, and some offer placement assistance for members. For example, the American Health Information Management Association (AHIMA) maintains job postings online for members. See Appendix A for a list of professional organizations and their contact information.

Keep in mind that new websites are continually being developed and old ones are merging, being deleted, or being moved to a different "address." Some of the addresses given in this book and in others may have changed by the time you try them. And it is certain that new websites will have been created. To locate current websites, use your browser to search with the phrase "websites with healthcare jobs."

Networking

LinkedIn and **Facebook** are social networking services that enable you to connect with others. LinkedIn is business-oriented, designed for people to expand their professional networks. According to Forbes, it is the largest professional social networking site and used by recruiters and hiring managers more than any other website to connect with job candidates.[1]

Facebook is used by many businesses and individuals to advertise their products and services. If you have an account, consider using it to let others know about your career goals. Putting pictures of yourself in uniform, performing volunteer work, and graduating are appropriate ways to help spread the word.

The Internet provides other opportunities for sharing information and ideas with others through mailing lists and newsgroups. **Mailing lists** (also known as *Listservs* and *e-mail discussion groups*) operate through e-mail. Each list is devoted to a specific topic: occupations, hobbies, health conditions, and so on. Once you have subscribed, you receive e-mail messages to which you can respond. Your e-mail is then sent to all other subscribers. Mailing lists offer a way to find out what other job seekers are doing and what's happening in your field around the country. Comprehensive directories of the thousands of mailing lists are available from CataList (www.lsoft.com/catalist.html) and Topica, Inc. (http://lists.topica.com). Another source of mailing list groups is available from Yahoo! (http://groups.yahoo.com).

Newsgroups offer another way to network online. A newsgroup is basically an online discussion group for a specific topic. Anyone can join and participate by reading and posting messages. Messages that address the same topic are called a "thread," and each time a different topic is introduced, a new thread is started. Most Web browsers have a search capacity called a "newsreader" that organizes the many newsgroups and enables you to post a message.

If you decide to use either mailing lists or newsgroups, it is important to learn the proper "netiquette" for participating. Experts suggest that you read a group's messages for at least two weeks before submitting anything. That way, you'll know the type and quality of material that is expected. It is also recommended that you check the "Frequently Asked Questions" (FAQ) section, if available, to avoid asking something that has already been covered. This is because all subscribers, not just you, receive the answer to your question and may find it annoying to receive information they already know and that is available elsewhere. When you do send messages, keep them short and to the point.

Web forums are another form of online discussion group offered through a variety of websites. You only need an e-mail address and Web browser to participate. You can ask questions, such as "How's the job climate in San Antonio?" and someone from that area may answer. Lists of discussion groups are available on the Internet. Using a browser, enter the keyword "forum" and a topic of interest to get a list of ongoing forums.

One important rule is never to send advertising or use these groups to ask for a job. You may, however, find someone in the group whom you can contact personally via e-mail for possible assistance, just as you would other professional contacts. Good people to write to are those who have posted messages demonstrating that they have knowledge of or work in the occupational area you wish to enter. In your e-mail to that person, identify yourself and the interests you have that seem related to what this person has said in his or her electronic messages to the group. Do *not* ask the person for a job. The purpose of this contact is to ask for—or better yet, share—information about something you have in common. Once a relationship is developed online, and this person seems to have useful knowledge and is willing to share it, it is appropriate to ask for information and career advice.

Finally, there are mobile apps that enable you to keep track of everything related to your job search, look for job postings, and post your resume. In addition to Monster.com that now has apps, you can check out the following:
- http://www.careerbuilder.com/s/cbmobile
- Indeed.com
- www.jibberjobber.com

Success Tips for Using the Internet

- **Learn more.** If you are not already proficient at using the Internet, take a class, find online help (see To Learn More at the end of this chapter), or get a copy of one of the many books available on how to use it. If your school does not offer instruction, look for adult education classes in your community. Many are offered free of charge.
- **Be patient.** The Internet is a developing technology and still has a few bugs. You may get bumped offline just as you find what you are looking for. A promising-sounding

website may have disappeared, but the wealth of information available is worth the time it takes to search.
- **Monitor where you are.** It's easy to get lost in a maze of links that takes you far from the original site. When you access a major site, write down its name and address so you can find it again.
- **Mark favorite sites.** Most Internet-access software allows you to create personalized lists of useful sites so you can find them later. Also, for any online groups you join, save information in your job-search notebook about how to unsubscribe and the name and e-mail address of the person who manages the list.
- **Watch the time.** Using the Internet can be addictive. You can wander for hours linking and looking and actually accomplishing very little. If you find sites that look interesting but are unrelated to the task at hand, write down or mark their addresses and return to them later.
- **Beware of scams.** Take care when posting your resume or sending out private information. If a website makes claims about jobs that seem too good to be true, this may simply be a means of getting personal information about you. Stick with major employment websites and the websites of employers whose existence you can verify in other ways.
- **Don't exceed 25%.** Remember, the Internet is only one tool for your job search. Use it wisely as a supplement to other methods. Some experts even recommend spending no more than 10% of your job-search time using the Internet.
- **Be careful what you post.** If you have pages on websites such as Facebook, be *very* careful about what you post. Photos of yourself that may be amusing but that don't show you at your best may damage your chances for employment. Many employers reportedly search potential employees on the Internet, and some admit not hiring based on what they find.[2] You could consider using the Internet to your advantage. For example, if you have volunteered for a community fundraiser or serve meals at a community center, include photos of yourself participating in these activities.

Internet Tracking Form

If you use the Internet to find information, post your resume, and/or participate in groups, take a little time to record your activities. Use the form in Figure 12-6 to track the job opportunities you find online. Make copies of the form, or set up one of your own to keep in your job-search notebook or on your computer or mobile device.

Responding to Job Postings and Ads

Regardless of the source—the Internet, a professional journal, or a newspaper—look under every category that may contain jobs for which you are qualified. For example, while "nursing assistants" are likely to appear under "nursing," they may also be listed under "medical" or "health care." If your training has prepared you for a variety of positions, be sure to check all the possible job titles. For example, graduates of

INTERNET TRACKING FORM

Name of website: _____

Website address: _____

Purpose of website:
- Job lists
- Resume posting
- Search scout
- Information, articles
- Newsgroup
- Mailing list
- Company website

My username: _____

My password: _____

Date resume posted: _____

Responses: _____

Employers identified: _____

_____

_____

Notes (information you provided the employer, version of resume submitted, etc.)

FIGURE 12-6 You are likely to conduct some of your job search using the Internet. *Print or put on your computer copies of this tracking form to keep yourself organized.*

health information programs may be qualified for the following positions: coding specialist, health information technician, medical records coordinator or supervisor, and patient records technician. New job titles are constantly being created to describe the many activities performed in the modern health care facility. Use the skill inventories you created for yourself to help you identify all the jobs for which you may qualify. Don't be discouraged if you find only a few postings or ads—or none—for your occupation. This may actually mean that there is such a shortage of applicants that employers have given up placing expensive ads.

When you respond in writing to a job opening, point out how you meet the employer's needs. You can do this in the cover letter, which will be discussed more fully in Chapter 13. For now, let's look at a couple of sample ads and see how to encourage the employer to read your resume and call you for an interview. Even very short ads contain information you can use. The ad for a medical assistant in Figure 12-7 lists three requirements and shows how they can be addressed in a cover letter sent with a resume. The response to the ad for a

dental assistant in Figure 12-8 is written in a different format, but still addresses the employer's needs. (The same advice applies to electronically posted openings.)

There is not one best way to write an effective response to an employer. Highlight your qualifications in a format that best suits the stated requirements. It isn't necessary—or even desirable—to repeat what's in your resume. A few quick highlights about how you meet the specific requirements are sufficient, along with a fuller description of why you, in particular, can help this employer.

Prescription for Success: 12-5 **Create a Targeted Response**

1. Find an employment ad, either a printed one or one on the Internet. Identify the employer's requirements and write a response that demonstrates how you meet these requirements. (Attach copy of the ad or computer printout.)

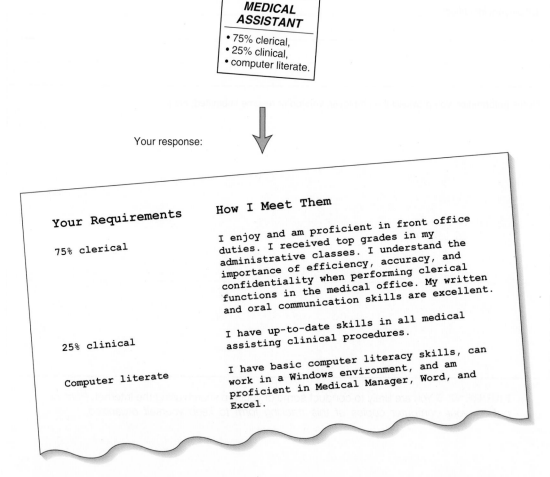

MEDICAL ASSISTANT
- 75% clerical,
- 25% clinical,
- computer literate.

Your response:

Your Requirements — **How I Meet Them**

75% clerical

I enjoy and am proficient in front office duties. I received top grades in my administrative classes. I understand the importance of efficiency, accuracy, and confidentiality when performing clerical functions in the medical office. My written and oral communication skills are excellent.

25% clinical

I have up-to-date skills in all medical assisting clinical procedures.

Computer literate

I have basic computer literacy skills, can work in a Windows environment, and am proficient in Medical Manager, Word, and Excel.

FIGURE 12-7 Example of a direct, point-by-point response to a job posting. *How does the applicant respond to the three requirements listed in the ad? Do you think the applicant does an effective job of responding to this ad? Why or why not?*

DENTAL ASSISTANT—RDA

We are looking for the best! If you understand quality, modern dentistry, appreciate excellent patient care and are dedicated to true teamwork, please fax your resume to...

Your response:

I am a registered dental assistant who recently completed a program of study at Dental Technical College in Health Town. My training program was patient-focused. In all courses, we learned the importance of considering the needs of each patient and delivering the best care possible. I also understand the importance of teamwork, having worked closely with other students throughout both the theory and lab portions of the program. During my clinical experience with Dr. Frank Samuels, I enjoyed sharing responsibilities with his five-member office staff.

FIGURE 12-8 Example of a paragraph that addresses the employer's stated needs. Compare this response with that in Figure 12-7. *Do you think this is as effective as the response in Figure 12-7? Consider how each response mirrors the format of the ad.*

Case Study 12-1

Linh was born in the United States shortly after her parents immigrated to California from Vietnam. Growing up in a close-knit community, she married the son of other immigrants when she was 20. While Linh's three children were growing up, she worked part-time as a teacher's assistant at the local preschool. Although she enjoyed the work, the pay was low and she and her husband were starting to think about paying for their children's college education, as well as saving for their own future retirement.

In high school, Linh had been interested in biology and chemistry. And true to the meaning of her name, which means "gentle spirit," she was a kind and giving person. When she brought up the subject of exploring career possibilities at an extended family dinner, her mother-in-law suggested nursing. Other family members agreed that Linh would likely be a good nurse and that she should look into it.

Linh contacted Cara, a family friend who was a nurse at a large hospital nearby. She conducted an informational interview to learn more about what's it like to be a nurse and was even allowed to job shadow Cara for a few days.

Linh knew that going to school for nurse's training would be challenging. She would have to be organized and balance her life as a mother, wife, and student. Her own mother agreed to spend time with the children after school most days of the week. Although supportive of her goals,

her husband was not enthusiastic about helping with the housework, but he did pick up a few extra chores.

A conscientious student, Linh did well in school. She had to work hard to master the extensive content, both theoretical and applied, that comprised nursing studies. But since graduating and passing her licensing exam, she has been struggling with her job search. Being somewhat shy, she is finding it difficult to make phone calls and approach people she doesn't know well. She has done some searching on the Internet and has reviewed the websites of local hospitals and clinics.

It has been a few weeks now, and Linh is becoming discouraged. She told her husband that she's really worried that the money they spent on tuition, books, and other school expenses was wasted. They discussed it one evening after dinner.

"Linh," said her husband, Bao, "I can't believe that after all your work it's just going to waste. Can't your school help you find a job?"

"I took the job-search workshop," replied Linh. "They emphasized that we had to take responsibility for our job searches, so I really didn't want to bother them again."

"Look," said Bao, "You did well in school. Go in tomorrow and see what they have to offer."

Linh took her husband's advice and made an appointment with the career services department at her school.

Continued

Mr. Bloom, the department director, met with her. He asked what she had done so far in looking for a job.

Linh described what she had done so far: reviewing the Internet and printed ads.

"Linh," said Mr. Bloom. "It sounds like you're missing some of the most effective ways of finding a job: networking and face-to-face contact."

"I'm sure you're right, Mr. Bloom," she responded. "But I just find that really difficult—approaching people I don't know and then actually asking them for something."

"You know, you don't have to start with people you don't know," explained Mr. Bloom. "You've been missing one of the most effective methods there is—networking. Do you know anyone who works in nursing? Have you contacted the people you worked with at the hospital where you did your clinical experience?"

Linh was embarrassed to admit she hadn't. She suddenly realized how obvious this was. She had begun her nursing education by contacting Cara; and she had received compliments on her skills from some of the health care workers in the hospital during her preceptorship. But asking for something—a job—didn't feel right for some reason.

When she explained this to Mr. Bloom, he pointed out that she wasn't asking anyone for a favor. She was offering her recent training, skills, and conscientious work habits to an employer who could benefit by hiring her. He encouraged her to get in touch with her contacts that he believed would not hesitate in helping her to find a job.

Questions for Thought and Reflection

1. Many recent graduates fail to realize what they have to offer an employer. Why do you think this is?
2. From what you've read, do you think Linh will be a good nurse? Why or why not?
3. What do you think of Mr. Bloom's advice to Linh?
4. Networking is one of the best ways to find a job. Why do you think this is true?
5. Do you know people who maybe willing to help you find a job?

Trouble Ahead? 12-1

Jacob was frustrated and angry when he entered the office of Mr. Gonzalez, director of career services at Health Career College. Jacob had graduated two months before he stopped by to see Mr. Gonzalez to tell him that he still hadn't received a job offer. In fact, he hadn't even had an interview.

"Hi, Jacob," Mr. Gonzalez greeted him. "I haven't seen you in awhile. What's going on?"

"Not much, to be honest," Jacob told him. "I'm not happy. I finished my externship two months ago and you guys haven't found me a job yet."

Mr. Gonzalez looked at Jacob for a moment and then said, "Well, I think there's been a misunderstanding. Our job is to *help* our students in their job search. We don't *get* them jobs."

"Look," says Jacob, "When I enrolled at this school I was told that the majority of students who graduated from my program get placed. I paid a lot of money to go here and the least you can do is find me a job."

"Let me ask you, Jacob, did you attend any of my job-search workshops?"

"Honestly, by the time I graduated, I'd had enough of school," Jason said. "I really didn't feel like coming back for more classes."

"I'm sorry you felt that way," responded Mr. Gonzalez. "The workshops are designed to help students carry out an effective job search. Let me ask you a few questions."

"Here we go," grumbled Jacob, as he flopped down into a chair.

"What have you done so far to look for a job?" Mr. Gonzalez asked.

"A lot! I went to those online job sites and looked for jobs for pharmacy techs," said Jacob. "But most of them were too far away, or didn't look very interesting, or didn't pay enough. I can't take just anything, you know. I've got student loans to pay."

"How about networking? Or visiting pharmacies where you might like to work?" asked Mr. Gonzalez.

"I thought I *was* networking by being a student here," explained Jacob. "My instructors know me, you know me. I didn't have time while I was a student to go out and meet a bunch of people. I thought that was *your* job. Going to meet employers and find us jobs."

"Jacob, I'm afraid that you're going to have to take more responsibility for conducting your own job search," said Mr. Gonzalez. "We can give you leads and connect you to employers who are interested in our graduates. But you haven't been in touch with us at all—not to attend the workshops or ask for help. That's our job, but you have to be willing to do your part."

"Well, I needed time to relax and just hang out after I graduated. And I can see it wouldn't have done any good anyway if *you're* not going to get me placed in a job I like—and that pays well."

Questions for Thought and Reflection

1. What mistakes is Jacob making in his job search?
2. What part do you think his attitude is playing in his failure to find a job?
3. What do you think about how Mr. Gonzalez handled being confronted by Jacob?
4. Do you think Jacob will have a successful career as a pharmacy technician? Why or why not?

Summary of Key Ideas

- Know yourself: what you want and need and what you have to offer an employer.
- Get to know the employment climate.
- Increase your chance of finding the right job by using a variety of different lead sources.

Positive Self-Talk for This Chapter

- I am confident and competent.
- I have valuable skills to offer an employer.
- I am organized and have a good job-search plan.
- I will find the job that's right for me.

Internet Activities

ⓔ For active links to the websites necessary to complete these activities, visit http://evolve.elsevier.com/haroun/career/.

1. Find an article on using networking to learn about job openings, and write a summary of what you learn.
2. Using websites that list job openings, find and list 10 jobs for which you might be qualified.
3. Read the article "How to Use the Internet in Your Job Search" on the Riley Guide website and create a list of the suggestions.
4. Explore the website of a professional organization related to your occupation. What kind of information does it contain? Job postings? Opportunities to network? Conference dates? Anything else?
5. Read the article "15 Myths and Misconceptions About Job-Hunting" from Quintessential Careers. Were you surprised by what you read? Why or why not? Were any of the myth-busters helpful to you?

Building Your Resume

1. Review and fill in the forms for Resume Building Blocks #6, #7, #8, and #9 in Chapter 2, which list the activities and skills that support your job search.

To Learn More

Bolles R.N.: What color is your parachute? A practical manual for job-hunters and job-changers, Berkeley, 2014, Ten Speed Press

www.jobhuntersbible.com

Bolles's book has become a classic job-search manual. The ideas are original, well researched, and reportedly very effective. The companion website is also packed with useful ideas, including hints on using the Internet effectively in the job search.

Career Builder

www.careerbuilder.com

Website includes job-search tools, career advice, a list of career fairs around the country, and a salary calculator.

The Riley Guide

www.rileyguide.com

Margaret Dickel is a librarian who has been tracking the Internet as a job-search resource for many years. Her book is excellent, or you can access lots of information from her website.

Quintessential Careers

General job-search and career information: www.quintcareers.com
Health care jobs: www.quintcareers.com/healthcare_jobs.html
This website contains information on every phase of the job search and career development in the form of articles, resources, and tutorials.

U.S. Department of Labor, Bureau of Labor Statistics

www.bls.gov
The BLS website contains information about economic conditions, wages, and unemployment rates.

References

1. Forbes, The 10 best websites for your career. Available at: http://www.forbes.com/pictures/mkl45hifd/1-linkedin-com/#gallerycontent.
2. Kate Lorenz, Warning: social networking can be hazardous to your job search. Available at: www.careerbuilder.com/Article/CB-533-Job-Search-Warning-Social-Networking-Can-Be-Hazardous-to-Your-Job-Search/?ArticleID=533&cbRecursionCnt=1&cbsid=920e95b94af84818bfb7a8e12af99ffd-288916701-R3-4.

Finalizing Your Employment Presentation Materials

1. Understand the building blocks and components of a resume.
2. Write an effective resume by choosing and assembling the building blocks that apply to you.
3. Distribute your resume and keep apprised of new developments with regard to resume distribution.
4. Write appropriate cover letters.
5. Fill out employment applications correctly and accurately.
6. Prepare a reference sheet and secure letters of recommendation to support your job-search efforts.
7. Create a professional portfolio that supports your qualifications.

Applications Forms containing questions and spaces for information you fill in that employers need to make a decision about your qualifications for a specific job.

Chronological Resume A resume that places emphasizes on the work history of a job applicant.

Combination Resume A resume that combines some detailed work history with a list of skills that apply to the targeted job.

Cover Letter A letter of introduction sent with a resume.

Functional Resume A resume that places the least emphasis on work history; the emphasis is on skills that relate to the targeted job.

Liability Responsibility, often financial, for damages and losses.

Objective Your job or career goal.

Portfolios Collections of items that provide evidence of job-related skills and capabilities.

Resumes Written documents that summarize professional skills and capabilities.

Targeted Objective An objective that matches the requirements of a specific employer.

Presentation: Putting Your Best Pen Forward

"The door of opportunity won't open unless you do some pushing."

Preparing high-quality written materials is an essential part of a successful job search. Some documents are designed to outline your qualifications and let potential employers know what you can do for them. These include **resumes**, cover letters, and **applications**. Other materials that serve to support your claims include reference sheets and **portfolios**.

Anything you submit in your bid for employment is a form of personal advertising. Written materials reflect who you are and what you can do, so apply your best organizing, writing, and spelling skills to their creation. Keep in mind that written materials are, in a sense, permanent. What's on paper stays there. You can't change, correct, or explain, "What I really meant to say was…." Once in the hands of prospective employers, a resume and cover letter are all they have to go by. So prepare all written materials thoughtfully and carefully so they represent you in the best way possible.

Prescription for Success: 13-1
First Impressions

1. Imagine yourself behind the employer's desk. You have placed an ad for a medical receptionist. You receive a large number of resumes, and among them you find the following:
   - Misspelled words
   - Pages lightly printed so that they are difficult to read
   - Lack of information about related training or experience
   - No telephone number for the applicant
   - Paragraphs misaligned
2. Answer the following questions:
   What is your impression of these applicants?
   What does each of these errors say about the person who submitted the resume?
   Would you call any of them for an interview? Which one(s)? Why or why not?
   Are the errors in the resumes more significant because this is a job in health care? Explain why or why not.

Your Resume: A Product Brochure

"The resume gets you the interview. The interview gets you the job."

Selling yourself as a qualified job candidate begins with a well-prepared resume. The purpose of a resume is to convince prospective employers to interview you. To accomplish this, you must show them you have the qualifications they need. Health care employers are looking for employees who will contribute to their success in caring for their customers.

(Yes, many employers think of their patients as customers.) Your well-constructed resume is one way to show them that you are the kind of person they are looking for.

Personal Reflection

1. Why do you think a resume is referred to as a "product brochure"?
2. Does thinking about your resume in this way influence how you will write it? If so, how?

Completing the Building Blocks of Your Resume

In the following sections, you will use the information you have been writing on the Resume Building Blocks provided in Chapter 2 to complete the various components of your resume. Then you will go through the steps to pull them all together into a completed resume that you can be proud to have represent you.

Many employers are using the Internet extensively in the hiring process. Some have started scanning all the resumes they receive and entering them into a computerized database. Each resume is then reviewed electronically, and key words are identified. When there is a job opening, the computer searches for resumes that contain key words that match those in the job description. Other employers only accept electronically sent resumes.

These new practices require thinking a little differently as you write your resume. Because of the key-word element, these are important considerations as you write the various sections. Start by preparing a list of key words that relate to your job target. Twenty to 60 words are recommended. Consider which key words most closely describe the jobs for which you want to be considered, as well as the types of skills and qualities employers are seeking. If possible, secure job descriptions from potential employers. Read ads or job announcements, and visit facility websites. The *Occupational Outlook Handbook*, a government publication that contains descriptions of thousands of jobs available online at www.bls.gov/ooh, is a good source. Good key words are nouns that name specific skills, such as "insurance billing," "laboratory tests," and "patient care."

Resume Building Block #1: Introduction

The introduction, or first section of your resume, can be written as a career **objective**, a professional or career profile, or as a summary of qualifications. The basic differences between the three is that a career objective states what you, the job applicant, are looking for; while a professional profile and summary of qualifications state or list what you have to offer the employer. A professional profile is a paragraph summarizing your qualifications for the job; a summary of qualifications is presented as a list of your qualifications and contains more detail than a profile. The following examples are for an applicant who is applying for a job as a medical assistant in a clinic that serves many Spanish-speaking patients:

Career Objective: Position as a medical assistant in a clinic in which I can contribute the skills from my recent training and my fluency in spoken Spanish.

Professional Profile: Certified medical assistant with recent training who has knowledge of the local community. Has experience working with people of all ages and able to communicate in both English and Spanish.

Summary of Qualifications:
- Recent, up-to-date training as a medical assistant
- Certification (CMA) from the American Association of Medical Assistants
- Skills include:
  - Scheduling appointments
  - Properly handling telephone calls
  - Maintaining medical records
  - Performing insurance coding
  - Performing billing and bookkeeping tasks
  - Taking vital signs
  - Preparing and administering medications
  - Performing venipunctures and ECGs
  - Assisting the physician in delivering patient care
  - Performing urinalyses, hematological tests, various specialty tests
- CPR certification
- Excellent attendance while attending school
- Successful completion of 160 hours of externship with Dr. Martinez at Good Health Clinic
- Good people skills acquired through previous work in customer service
- Fluent in spoken Spanish

If you write a Summary of Qualifications instead of an Objective, include the name of the job for which you are applying in your cover letter. You could also place the title of the job you are seeking (medical transcriptionist, dental assistant, etc.) centered at the top of your resume, between your contact information and summary of qualifications.

If you do decide to write an objective, consider writing one that is targeted for a specific job. This type of objective mirrors the employer's language and draws attention to how you fit that particular job. The following example shows how to write a targeted objective:

Ad: "X-ray tech with strong patient-relations skills for orthopedic practice. Great opportunity to join an established team environment."

Key words in the ad: "x-ray tech," "patient relations skills," "orthopedic," "team."

Targeted objective: Position as an x-ray tech in an orthopedic office where I can apply my excellent human-relations skills working with patients and fellow professionals.

If you create and print your own resume on a computer, you can change your objective slightly for each job you

apply for. An alternative approach is to omit the objective in your resume, but include information from the ad in your cover letter—in other words, point out how you fit the requirements of the position and can meet the needs of the employer.

Prescription for Success: 13-2 Writing a Targeted Objective

1. Find an advertised position in your occupational area.
2. Underline the portions of the ad or posting that describe what the employer is looking for.
3. Write a targeted objective that responds specifically to the stated needs of the employer.

NOTE: Although you may decide not to use an objective in your resume, you should be aware of the employer's needs and how you can help address them as an employee. This will help you in writing an effective cover letter and responding to questions at the job interview.

Prescription for Success: 13-3 Write Your Introduction

Use Resume Building Block #1 to write a general objective to use on your resume OR write a Summary of Qualifications OR write a Career Profile.

Resume Building Block #2: Education

Up-to-date training is likely to be one of the strongest employment qualifications of recent graduates who don't have previous experience in health care. The Education section can contain more information than simply a list of the schools you have attended. The following items are examples of what you can include:
- Name of the health care program you completed
- Degree, diploma, or certificate earned
- Grade point average, if at least 3.0 (on a 4.0 scale)
- Licenses, special certifications, and other documentation of training and skills
- Additional courses, workshops, seminars, and special training you have completed
- Special projects that demonstrate your qualifications

Some program titles do not clearly communicate the types of skills acquired by students. For example, the program entitled "Patient Care Assistant" varies in content from school to school throughout the country. In cases like this, it is a good idea to list the courses you have completed. This gives the employer a better idea of your skills. (If this takes up too much space on the resume, consider including a list of courses or a copy of the curriculum in your portfolio.)

The following is an example of an Education section:

Mental Health Technician Certificate, 2012
Wellness College, Salem, OR
- Graduated with Top Honors
- Grade point average 3.7 on a 4.0 scale
- Received Perfect Attendance Award

Nursing Assistant Certificate, 2010
GetWell Health College, Portland, OR
- Grade point average 3.8 on a 4.0 scale
- Maintained perfect attendance
- Completed CPR training
- Organized musical program presented by students at Christmas to local extended-care residents

Workshops completed 2013-2014
Sunnyville Psychiatric Institute, Salem, OR
- Review of Research on Depression (25 hours)
- Suicide Prevention Measures (20 hours)
- Managing Assaultive Patients (25 hours)

> **Prescription for Success: 13-4 Write Your Education Section**
>
> Use Resume Building Block #2 to complete the Education section of your resume. List all the schools you have attended, starting with the most recent one.

Resume Building Block #3: Professional Skills and Knowledge

Note: To avoid duplication, include this section *only* if you did not introduce your resume with a Summary of Qualifications. You may also omit it if you plan to list or summarize your skills and classes in the Education section.

Occupational skills acquired through both training and work experience are listed in the Professional Skills and Knowledge section. Recall from Chapter 2 that these may be listed individually or in clusters of related skills. Take a look at the following examples:

Example 1: Creating skill clusters
Medical assistant skills
- Administrative skills
- Scheduling appointments, handling telephone calls, greeting patients, maintaining medical records, coding and filling out insurance forms, performing billing and bookkeeping functions
- Clinical skills
Assisting the physician, preparing and administering medications, performing venipunctures and ECGs, taking vital signs, practicing aseptic techniques
- Laboratory skills
Performing urinalyses, hematological tests, and various specialty tests
- Computer skills
Medical Manager, Microsoft Word, Excel, PowerPoint
Example 2: Listing individual skills
Medical insurance technician skills

- Abstracting medical information from patient records
- Coding diagnoses and procedures accurately
- Completing insurance forms correctly
- Submitting and monitoring insurance claims
- Processing payments

> **Prescription for Success: 13-5 Write Your Professional Skills and Knowledge Section**
>
> If this section applies to you, complete Resume Building Block #3.

Resume Building Block #4: Work History

A record of your previous employment, this section can be more than a simple listing of jobs and the duties you performed. As discussed in Chapter 2, your Work History section can be strengthened by including your accomplishments and emphasizing transferable skills that relate to the health care job you want now.

Use action verbs when describing job duties and achievements. For example, saying "Taught students of all ages to swim" is a stronger and more effective statement than "Responsible for teaching swimming." Even better is "Successfully taught students of all ages to swim so that 97% passed the Red Cross Swim Test for their level." See Box 13-1 for a list of suggested action verbs.

Military service and your externship can also be included in this section. Just be sure to make it clear that the externship experience was an unpaid position and that you were a student. It is not necessary to include very short-term or part-time jobs unless they are directly related to your job target. Do not state your reasons for leaving each job. You may find this question on employment applications, but it should not be included on your resume.

Here is an example of a Work History entry:

Cashier, Petamerica
Bigdog, GA
- Assisted customers and informed them about products
- Performed cashier duties
- Closed out registers at end of day
- Named "Most Helpful Employee" for 2013
- Maintained perfect attendance for two years
- Promoted to head cashier after one year
- Selected to train newly hired cashiers

Although this list does not include health care duties or skills, the items on it demonstrate responsibility, reliability, and communication skills.

> **Prescription for Success: 13-6 Write Your Work History Section**
>
> Use Resume Building Block #4 to complete the Work History section of your resume, starting with the most recent job held.

BOX 13-1 Examples of Action Verbs to Use on Your Resume

Achieved	Educated	Launched	Recorded
Administered	Encouraged	Led	Regulated
Assisted	Established	Maintained	Repaired
Billed	Expanded	Managed	Reported
Budgeted	Generated	Monitored	Represented
Calculated	Greeted	Motivated	Revised
Cared for	Handled	Negotiated	Scheduled
Coded	Helped	Obtained	Secured
Communicated	Hired	Operated	Set up
Composed	Implemented	Ordered	Showed
Constructed	Improved	Organized	Sold
Controlled	Increased	Participated	Supervised
Coordinated	Influenced	Performed	Taught
Created	Informed	Planned	Tested
Demonstrated	Initiated	Prepared	Trained
Designed	Inspired	Presented	Verified
Developed	Instructed	Produced	Word processed
Directed	Introduced	Provided	Wrote
Documented	Justified	Purchased	

Resume Building Block #5: Licenses and Certifications

Include a Licenses and Certifications section on your resume only if this information is not listed in the Education or any other section. Wherever you put it, be sure the dates and numbers are accurate.

Examples of ways to present certifications:

- Certified Occupational Therapist Assistant, 2014
  American Occupational Therapy Association
- Registered Nurse
  California State Nursing License, #123456
- Certified Medical Assistant, 2013
  American Association of Medical Assistants

> **Prescription for Success: 13-7 Write Your Licenses and Certifications Section**
>
> If this section applies to you, complete Resume Building Block #5.

Resume Building Block #6: Honors and Awards

Honors and awards can be from organizations other than your school. Include information about why you received them if this is not clear from their titles. (These could be listed under Summary of Qualifications, Education, or Professional and Community Organizations. Choose where they fit best; just make sure to list them only once.)

Examples:

- Parent Volunteer of 2012 for James Madison Middle School
- Recognition for organizing activities that raised over $150,000 to purchase instructional equipment, such as computers and library books
- Perfect Attendance Award, Wellness College, 2011

> **Prescription for Success: 13-8 Write Your Honors and Awards Section**
>
> If this section applies to you, complete Resume Building Block #6.

Resume Building Block #7: Special Skills

Do you have skills that don't fit in any other section but add to your value as a health care employee? This section gives you the opportunity to include and even highlight them.

> **Prescription for Success: 13-9 Write Your Special Skills Section**
>
> If this section applies to you, complete Resume Building Block #7.

Resume Building Block #8: Volunteer Work

Service and volunteer work do not have to be directly related to health care. For example, work in which you demonstrated responsibility, the willingness to contribute to society and help others, and/or your teamwork skills is appropriate to include. You may have done this at school, through a religious organization, or with any group devoted to promoting the good of the community. Write brief phrases to describe what you did, if necessary. Use action verbs as you did in the Work History section. Do not list activities you already included in the Education section or elsewhere.

Here are some examples:

- March of Dimes, 1999 to present
  Participated in annual fund drives
- Boy Scout Troop Leader, 1997-2003

Resume Building Block #9: Professional and Civic Organizations

In the Professional and Civic Organizations section, list the organizations to which you belong. Briefly describe any organizations that may not be familiar to prospective employers. If you take or have taken an active part, such as serving on a committee or as an officer, state what you are doing or did. On your resume, this heading can also be called "Memberships" or "Affiliations."

Examples include the following:
- Florida Association of Medical Assistants, Tampa Chapter Chair of membership drive, 2002
- Member of Continuing Education Planning Committee, 2008 to present

(**Note:** It is best not to include organizations that are highly political or are generally considered to hold radical views. If you are in doubt about what to include on your resume, check with your instructor or your school's career services' office.)

Resume Building Block #10: Languages Spoken

If you are able to communicate in a language other than English and have not included it in any other section, it can go in a Languages section. Include a little information about your skills and level of ability, as in the **following examples:**

Spanish: Speaking and reading: good; writing: fair.
Vietnamese: Very basic conversational ability. Some knowledge of health care terms for conducting patient interviews.

Pulling It All Together

You are now ready to gather the information in your Resume Building Blocks to construct a finished product. These blocks, contained in your Prescriptions for Success 13-3 through 13-12, can be put together in a variety of ways. The steps described in this section will help you to create a document that best highlights your qualifications.

You will see as you progress through this chapter that there is no one best way to write a resume. Everyone has different talents and experiences. Even students who complete the same program at the same time come from a variety of backgrounds that can be presented in different ways. For example, a young person who graduated from high school shortly before beginning a dental assisting program will most likely benefit from emphasizing different areas than a classmate who worked in sales for 20 years before entering the same program.

Local customs and employer preferences also apply to resumes. Seek the advice of your instructors, school career service personnel, and professional contacts. They keep in touch with employers and can offer sound advice.

At this busy time in the job-search process, you may be tempted to use a standard resume format. Filling in the blanks on a "one-type-fits-all" resume may seem to be a quick and easy way to complete this task. However, the time spent customizing your resume can pay off in several ways. For example, you will do the following:

1. Better recognize and review your own qualifications
2. Respond to employers' specific needs
3. Be prepared to support your claims with examples
4. Demonstrate your organizational skills
5. Show your initiative and creativity

Note: Your school may require or recommend that you use a format it has developed. In this case, it may be best to use what is provided.

An effective way to increase your efficiency when putting together your resume is to use word-processing software. This gives you several advantages because you can:

- Try different layouts and formats
- Change and reorganize content quickly and easily
- Check for (most) spelling errors
- Vary your summary of qualifications or objective to address specific employer needs
- Use special features such as bolding and changing the size and style of the letters
- Send your resume as part of an e-mail and/or post it on the Internet (this will be discussed later in this chapter)

If you don't know how to use a word-processing program, now is a good time to learn if you have a little time. Today's software is quite easy to learn and even non-typists can produce great-looking documents by learning a few basic commands. Spacing, bolding, underlining, moving text, and printing can be accomplished with the click or two of a button. If you can spend a few hours to learn the basics of a word-processing program now, it will be a good investment of your time. Not only will this skill support your job-search effort, it will provide you with a valuable workplace skill. Even health care professionals who dedicate most of their time to hands-on patient activities can benefit from knowing how to word process. Today, computer skills are considered essential for most health care jobs.

10 Steps for Assembling Your Resume

Whether you create your resume on a computer or not, following a step-by-step process can help you assemble a resume to fit your needs. Box 13-2 summarizes the steps that are explained in the following sections.

Step One: Prepare the Heading

It is not necessary to write the word "Resume." Instead, clearly label the top of the page with your name, address, telephone number, and e-mail address. Centering your name is good for both appearance and practicality. Placing it on the far left side makes it more difficult for the employer to find if it is placed in a stack of other resumes or in a file. (You might even put your heading justified right.) Capitalizing your name and/or using a slightly larger font (letter) size than the rest of the document helps it to stand out.

JAIME RAMIREZ
3650 Loma Alta Lane
San Diego, CA 92137
(619) 123-4567
jrnurse@gmail.com

Capitalize and boldface your name and consider using a larger size font. Include your ZIP code and area code. Be sure all numbers are correct. Include your e-mail address if you have one.

The following format is an option if your resume is long and you are trying to save space:

JAIME RAMIREZ
3650 Loma Alta Lane, San Diego, CA 92137
(619) 123-4567 jrnurse@gmail.com

Step Two: Add the Introduction

The introduction (summary of qualifications or objective), from Resume Building Block #1, helps prospective employers quickly see whether there is a potential match between your qualifications and their needs. This part of the resume may change slightly, as discussed previously, if you are trying to match your objective or select among your qualifications those that best match the stated needs of each employer. Your objective will not change if you have specific requirements you are not willing to change, if you have written a very general objective that meets a number of job targets, or if your objective simply states a job title such as "surgical technologist."

Step Three: Select the Best Type of Resume for You

The three basic types of resumes are chronological, functional, and combination. They provide different ways to present your work history and professional qualifications. Your particular background and qualifications determine which type you should choose.

Chronological Resume

The **chronological resume** emphasizes your work history. It shows the progression of jobs you have held to show how you have gained increasing knowledge, experience, and/or responsibility relevant to the job you want now. This type of resume is recommended if you have:

- Held previous jobs in health care
- Had jobs in other areas in which you had increases in responsibility or a strong record of achievements
- Acquired many skills that apply to health care (transferable skills)

In the chronological resume, each job you've had in the past is listed, followed by the duties performed and your achievements. The Work section is well developed and likely to be longer than most other parts of your resume. Figure 13-1 shows an example of the Work History section for a nurse's chronological resume.

Functional Resume

A **functional resume** emphasizes skills and traits that relate to the targeted job but that weren't necessarily acquired through health care employment. They can be pulled from both work and personal experiences. For example, if you cared for a sick relative for an extended period of time, this is an experience you may decide to include. Review Prescription for Success 1-4 and your transferable skills, discussed in Chapter 2. Once you have identified and listed the qualifications that fit your target jobs, organize them into three or four clusters with descriptive headings. Figure 13-2 shows three clusters developed by a graduate who wants to find a job in health information technology. She has drawn from her experiences as a parent, active member of her community, and bookkeeper.

Functional resumes are advantageous in the following situations:

- You are entering the job market for the first time.
- You have held jobs unrelated to health care.
- You have personal experiences you can apply to health care work.

| WORK HISTORY | **Registered Nurse III, Surgical Unit** | 2008-Present |
| | **Gladstone Hospital, Happy Valley, OR** | |

- Serve as charge nurse, providing high quality nursing care without supervision

- Develop and implement patient care plans based on individual needs

- Evaluate and revise plans as needed

- Conduct patient care conferences with care team members

- Serve as a patient advocate to ensure provision of appropriate and high quality care

- Teach and counsel patients and their families to perform home care procedures and maximize wellness

- Serve as preceptor for ADN and LPN nursing students

Registered Nurse II, Surgical Unit   2005-2008
Gladstone Hospital, Happy Valley, OR

- Identify patient care problems

- Implement nursing interventions and evaluate the results

- Administer medications without error

- Teach patients preoperation and postoperation procedures

- Carry out procedures as ordered by physician

- Communicate clearly to patients, their families, co-workers, and physicians

- Orient new employees

Staff Nurse   2000-2005
Sunnyville Community Hospital, Sunnyville, OR

- Provide direct patient care

- Carry out nursing care plans

- Complete prescribed treatments

- Give medications

- Document all care given on patient charts

- Call physicians as needed in response to patient's conditions

FIGURE 13-1 Work history section of a chronological resume for an experienced applicant seeking a nursing position. The most recent job is listed first. As you read from the bottom up, note the increasing complexity of tasks and levels of responsibility. For example, in his first job, he carried out nursing plans. In his most recent job, he developed the plans.

The Work History section of a functional resume consists of a simple list of job titles with each employer's name, city and state, and your dates of employment. See Figure 13-2 and note how this is done. A functional resume may take more time to develop than a chronological one, but the extra effort can really pay off because it allows you to highlight the qualifications that are your strongest bid for employment.

Combination Resume

The **combination resume**, as its name implies, uses features of both the chronological and functional types. The details of the job(s) held in health care or those closely related to it are listed, along with clusters of qualifications or a list of supporting skills. This resume is appropriate in the following situations:

- You have held jobs in health care *and*

COMPUTER SKILLS

- Created electronic spreadsheet to track fund-raising for Lewison Elementary School PTA

- Taught self to effectively use leading brand software programs in the following areas: word processing, database, spreadsheets, and accounting

- Set up and managed electronic accounting system for family construction business

- Teach computer classes at Girl Scout summer day camp

ORGANIZATIONAL SKILLS

- Created system to monitor all church collections and fund-raising projects

- Initiated and developed computer career awareness program for Girl Scouts

- Secretary for college HIT student organization

- Completed HIT associate degree program with record of perfect attendance while working part-time and managing family life

CLERICAL/ADMINISTRATIVE SKILLS

- 7 years bookkeeping experience

- Keyboarding speed of 78 wpm

- Excellent written communication

WORK HISTORY

Bookkeeper 2011-Present
Buildwell Construction Company, Yuma, AZ

Bookkeeper 2006-2011
Perfect-Fit Cabinetry, Yuma, AZ

Secretary 2002-2006
Caldwell Insurance Company, Yuma, AZ

FIGURE 13-2 **Work history section of a functional resume for a recent graduate seeking a health information technology (HIT) position.** The graduate does not have experience in this field, so she has clustered other skills that support work in HIT, such as bookkeeping and tracking details.

- You have related qualifications you gained through other, non–health care jobs and experiences *or*
- You have held a number of jobs in health care for which you performed the same or very similar duties

Let's look at how a recent occupational therapy assistant graduate who worked for four years as a nursing assistant and for three years as a preschool aide creates a combination resume. She decides to do the following:

- Include a list of the duties she performed in the nursing assistant job.
- Create clusters to highlight her teaching and interpersonal skills, both important in occupational therapy.
- List skills from her teaching and other experiences under each cluster heading.

Figure 13-3 illustrates how she organized her material to best show her qualifications.

Choosing the Best Resume for You

Review your skills and experiences and use the guidelines in this section to choose the best type of resume for you. If you decide to use a chronological presentation, copy what you prepared for your Work History in Building Block #3.

If a functional resume would serve you better, use the following guidelines to create the clusters:

1. Consider the current needs of employers. Check your local help-wanted ads and job announcements, the National Healthcare Foundation Standards, and the SCANS competencies for ideas.

NURSING ASSISTANT　　　　　　　　　　　　2008-2012
GoodCare Nursing Home, Denver, CO

- Encourage patients to achieve their maximum level of wellness, activity, and independence
- Demonstrate interest in the lives and well-being of patients
- Assist patients with prescribed exercises
- Organize and participate in activities with patients
- Help patients carry out basic hygiene and dressing

TEACHING SKILLS

- Teach swim classes to all ages at YMCA
- Conduct CPR instruction for the American Heart Association
- Organize holiday programs and outings for nursing home residents (volunteer)
- Planned and supervised craft and play activities for preschool children
- Tutored ESL students at Salud College while in OTA program

INTERPERSONAL SKILLS

- Provided daily care for parent with Alzheimer's disease for 18 months
- Answered telephone, directed calls, and took messages for busy sporting goods manufacturer
- Received Connor Memorial Award for graduating class for making positive contributions and assisting classmates at Salud College

WORK HISTORY　　　　**Preschool Aide**　2005-2008
　　　　　　　　　　　　Bright Light Preschool, Denver, CO

　　　　　　　　　　　　Swim Instructor　2002-Present
　　　　　　　　　　　　YMCA, Denver, CO

　　　　　　　　　　　　Receptionist　2002-2005
　　　　　　　　　　　　Sportrite Manufacturing Co., Denver, CO

FIGURE 13-3 **Work history section of a combination resume for a recent graduate seeking an occupational therapy assistant position.** She details the one health-related job she has held while organizing into clusters other skills that support the new career goal.

2. Think about the skills and traits that will contribute to success in your occupation.
3. Look over your work history, externship experience, personal experiences, volunteer activities, and participation in professional organizations.
4. Refer to your completed Prescriptions for Success 1-4 and 12-1 for the skills and characteristics you can use in clusters.
5. Create three or four headings for clusters that support your job target and give you an opportunity to list your most significant qualifications. The following list contains examples of appropriate clusters for health care occupations:
- Communication Skills
- Organizational Skills
- Teamwork Skills
- Interpersonal Relations
- Computer Skills
- Clerical Skills
6. List the appropriate specific skills under each heading.
7. If you wrote a Summary of Qualifications for your introduction, take care not to repeat what you listed there in this section.

Step Four: Summary of Qualifications

Decide whether to include a Summary of Qualifications Section (if you didn't include one in your introduction). This is an optional section. Its purpose is to list the skills that support you as a product, but that don't fit well in other sections. It can also serve to highlight how you will benefit the employer and encourage the reader to look over the rest of your resume. In other words, it can serve as an appealing introduction to you and your resume.

You may have decided to use a chronological resume, but have additional experiences that don't belong in the Work History section. Or maybe you have designed a functional resume, but have single experiences worth mentioning that don't fit any of the headings, as in the following examples:

- Excellent time-management skills
- Works calmly under pressure
- Proven problem-solving ability
- Cost-conscious
- Enthusiastic team player
- Works well without supervision
- Enjoys learning new skills

A Qualifications section can also serve as a summary of highlights to draw attention to your most significant features. Such a summary might look like this:

- Eight years' experience working in health care
- Up-to-date administrative and clinical medical assisting skills
- Current CPR certification
- Fluent in spoken Tagalog
- Excellent communication skills

Review the same information sources recommended in Step Four for preparing functional clusters. The difference in preparing the Qualifications section is that you can combine different kinds of characteristics. They don't have to fall into neat categories, but only have to demonstrate the capabilities, traits, and special skills that relate to the job you want.

Note: If you wrote a Summary of Qualifications for your introduction, do not include this section. Also, if you have created clusters and are using them in a functional or combination resume, you need not create this section. The important thing is *not to repeat* information in your resume. Step Five talks more about deciding what to include.

Step Five: Choose Which Resume Building Blocks to Include

You want your resume to be comprehensive, but at the same time you don't want to repeat information. For example, if you are using a functional format and have listed a special skill in one of your clusters, don't repeat it under another heading. Group as much as fits well into each Resume Building Block instead of having many headings with just one item listed. Think about which items fit together. The following are the most appropriate to combine:

1. Licenses and certifications can be placed in their own section, can be listed in the Education section, or can be listed as a Professional Qualification.
2. Honors and awards earned in school can be listed under Education. However, if you have a variety of types of awards, it might be better to highlight them by listing them in their own section.
3. Memberships can go under Education if they are related to school groups or your health care professional organization.

If you have been active in the organizations and want to state what you've done or are involved in several organizations, they may fit better in their own section.

4. Externship experience can be listed under either Education or Work History. Wherever you place it, include some information about the duties you performed. For career changers and recent graduates, this may be a significant part of your work history. Be sure to indicate clearly, however, that the work was unpaid and part of an educational program.
5. Languages you speak other than English can be listed under Summary of Qualifications, Special Skills, or Languages Spoken.

Step Six: Plan the Order of Your Building Blocks

Place the sections that contain your strongest qualifications first. For example, if you are changing careers and recent education is your primary qualification, list that section before Work History.

Step Seven: Decide Whether You Want to Add a Personal Statement

In their book *Career Planning*, Dave Ellis and coauthors suggest adding a positive personal statement at the bottom of your resume.[1] This gives you an opportunity to make a final impression and add an original touch. It is a way to say, "Here is something personal and interesting about me that might help you, the employer." If you decide to write a personal statement, be sure it is a sincere reflection of you and not simply something that sounds good.

And, as with the entire resume, be sure it relates to your job target. Here are a couple of examples:

- "I enjoy being a part of a team where I can make a positive contribution by using my ability to remain calm and work efficiently under stressful conditions."
- "I get great satisfaction working with people from a variety of backgrounds who need assistance in resolving their health care problems."

If you do decide to include a personal statement, review your reasons for choosing a career in health care along with what you believe are your best potential contributions to prospective employers. It is also a good idea to have someone else, such as your instructor, review your statement. If you are unsure about what to say, it is best to simply omit this extra piece.

Another trend is to include a positive statement about you or your work from a reference, such as your externship supervisor or a former employer, at the conclusion of your resume. If you decide to include this, be sure to *secure the permission of the person who made the statement.*

Step Eight: Leave Out Personal Information

Do not include personal information such as your age, marital status, number of children, and health status. And never include false statements about your education or experience.

If these are discovered later, they can be grounds for dismissal from your job.

Although it is important to have a Reference Sheet (list of references) available for potential employers who request it, it is not necessary to write a statement such as "References Available upon Request."

Step Nine: Plan the Layout

Each section of your resume, except the heading at the top and personal statement (optional) at the end, should be labeled: Objective, Education, Work History, and so on. Headings can be flush (aligned) with the left margin, with the content set to the right, as follows:

SUMMARY OF QUALIFICATIONS
XXXXXXXXXXXXXXXXXXXX
XXXXXXXXXXXXXXXXXX
EDUCATION   XXXXXXXXXXXXXXXXXXXXX
                 XXXXXXXXXXXXXXXXXXX

Alternatively, you can center your headings and list the information beneath and flush left.

SUMMARY OF QUALIFICATIONS
XXXXXXXXXXXXXXXXXXXXXXXXXXXXXXX
XXXXXXXXXXXXXXXXXXXXXXXXXXXXX
EDUCATION
XXXXXXXXXXXXXXXXXXXX
XXXXXXXXXXXXXXXXXXXXXXX
XXXXXXXXXXXXXXXX

The information you list under the headings can be arranged in a variety of ways. The design should be based primarily on whether you need to use or save space on the page. The second consideration is personal preference. However you choose to lay out your resume, strive for a balanced, attractive look. Note the varied use of capitalization and boldface to draw attention to the job title in the following examples:

WORK HISTORY   Medical Transcriptionist
                   2010 - Present
                   Hopeful Medical Center
                   Better Health, NJ
OR

                   MEDICAL TRANSCRIPTIONIST
                   2010 - Present
                   Hopeful Medical Center
                   Better Health, NJ
OR

                   Medical Transcriptionist
                   2010 - Present
                   Hopeful Medical Center
                   Better Health, NJ

Step Ten: Create an Attractive and Professional-Looking Document

Selecting and organizing content takes time and effort, so don't waste your efforts by failing to attend to the details of appearance. A poor appearance can land a resume in the wastebasket without even a review. The following tips will help you achieve a professional look:

- Leave enough white space so the page doesn't look crowded. Double space between the sections.
- It is recommended that you limit your resume to one page. It is better to use two pages, however, than to crowd too much information onto one page. If you do use two pages, write "More" or "Continued" at the bottom of the first page and your name and contact information and "Page 2" or "Page Two" at the top of the second.
- Capitalize or bold the headings.
- Use bullets to set off listed items.
- Try using boldface for emphasis.
- Make sure your spelling and grammar are perfect.
- Leave at least a 1-inch margin on all sides.
- Use good-quality paper in white, ivory, or very light tan or gray.

Whether printing from the computer or using a copy machine, make sure the print is dark and clear. If you don't have access to a computer printer or a good copy machine, consider paying to have your resume printed. Although this limits your flexibility in customizing the resume for various employers, it will provide professional-quality copies.

See Box 13-3 for a checklist to ensure you have a comprehensive and high-quality resume that represents you well. Your basic resume can serve you throughout your health care career. Think of it as a living document on which you continually record your experiences and new skills.

Figures 13-4, 13-5, and 13-6 show examples of completed resumes. Yours will look different, of course, but these will give you some ideas.

Prescription for Success: 13-13 Write Your Resume!

Using the information from the Resume Building Blocks and what you have learned in this chapter, put together your resume. Have your instructor, someone in your career services department, or someone with good proofreading skills look it over for you. (A good hint for proofreading you can try is to read your resume backwards. That way, you don't anticipate the words, and "correct" mistakes with your eyes.)

BOX 13-3   Resume Checklist

_____ Dates and numbers are complete and accurate.
_____ Your phone number(s) and e-mail address are included.
_____ Content is organized in order of importance.
_____ All important qualifications are included.
_____ Information is not repeated.
_____ Spelling is perfect.
_____ Grammar is correct.
_____ Layout is consistent.
_____ Page is attractively laid out.

Distributing Your Resume

Make the best use of your printed resume by distributing it to people who may have job openings—employers—and people who might know about jobs. Here are some suggestions to get you started:

- Employers who place help-wanted ads or post job openings on the Internet or elsewhere
- Employers who have unadvertised openings you have heard about from other sources
- Facilities where you want to work
- Your networking contacts
- Friends and relatives
- Anyone who indicates that he or she knows someone who might be hiring
- Your school's career services department

Keep enough copies of your resume on hand to respond to unexpected opportunities. Take copies to interviews (even if you have sent a copy in advance), career fairs, and the Human Resource departments of health care facilities. Be sure to have plenty on hand if you decide to drop in on employers as described in Chapter 12. A well-prepared resume in many hands is an effective way to get the word out that you are a serious job candidate.

It is usually not recommended, however, that you send resumes to dozens of employers in the hope of locating

---

RUDY MARQUEZ
1909 Franklin Blvd.
Philadelphia, PA 19105
(610) 765-4321   MAmarquez@aol.com

CAREER PROFILE
- 14 years experience as a certified medical assistant
- Current certifications in CPR and Basic Life Support
- Proven ability to communicate with patients and staff
- Proactive employee who anticipates office and physicians' needs
- Fluent in Spanish and Italian

WORK HISTORY
Medical Assistant   2007-Present
Founders Medical Clinic   Philadelphia, PA 19106
- Perform clinical and laboratory duties
- Assist physicians with exams, procedures, and surgeries
- Reorganized patient education program, including selection of updated brochures, audio-visual materials
- Provide patient education and present healthy living workshops
- Selected by physicians to train and supervise new medical assistants
- Maintained perfect attendance for six years

Medical Assistant   2003-2007
North Side Clinic   Pittsburgh, PA
- Performed clinical and laboratory duties
- Developed system for monitoring and ordering clinic supplies that resulted in annual savings of over $25,000
- Received commendation for providing outstanding patient service

Medical Assistant   2001-2003
Dr. Alan Fleming   Erie, PA
- Assisted Dr. Fleming with procedures and minor office surgeries
- Prepared treatment and examining rooms
- Took vital signs and administered injections
- Performed routine laboratory tests
- Handled computerized recordkeeping tasks
- Assisted in researching and purchasing new office computer system

EDUCATION
Associate of Science in Medical Assisting   2001
Emerson College of Health Careers, Erie, PA

Recently Completed Workshops and Continuing Education Courses
- Health Care Beliefs of Minority Populations
- Medical Spanish
- New Requirements for Maintaining Patient Confidentiality

ORGANIZATIONS
American Association of Medical Assistants (AAMA)
Pennsylvania Association of Medical Assistants
Philadelphia Lions Club

FIGURE 13-4 Example of a chronological resume. This type of resume, which includes a detailed work history, is recommended for applicants who already have experience working in health care.

HEATHER DIETZ
10532 Cactus Road
Yuma, AZ 85360
(520) 321-7654   thedietz@linkup.com

SUMMARY OF QUALIFICATIONS	Recent graduate with up-to-date skills in health information technology with emphasis on current trends in electronic health records. Previous experience in employment and volunteer positions that required computer expertise, accuracy, and good organizational skills.
EDUCATION	Associate of Science in Health Information Technology 2014 Desert Medical College Yuma, AZ

COMPUTER SKILLS
- Created electronic spreadsheet to track fund raising for Sage Elementary School PTA
- Taught self to efficiently use leading brand software programs in the following areas: word processing, database, spreadsheets, and accounting
- Set up and managed electronic accounting system for family-owned construction business
- Teach computer classes at Girl Scout summer day camp

ORGANIZATIONAL SKILLS
- Created system to monitor all church collections and fund raising projects
- Initiated and developed computer career awareness program for Girl Scouts
- Secretary for college HIT student organization
- Completed HIT associate degree program with perfect class attendance while working part-time and managing family life

CLERICAL/ADMINISTRATIVE SKILLS
- 7 years bookkeeping experience
- Keyboarding speed of 78 wpm
- Excellent written communication skills

WORK HISTORY	Unpaid Internship at St. John's Medical Center, Yuma, AZ 2013 Medical Records Department
	Bookkeeper 2007-2011 Buildwell Construction Company, Yuma, AZ
	Bookkeeper 2004-2007 Perfect-Fit Cabinetry, Yuma, AZ
	Secretary 2000-2004 Caldwell Insurance Company, Yuma, AZ
ORGANIZATIONS	American Health Information Management Association Desert Medical College Health Information Technology Student Organization, Secretary Sage Elementary School PTA, Treasurer Faith Community Church, Member of Social Service Committee

FIGURE 13-5 Example of a functional resume. This type of resume, which lists skills from various sources that support the targeted job, is recommended for applicants who have not previously worked in health care.

one that has a job opening. One exception is when there are more job openings than applicants. This can occur when there is a shortage, such as the current nationwide shortage of registered nurses. When there is a shortage, you are more likely to receive responses to unsolicited resumes. A second exception is when you are moving to a new area. Sending out a large number of resumes, along with a cover letter explaining that you are relocating, may be more economical and productive than calling many potential employers.

If you have business cards with your contact information, consider clipping one to your cover letter and resume for a professional presentation.

New Developments in Resumes

The computer's capability to sort and organize data, along with the speed and convenience of the Internet, has resulted in new forms of resumes and ways for job searchers and employers to connect.

EMILY COLLINS
8215 Mile High Drive
Denver, CO 80201
(303) 987-6543

SUMMARY OF QUALIFICATIONS	• Recent training and fieldwork experience in occupational therapy • 4 years experience working with a variety of patients in a skilled nursing facility • Proven ability to effectively communicate with people of all ages • Successful teaching experience in a variety of settings

EDUCATION

Associate of Science   Occupational Therapy Assistant   2015
Salud College   Denver, CO
Graduated with Honors
Passed national certification exam
Fieldwork completed at Central Rehabilitation Hospital

Certificate   Nursing Assistant   2008
San Juan Medical Center   Denver, CO

HEALTH CARE WORK EXPERIENCE

Nursing Assistant   2008-2012
GoodCare Nursing Home, Denver, CO
• Encouraged patients to achieve their maximum level of wellness, activity, and independence
• Demonstrated interest in the lives and well-being of patients
• Helped patients to perform prescribed physical exercises
• Organized and participated in activities with patients
• Assisted patients with basic hygiene and dressing

INTERPERSONAL SKILLS

• Provided daily care for parent with Alzheimer's disease for 18 months
• Answered telephone, directed calls, and took messages for busy sporting goods manufacturer
• Received Connor Memorial Award from Salud College for making positive contributions and assisting classmates

TEACHING SKILLS

• Teach swim classes to all ages at YMCA
• Conduct CPR instruction for the American Heart Association
• Organize holiday programs and outings for nursing home residents (volunteer)
• Planned and supervised craft and play activities for school-age children
• Tutored ESL students at Salud College

WORK HISTORY

Preschool Aide   2006-2007
Bright Light Preschool, Denver, CO

Swim Instructor (part-time)   2002-Present
YMCA, Denver, CO

Receptionist   2002-2006
Sportrite Manufacturing Co., Denver, CO

ORGANIZATIONS

American Occupational Therapy Association
American Heart Association, Chair of Local Fundraising Committee

FIGURE 13-6 Example of a combination resume. This type of resume is recommended for applicants who have some experience working in health care, but who also want to highlight other skills that support their targeted job.

E-Resumes

You will need to modify your resume if you are sending it to an employer electronically, if it will be scanned, or if you are posting it on an Internet site. This is to ensure that it transmits and scans properly. You will note that some changes require you to do exactly the opposite of the directions given in the previous sections to create an attractive printed resume! But this doesn't mean destroying or not using your original version—it means creating an additional version.

Start by converting your resume to what is called "plain text." If you created your resume using MS Word (on either a PC or a Mac), use the "save as" command and choose the plain text format (the ending will be .txt). This format strips your document of all special formatting—things like bullets, boldface, and italics. The instructions embedded to create these "special effects" do not translate well electronically, and your resume can become scrambled or interspersed with odd-looking characters.

Once you have created a plain-text version, do the following[2]:

1. Proofread it for oddly wrapped lines, scrunched up words, and similar problems that can happen when text is converted.
2. Delete "continued" and "page 2" if these are on your pages.
3. Use capitals to emphasize words that otherwise would have been boldfaced or italicized—your name, for example.
4. Replace bullets with standard keyboard symbols such as *, +, --, or ~. (Bullets may have converted to little boxes or other odd characters.)
5. If you need to add spaces, use the space bar, not the tab key.
6. If you use quotation marks anywhere, these only convert if they are straight, not curly (curly quotation marks are also called "smart quotes"). Check your word-processing program to see how to do this.

Just as in the case of the original version of your resume, it is critical for this version to be free of errors. Once sent or posted online, it is there for potentially millions of people to view.

If you send your resume as an e-mail attachment, you do not need to change to format (from Word, for example). However, include your name when you name the file. That is, it should not simply be titled "Resume," because this will not distinguish it from other resumes the employer may receive.

Posting Your Resume on the Internet

There are many types of websites on which you can post your resume. Some are general employment sites, such as Monster. Others are specific to health care. And still others are employer websites that allow—or even require—you to apply electronically for specific job openings. Deciding whether to place your resume on the Internet and which type of website to choose depends on your job target and the type of employer you are seeking (large hospital, single-physician office, etc.). Although many websites allow job searchers to post their resumes free of charge, they charge employers to place help-wanted ads online and to view the resumes in their databases. Therefore, larger organizations are the ones most likely to pay for this service. A physician's office or small clinic may not be able to justify the expense for its relatively small number of hires. Organizations with many employees, such as Kaiser Permanente or even a single hospital, may have their own websites and online application capabilities.

Spend some time considering whether to post your resume on the Internet. Although posting on a large website makes your resume available to millions of viewers, you are also competing with millions of other job seekers. Experts suggest that posting your resume on a few carefully chosen sites is worth some of your time, but is not as likely to help you find a job as methods such as networking and applying directly to specific employers.

In general, experts recommend that you should not pay to have your resume distributed. Many of these "services" simply send out mass e-mails containing the resumes of anyone who pays them. The resumes may or may not match the jobs posted (if indeed, the targeted employers even have job openings), and it is reported that resumes are often sent without contact information, such as your name and telephone numbers, so employers cannot reach you even if they are interested in learning more about you. You must explore websites for yourself, but starting with the recommendations of well-known job-search experts will help you avoid unreliable websites. The following two sites are well-established and appear on all "recommended" lists:

1. Monster.com
2. CareerBuilder.com

In addition, check sites dedicated to health care or your particular occupation, and the website of your professional organization. (See the information on health-specific websites in Chapter 12.)

The following suggestions can help you choose an appropriate website[3]:

- Do not use websites that won't allow you to review at least a sample of their job lists before you provide any personal information or your resume.
- Read the privacy policy! Some websites sell or give your information to other businesses. Important: *Never* put your social security number on your resume.
- If you are currently employed, do not use your work e-mail address for responses. Also, you may want to make your contact information confidential—not displayed—in case your current employer views the website. (Check the website's procedures on how to do this.)
- Check the wording. Do the lists provided include real jobs, or are they examples of what the website claims to be trying to fill?
- Check for currency. Are there dates on the jobs listed? Are they recent?
- Look for information about who sponsors the site. Do they have credentials and/or experience in the job-search industry?
- If you do not get any responses to your resume within 45 days, remove it and find another website on which to post it.

As a courtesy to those who are looking for applicants, remove your resume from all the websites on which you have posted it once you become employed. Another consideration is that your new employer may see your resume online and wonder if you are looking for a better deal.

Introducing Your Resume: Cover Letters

Send a **cover letter** along with your resume, whether it goes by conventional ("snail") mail or is sent electronically. The purpose of a cover letter is to provide a brief personal introduction. It should be short, informative, persuasive, and polite. The fact that you write a letter can be persuasive in itself. It shows that you took the time and made the effort to consider why and how you meet this particular employer's qualifications. You did more than simply put a resume in an envelope or send it electronically.

Cover letters can be customized for different circumstances. Before discussing the different types, let's look at a few how-tos common to all cover letters:

1. Use a proper business letter format. Figure 13-7 illustrates this form.
2. Be sure your spelling and grammar are error-free.
3. Direct your letter to a specific person whenever possible. Look for a name in the employment ad, ask your contact for the name of the appropriate person, or call the facility and ask. If you are writing in response to an unadvertised position, having a name on your correspondence is especially important. Letters without names can get misdirected or discarded. Busy facilities don't have time to determine to whom to direct your inquiry.
4. Write an introduction. State who you are, why you are writing, who referred you, or what ad you are responding to, and what position you are applying for. Employers may have more than one position open, so don't assume they will know which job you are applying for.
5. Develop the body of the letter. Explain why the employer should interview you—that is, what you have to offer and how you can help him or her. Summarize your qualifications for the job. Do your best to match them with what you believe the employer is seeking. At the same time, don't simply repeat the same information that is on your resume.
6. Include a closing paragraph. Ask the employer to call you for an interview or state that you will call for an appointment.
7. If you are sending your cover letter electronically (in the body of an e-mail, for example), keep the format simple: don't use bolding, bullets, or other special features and use the space bar rather than tabs to indent text.

	Your address and the date	1234 Graduate Lane Collegeville, CA 90123 June 6, 2015
Samantha Ernest, Office Manager Good Health Clinic 922 Wellness Avenue Cassidy, CA 91222	Receiver's name, title, and address	
Dear Ms. Ernest:	Salutation. Note use of colon.	
Introductory paragraph	Identify yourself, why you are writing, and the source of your information.	
Body of letter	Explain how you meet the employer's requirements. Provide examples.	
Closing paragraph	Request an interview, state that you will call, etc. Offer thanks for employer's time and consideration.	
Sincerely, *Gwen Graduate* Gwen Graduate	Closing Written signature Typed name	

FIGURE 13-7 Format for a business letter, recommended for writing cover letters. You should always include a cover letter with your resume.

Letter for an Advertised Position

In Chapter 12, we discussed responding to employment ads in a way that demonstrates how you meet the employer's needs. Use language in your letter that mirrors the words used in the ad, or job announcement, and explains how you meet the employer's needs. Review the examples in Figures 12-7 and 12-8; then take a look at Figure 13-8 for an example of a complete cover letter.

Prescription for Success: 13-14 Respond to Some Advertised Positions

1. Find three ads or postings for health care jobs.
2. Write complete cover letters, in sendable form (containing all the features mentioned in this chapter and having no errors), that respond to the requirements stated in each ad. (Attach the ads to your letters.)

1234 Graduate Lane
Collegeville, CA 90123
June 6, 2015

Samantha Ernest, Office Manager
Good Health Clinic
922 Wellness Avenue
Cassidy, CA 91222

Dear Ms. Ernest:

I was excited to see your ad in the Cassidy Times on June 5 for a medical assistant. As a recent graduate of Medical Career College, I believe I can make a positive contribution to your health care team. In addition to submitting my resume for your review, I would like to point out how I believe I meet your needs for this position.

Your requirements:	How I Meet Them:
75% clerical duties	I enjoy and am proficient in front office duties. I received top grades in all my administrative classes. I understand the importance of efficiency, accuracy, and confidentiality when performing clerical functions in the medical office. I have very good written and oral communication skills.
25% clinical duties	I have up-to-date skills in all medical assisting back-office procedures.
Computer literate	I have basic computer literacy skills, can work in a Windows environment, and am proficient in Medical Manager, Word, and Excel.

I am an energetic, detail-oriented person with good interpersonal skills. I understand the need to maintain high-quality patient relations in today's health care environment and know I am capable of providing efficient, caring service.

Good Health Clinic has an excellent reputation in Cassidy and it would be a privilege to have the opportunity to discuss my qualifications with you in person. I will call next week to schedule an appointment or you can contact me at (760) 123-4567. Thank you for your time and consideration.

Respectfully,

Gwen Graduate

FIGURE 13-8 Example of a cover letter for an advertised position. Note how the writer responds to the specific qualifications the employer is seeking.

5687 Success Avenue
Schoolville, MI 48755
September 10, 2015

Joseph Featherstone, Laboratory Supervisor
North Valley Medical Laboratory
4657 Flanders Road
Schoolville, MI 48757

Dear Mr. Featherstone:

Kim Lee, the academic director of the Laboratory Technician Program at High Tech Institute, told me that your facility has an opening for a laboratory technician. North Valley has an excellent reputation for performing high-quality work and providing learning opportunities for employees. As a recent graduate of High Tech, I am enthusiastic about starting my career in an environment in which I can make a positive contribution and at the same time, continue to acquire new skills.

I am dedicated to performing my work accurately and efficiently. High standards are important to me and I earned top grades in all my classes at High Tech. At the same time, I maintained near-perfect attendance and served as president of the student council.

My resume is enclosed for your review. Because a resume can only partly communicate my qualifications, I would appreciate the opportunity to meet with you personally. I will call you on Friday to arrange a time that is convenient for you. I can be contacted at (906) 123-4567.

Sincerely,

Sandy McDougal

Sandy McDougal

FIGURE 13-9 Example of a cover letter for an unadvertised position identified through professional networking. Note how the writer includes general qualifications that would be important for any job in health care.

Letter for an Unadvertised Opening

You may learn about unadvertised job openings through your school or from your networking contacts. Mention your source of information in the introduction of your cover letter. (Be sure to obtain permission from the contact person before using his or her name!) Before writing the letter, find out as much as possible about the job. Sources of information include the person who told you about it, the employer's website, or an inquiry call to the facility. Figure 13-9 shows an example of this kind of letter.

Letter of Inquiry

There may be a facility where you would like to work, but you don't know if it has any job openings. Perhaps you have a

10752 Learning Lane
Silver Stream, NY 10559
July 22, 2015

Ms. Sandra Walters, Manager
Caring Clinic
7992 Oates Road
Greenville, NY 10772

Dear Ms. Walters:

I am writing to inquire about job openings at Caring Clinic. My husband and I are relocating to Greenville in September and I am looking for a position in which I can apply my up-to-date skills as a phlebotomy technician. Caring Clinic has a reputation for excellent service to the health needs of the Greenville community and I would be proud to be a contributing member of your team.

As a recent graduate of Top Skill Institute, I had the opportunity to perform my internship at Goodwell Laboratory Services, an affiliate of Caring Clinic. I understand the importance of combining technical excellence with attention to customer service. While at Goodwell, my technical skills were highly praised by my supervisor, Mr. Jaime Gutierrez. In addition, I consistently received top ratings on patient satisfaction surveys.

My resume is enclosed for your review. I will call you in early September to see if I can set an appointment to meet with you. Thank you for your consideration.

Respectfully,

Carla Martinez
Carla Martinez

FIGURE 13-10 Example of a cover letter used to inquire about possible job openings.

friend who is happily employed there and has recommended it as a great place to work. Or it may have a reputation for excellent working conditions and educational and promotional opportunities. When you are not responding to a specific job opening, state your general qualifications that meet the current needs in health care. Explain why you are interested in working at the facility. Find out as much as possible about the facility so you can emphasize any specific contributions you can make (Figure 13-10).

Prescription for Success: 13-15 Inquire About the Possibilities

1. Select a facility where you might like to work.
2. Learn as much about it as possible. Sources of information include networking contacts, the Internet, acquaintances who work at the facility, school personnel, and published information such as brochures and newspaper articles.
3. Write a complete inquiry cover letter in mailable form.

Applications

Applications are commonly requested of job applicants, even if they have submitted a resume. Applications provide the employer with complete, standardized sources of information. Once you have been hired, the application is placed in your personnel file and can serve as a legal document and record of information about you and your previous employment.

Some applications contain important statements you are required to read and sign. For example, employers of home health care workers may protect themselves from **liability** if employees have an accident when they are driving to and from job assignments. Read all the statements carefully before signing. Applications and employment contracts may contain legal language and unfamiliar words. Don't hesitate to ask for an explanation of anything you don't understand.

After the work of constructing a resume, filling out an application may seem easy. But don't take it for granted. Take time to read the instructions, and fill it out as accurately, and neatly, as possible. This is especially important when applying for health care positions because neatness and accuracy are job requirements. Use this opportunity to demonstrate that you meet these requirements. A sample application is shown in Figure 13-11.

Success Tips for Filling Out Job Applications

- Read the entire application before you begin to fill it out.
- Fill out all the sections completely. Do not leave blanks or write in "See resume."
- Use black or blue pen, never pencil.
- Print neatly.
- Go to interviews prepared to fill out an application. Take the following information with you:
  - Social security number
  - Education, including dates, and locations
  - Work history, including names of employers, and dates of employment
  - Military service
  - References
- Proofread what you have written before submitting it.
- Be honest when answering questions. Giving false information can be grounds for dismissal if you are hired.
- For questions that don't apply to you, write "N/A" instead of leaving them blank. This way it is clear that you saw the question and didn't accidentally skip over it.
- Some jobs have a set salary. If the one you are applying for does not, it is best to write "negotiable" when asked for your salary requirements.
- Be sure to sign and date the application.

Electronic Applications

Many employers now have application forms on their websites. When applying electronically, it is especially important to follow the directions and check your entries carefully before pushing the "send" button. Once the application has been sent, it is difficult to change incorrect information. In some cases, an online application takes the place of sending a resume. As with traditional, written materials, what you submit is a reflection of you as a professional. In fact, some employers use electronic applications to test the computer skills of potential employees.

Use the Internet tracking form provided in Chapter 12 to record to whom you sent electronic applications, your password (if any), and the specific information you sent (for example, some applications ask for your salary requirements). If possible, print out your completed application and place it behind the tracking form in your job-search notebook.

Prescription for Success: 13-16 Preparing Your Reference Sheet

Contact possible references, gather the data you need about each, and put together your reference sheet.

Q&A with a Health Care Professional

Rick Baird

Rick Baird is the former Chief Human Resources Officer at Bend Memorial Clinic in Bend, Oregon. Rick discusses how resumes and applications are handled at Bend Memorial Clinic.

Q How much of the application process at this clinic is done electronically?

A Actually, we accept only electronic applications. We also prefer that resumes be submitted electronically, either typed into the electronic application or sent as an attachment. There are a couple of reasons for this. One is that people who work here must have computer skills, so the application process requires that they demonstrate these skills. The second reason is so we can maintain an electronic database of applicants. If someone submits an application and resume today, we may not have a job that matches their skills. But an opening may come in a month. Then we can electronically review the resumes that we've scanned into our database and quickly identify potential candidates.

Q Does this mean that applicants shouldn't bother to prepare printed resumes?

A No, no. They should still have them. In fact, they should always bring extra copies to an interview, in case they're needed.

Q Do you recommend any particular type of resume?

A No, the standard resumes—chronological and functional—are still acceptable. One thing a resume should demonstrate is the applicant's computer skills. Its appearance is important, too; proper alignment, consistent fonts, that kind of thing. Resumes should also show that candidates have thought about where they want to go in their careers.

Q How do applicants access an application?

A They can go to our website. We list all current job openings on the site along with our general application. For applicants who don't have computers, we have one they can use in the Human Resources office.

Wellness Plus Physicians Group

Employment application

This facility is an equal opportunity employer that accepts applications and employs persons based on their qualifications without regard to age, sex, race, color, national origin, religion, veteran status, or disability. The facility makes reasonable accommodations to the needs of disabled applicants and employees. The receipt of this application does not mean that job openings currently exist. Thank you for your interest in Wellness Plus Physicians Group.

Please print requested information in ink

PERSONAL INFORMATION

Name _____ Social security number _____

Address _____

Home telephone _____ Cell phone _____

Have you previously been employed by Wellness Physicians Group? ☐ Yes ☐ No
If yes, give dates of employment _____

Have you ever been convicted of a felony? ☐ Yes ☐ No
If yes, please explain.

If hired, can you provide documentation verifying eligibility to work in the U.S.? ☐ Yes ☐ No

If hired, can you furnish proof that you are at least 18 years of age or have a permit to work? ☐ Yes ☐ No

AVAILABILITY

Position applying for: _____ Date available for work: _____

Days and hours available for work: _____

Type of employment desired: ☐ Full-time ☐ Part-time ☐ Temporary

EDUCATION

	Schools Attended	City and State	Years Completed	Certificate/Diploma/Degree
High School				
Technical/ Vocational/ Military training				
College or University				
Graduate School				
Other				

PROFESSIONAL LICENSES AND/OR CERTIFICATIONS

Type	State/Organization Issued	Date	Number
Type	State/Organization Issued	Date	Number
Type	State/Organization Issued	Date	Number

FIGURE 13-11 Example of an employment application. Be sure to fill out applications accurately and completely.

EMPLOYMENT HISTORY

List current or most recent employer first. If you were employed under a different name, please enter it under the employer's name.

Employer Name	Employer Address	Employer Telephone ( )
Name of Supervisor	Employed (Month and Year) From _____ To _____	Reason for Leaving
		May we contact this employer? ☐ Yes ☐ No

Position and Duties

Employer Name	Employer Address	Employer Telephone ( )
Name of Supervisor	Employed (Month and Year) From _____ To _____	Reason for Leaving
		May we contact this employer? ☐ Yes ☐ No

Position and Duties

Employer Name	Employer Address	Employer Telephone ( )
Name of Supervisor	Employed (Month and Year) From _____ To _____	Reason for Leaving
		May we contact this employer? ☐ Yes ☐ No

Position and Duties

Employer Name	Employer Address	Employer Telephone ( )
Name of Supervisor	Employed (Month and Year) From _____ To _____	Reason for Leaving
		May we contact this employer? ☐ Yes ☐ No

Position and Duties

REFERENCES

List three professional references (no relatives) we may contact.

Name	Position	Complete address	Telephone
Name	Position	Complete address	Telephone
Name	Position	Complete address	Telephone

I hereby state that the information given by me in this application is true and correct. I authorize this facility to contact references, current and past employers, schools, law enforcement agencies, and any other sources of information that may be relevant to my application for employment.

Signature _____ Date _____

FIGURE 13-11, cont'd

Reference Sheets

As we discussed in Chapter 2, references are people who will vouch for your qualifications and character. Good references can be a key factor in tipping the hiring scales in your favor. Give careful consideration who you ask to be a reference. They must be considered believable. Take care not to ask people who may be competing for the same jobs. Friends and relatives are not generally accepted as good work references, but they are often acceptable if you are asked to provide character references. In addition to being credible, references must have the following characteristics:

- Have the time and willingness to speak on your behalf to potential employers
- Be able to speak positively about you
- Have the ability to speak clearly and in an organized way

As suggested in Chapter 2, the following people are good candidates to be work references:

- Instructors
- Other school personnel
- Externship, clinical, internship, or fieldwork supervisor(s)
- Previous employers
- Supervisors at places where you have performed volunteer work
- Professionals with whom you have worked on committees or projects

Contact each person you want to serve as a reference. Do this before you begin your job search. Never give out a name and then ask the person for permission afterward. This can put the person on the spot and makes it difficult if he or she would prefer not to be a reference. Inform your references about the types of jobs you are applying for and what qualifications are important. This will enable them to be prepared to answer the potential employer's questions.

Create a list of at least three references. At a minimum, include their names, titles, telephone numbers, and e-mail addresses. Ask them if they can be contacted at work. If not, provide recommended times to call. It is essential for the telephone numbers to be current and accurate. If you list a work number and the person is no longer employed there, your credibility may be questioned. Potential employers don't have time to call you back or make numerous calls trying to locate your references. Make it easy for them. This makes it easier for them to hire you.

Organize your reference list in an easy-to-read format, and print it on the same kind of paper as your resume. Write "References for (your name)" at the top of the page. The reference sheet should not be mailed with your resume unless it is specifically requested. Take copies with you to interviews to give to potential employers who ask for it. If you are visiting a Human Resource department, take a copy with you, because many employment applications have a section for listing references.

Be sure to let your references know when you are hired. Thank them for their willingness to assist you. Keep them posted about your career progress. In the future, you may be in a position to help them, and that is what true networking is all about—mutual career support.

Letters of Recommendation

Another type of reference is provided through letters of recommendation. These letters are usually written by supervisors or people in authority, such as instructors, who write statements about your work record, skills, and personal qualities. It is a good idea to request reference letters from employers throughout your career because they can serve as a record of endorsements and your achievements over the years. As you leave each job (on good terms, it is hoped!), ask for a letter of recommendation from your supervisor.

Make copies of your letters of recommendation to place in your portfolio and/or give to potential employers who request them. It is appropriate at interviews to mention that you have them available.

As with other references, be considerate. Ask only those people who you believe can write a positive letter. Also, try to give people enough time to compose a letter. Avoid giving only a day's notice. Finally, let your references know what kind of job you are seeking, so they can phrase their letters appropriately.

The Portfolio: Supporting What You Say

Look over the items you have been collecting to put in your portfolio. (Review the suggestions given in Chapter 2.) Choose the ones that represent your best work and support the qualifications needed for your target jobs. Think about others you can include. For example, you could add a list of the courses you have taken.

Organize your materials in a logical order, grouping related items together in sections. Place them in a binder or presentation folder using plastic protection sheets. It is not necessary to go to a lot of expense, but the folder should be well made and in a plain, conservative color. Prepare a title page labeled "Professional Portfolio" and include your name, address, and telephone number. If you have a large number of items, number the pages and prepare a table of contents.

You need to make only one portfolio if it is rather large; if it consists of only a few pages, make a few copies in case a potential employer asks you to leave it with him or her after the interview. Portfolios are not generally sent with your resume, but are taken to interviews. You may mention to the interviewer that you have a portfolio. Don't simply hand it to the employer and expect him or her to read it (unless you are asked for it, of course). It is to be used during the interview to demonstrate your capabilities. For example, if you are asked about your knowledge of coding, you could show assignments in which you accurately coded a variety of diagnoses and procedures. Chapter 14 contains a section on using your portfolio at interviews.

Using the items you have gathered and the information in this chapter, put together a portfolio that demonstrates your qualifications for the kind of job you want.

Summary of Key Ideas

- Preparing high-quality written materials is a key part of a successful job search.
- Your resume is a major method for advertising your qualifications.
- The main purpose of a resume is to secure an interview.
- Good cover letters increase the effectiveness of your resume.
- Written materials for health care jobs should reflect the job requirements of accuracy, neatness, and orderliness.
- Good references are vital links to future employment.
- A portfolio is a tool to support your qualifications.

Positive Self-Talk for This Chapter

- My resume is a good representation of my skills and qualifications.
- I write effective cover letters.
- I fill out applications accurately and neatly.
- My portfolio supports my claims and qualifications.

Internet Activities

ⓔ For active links to the websites needed to complete these activities, visit http://evolve.elsevier/Haroun/career/.

1. Locate two employment websites on which resumes can be posted. List the name and address of each website. Explain what you must do to post a resume (to register, etc.).
2. Find three health care employer websites that include electronic applications for job applicants. List the names of the employers and their website addresses.

3. Use key words such as "professional portfolio" and "employment portfolio" to find information about employment portfolios. Report on any suggestions you find useful for creating an effective portfolio or using a portfolio at interviews.
4. The Job Hunt website contains articles about protecting your privacy when posting your resume on the Internet. Read one of the articles and write a list of dos and don'ts for people who want to post their resumes.

To Learn More

Online Writing Lab—Purdue University

http://owl.english.purdue.edu/owl

A very comprehensive source of help for all types of writing, including resumes and cover letters. Click on the tab entitled "Job Search Writing."

Quintessential Careers

"Resume and CV Resources and Tools for Job-Seekers"
http://www.quintcareers.com/resres.html
"Researching Key Words in Employment Ads"
http://www.quintcareers.com/researching_resume_keywords.html

The Riley Guide

www.rileyguide.com

The *Guide* has links to dozens of online resume-writing resources. All have been reviewed and evaluated for content and quality. Click on the tab entitled "Making Contact."

References

1. Ellis D, Lankowitz S, Stupka E, Toft D: *Career planning*, ed 2, New York, 1997, Houghton Mifflin.
2. Ireland S: How to email your resume. Available at: susanireland.com/resume/online/email.
3. Dickel MR, Roehm F: *Guide to Internet job searching 2008-2009*, Columbus, Ohio, 2008, McGraw-Hill.

CHAPTER 14

The Interview

1. Explain why an interview should be considered a "sales opportunity."
2. Identify the needs of potential employers and understand the interviewer's point of view.
3. Know what to expect during an interview and prepare to answer questions in ways that demonstrate what you can offer an employer.
4. Come prepared to the interview and demonstrate appearance and behavior that create a positive first impression.
5. Communicate courteously and effectively.
6. Use your portfolio to support your qualifications.
7. Deal appropriately with difficult situations, including illegal questions.
8. Focus on the positive during an interview and distinguish between appropriate and inappropriate questions to ask.
9. Leave graciously when the interview is over.

KEY TERMS AND CONCEPTS

Behavioral Interview Job applicants are asked to describe how they handled specific situations in the past.

Discriminate Using unfounded bias as a reason for not hiring someone.

Illegal Questions Requests for information from a job applicant that cannot be used to make a hiring decision.

Interview A meeting, usually in person, in which a job applicant and an employer or representative exchange information.

Mirroring A communication technique, in which you match your communication style to that of the other person for the purpose of increasing mutual understanding.

Situational Questions Job applicants are given workplace scenarios and asked how they would act and/or resolve the situation.

The Interview—Your Sales Opportunity

"You don't have to be perfect. Just be the best for the job."

—Rick Baird

Finally! The words you have been hoping to hear: "When can you come in for an **interview**?" Your job-search efforts are paying off. But wait a minute! You begin to worry: "What if I can't think of anything to say?" "What if I don't have the skills they are looking for?" "What if they ask me about…?"

The purpose of this chapter is to help you put the "what ifs" to rest and see the interviewing process as an opportunity to present yourself at your best. In Chapter 3 we discussed the power of attitude and how, with practice, you can choose your reaction to any situation. Many applicants view interviews as opportunities to be rejected. But you have another choice. You can view an interview as an opportunity to determine an employer's needs and to show how you meet them.

Think about it. Employers are busy people who don't have time to conduct interviews with people who are unlikely job candidates. You obviously meet the minimum qualifications. The interviewer wants to see whether you are a person who can back up your qualifications, communicate well, and contribute to the organization.

By learning what will be expected of you at an interview and practicing your presentation skills, you can attend each interview with confidence and enthusiasm. A common reason for not being hired is lack of preparation for the interview. And this is a factor over which you, not the interviewer, have control.

The Customer's Needs

Good sales presentations are based on showing customers—employers—how they can benefit by buying a product—in this case, by hiring you. Recall from Chapter 1 that identifying the employer's needs is an important step for students who are beginning a program of career preparation.

In the same way, if you attend an interview without knowing anything about what the employer is looking for, you put yourself at a disadvantage. To be your best during the interview, you must prepare in advance by doing the following:

- Identify possible needs of the employer.
- Think of ways you might meet those needs as an employee.
- Anticipate what types of questions might be asked.
- Practice answering them.
- Create examples to demonstrate your qualifications.
- Prepare appropriate questions to ask.

All employers have general qualities they look for in applicants such as the ones identified in the SCANS report. And health care employers have expressed their needs through the National Healthcare Foundation Standards discussed in Chapter 1. In addition, individual employers have more specific requirements based on factors such as patient population, services offered, size of facility, budgets, and so on. It is important for you to learn as much as possible before

attending the interview. Here is a checklist of possible sources of information:

- Direct contact by phone or in person: ask questions, request a job description, observe the facility
- Brochures produced by the organization
- People who work there, such as friends, classmates, or networking contacts
- The local newspaper: large facilities are sometimes the subject of news articles
- The employer's website
- Your school's career services department
- The Chamber of Commerce and other organizations that have information about employers
- The local chapter of your professional organization
- Information gathered at career fairs and employer orientation meetings
- Employment advertisement if the position was advertised

If the facility is small, such as a one-physician office, you should know, at a minimum, the type of specialty practiced and the patient population served. If you are unable to learn very much before the interview, it is especially important that you listen carefully to the employer during the interview and ask good questions. How to do this is discussed later in this chapter.

> **Prescription for Success: 14-1**
> **Be Prepared**
> 1. Select a facility where you might want to work.
> 2. Use the resources suggested in this chapter to learn as much as possible.
>   - What type of work do they do?
>   - What is their patient population or client base?
>   - What is the size of the staff?
>   - What are the duties and responsibilities of the job(s) for which you might apply?
>   - What is the mission of the organization? How does the organization describe its core values?

The Interviewer Is Human Too

"Research into interviewing shows that the person conducting the interview is often more stressed than the candidate."

—Allan-James Associates

In addition to knowing the employment needs of the employer, consider the personal situation of the interviewer. Many applicants view the interviewer as a confident person who has all the power in the hiring process. Applicants mistakenly see themselves as the underdogs in a game they have little chance of winning. In reality, interviewers may be experiencing a number of pressures:

- Concern about finding the right candidate who can perform the job as needed
- An extremely busy schedule
- Lack of interviewing skills
- A demanding supervisor who will hold them responsible for the performance of the person who is hired

- Concern about finding the time and resources to orient and train a new employee

Understanding the interviewer's point of view requires empathy—attempting to see the world through the eyes of others (see Chapter 10). This may not seem easy in a job interview when you are nervous and concentrating on presenting yourself well. But it is this very shift of focus—from you to the interviewer—that leads to a more successful interviewing experience. It is through this attempt to understand and then show how you can help solve the employer's problems that you best present yourself as the candidate for the job.

Heads Up! Knowing What to Expect

Some interviews are highly structured, meaning that each candidate is asked the same set of prepared questions. Others are more like a conversation, with topics and questions generated freely. Most interviews fall somewhere between these patterns, with interviewers preparing at least a few questions in advance. The style of the interview and types of questions most likely depend on the size of the organization. Large health care systems, hospitals, and clinics usually have dedicated personnel to conduct initial interviews. As human resource professionals, they have the time and expertise to study the latest hiring practices and develop their interviewing skills. They are most likely to conduct **behavioral interviews**, described later in this chapter. A physician who has a single practice is more likely to focus on what skills you have acquired through your education and experience—specific skills he needs, for example, in a clinical medical assistant or receptionist.

In any case, always base your answers on the needs of the health care industry in general and the specific needs of the employer. Your purpose is to demonstrate how *you* can contribute to *their* success.

Traditional Interview Questions

There are many "golden oldie" questions that interviewers have been using for years. Here are a few examples:

1. How would you describe yourself?
2. What are your long-range career objectives?
3. Why did you choose this career?
4. What makes you qualified for this position?
5. How well do you work with people?
6. What motivates you to go the extra mile on a job?
7. How do you define success?
8. What characteristics would a past supervisor say are your strongest? Your weakest?
9. Why should I hire you?

You can see that these questions are very open-ended. You can answer them in many ways, which actually can present a problem if your answers are too vague or not related to the job under consideration. In each case, what employers want to know is how your answer applies to *them*. For example, in explaining why you chose a career in health care, focus on what it is about you that relates to the job you are applying for. Be specific. Saying, "I've always been a people person"

doesn't give much information. Saying, "I've been interested in health care since I was 11, when I spent time playing chess with my grandfather after he had his stroke. I noticed how he really perked up when he played, and I became fascinated by how the brain works better when stimulated with an enjoyable activity. This led me to explore a career in occupational therapy" is more specific and gives the interviewer more insight into who you are and what this means in terms of health care employment. When answering, "Why should I hire you?" mention specific skills and personal and professional qualities that will make a positive contribution to the physician's practice, the department's success, patient satisfaction, and so on.

Prepare for traditional interview questions by reviewing your inventories of skills and qualities, along with specific supporting examples, and then thinking about how you can incorporate them into your answers.

> **Prescription for Success: 14-2 Answering Traditional Interview Questions**
>
> 1. Think of five traditional questions you might be asked in an interview.
> 2. Choose a specific job and facility (real or imaginary) and prepare an appropriate response for each question.
> 3. Say your answers aloud.
> 4. Continue to practice the exercise aloud until you can answer the questions smoothly, but without sounding "canned" or phony. You may not be asked these same questions, but this exercise will give you practice thinking quickly and creating targeted answers.

Behavioral Interview Questions

Behavioral interviews have been part of the hiring process in many large organizations since the 1970s, and are being increasingly used in the health care industry. In this type of interview, applicants are asked questions about their past performance—how they handled specific situations. Behavioral interviews are based on the premise that past performance is a good indicator of future performance.

Interviewers prepare in advance by listing the key qualifications for the jobs they post. Then they develop questions to help determine whether applicants possess the desired characteristics. Here is an example: suppose that getting along with others is very important. A question might be, "Describe a time when you had to work with someone with whom you found it difficult to get along." As you tell your story, the interviewer follows up with additional questions, such as "In what ways was this person difficult?" "What was it you needed to do together?" "What did you say to this person?" "Did you get the job done in spite of the difficulties?" "How did you feel about this situation?" "What did you learn from this?" There may be additional probing questions from the interviewer to get more detail as you tell your story and verify that this is an experience you really had. In the case of the difficult person, these might be,

TABLE 14-1
Behavioral Interview Questions

Qualifications	Sample Questions
Interpersonal skills	Tell me about a time when someone disagreed with you about a major decision. What did you say or do? How was the decision ultimately made? Describe a situation in which you were able to use persuasion to successfully convince someone to consider your ideas.
Flexibility	Describe a situation in which you were required to conform to a work policy you really didn't agree with. What was the policy? Why didn't you agree? How did you feel about the situation? Give me an example of a job in which your working conditions frequently changed. How did you adapt to these changes? Tell me about a time when you had to reorganize your schedule in order to help a coworker meet a deadline. How did you help? What was the result?
Communication	Give me a specific example that shows how you typically deal with conflict. Describe a time when you had to communicate something difficult to your supervisor. What was the situation? How did you plan your communication? What did you say? What was the result? Describe a situation in which you felt you didn't communicate well. How did you follow up? What did you learn? How did you respond the last time a supervisor critiqued your work?
Customer service skills	Tell me about a time when you had to deal with a very upset customer or patient. How did you handle the situation? What was the result? Give me a few examples of what you have said to customers or patients who have approached you for help. How did you decide the appropriate way to work with each one? Describe something you did to help an employer improve customer service.
Stress management	Describe a stressful situation in which you applied your coping skills. What specifically caused the stress? How were you feeling at the time? What techniques did you use? How was the situation resolved?
Problem solving	Describe a time when you anticipated a potential problem and developed preventive measures. How did you identify the problem? What were the signs? How did you decide on ways to prevent it? How did others feel about your actions? What was the final result? Describe a time when you were asked or assigned to do a task you didn't feel qualified to handle. What did you do?
Dependability	How do you handle situations that might cause you to be tardy or absent from work?
Integrity	Describe an incident in which you made a serious mistake. How did you handle this with your supervisor and/or coworkers? Tell me about a time when you had to make an unpopular decision. What were the circumstances? Why were others unhappy with the decision? Why did you believe you were making the right decision?
Initiative	Give an example of something you did at work without being asked.

"How did these difficulties affect others, such as coworkers and customers?" "Did your supervisor become involved?" Table 14-1 contains examples of behavioral interview questions.

It has been shown that this kind of questioning about real events is more difficult for applicants to answer because they must be supported by facts. For this reason, behavioral interviewing has been found to be 55% predictive of future behavior on the job as compared with traditional interviewing, which is 10% predictive.[1]

Preparing to answer behavioral questions generally takes more preparation than for traditional questions. However, if you have been collecting examples of your skills and qualifications, as was first suggested in Chapter 2, you are already getting ready. The key is to anticipate the kinds of qualifications an employer wants and then search your inventory—and memory—for experiences you've had that illustrate that qualification. Examples can come from any area of your life. You may never have worked in health care. In fact, you may have limited work experience of any kind. But perhaps you have raised children. That experience may help you answer questions about making an unpopular decision. These were likely based on good judgment, your values, even ethics and morality. Employers want to know you can make decisions that are guided by what is right rather than by what is popular. In addition to family life, there are other experiences you can draw from, such as the following:

- Externship experience
- Previous work experience
- School: classes, labs, extra activities
- Community and service work

In a behavioral interview, it is essential to *listen carefully*. Not only must you understand the question, you need to understand *what it is the interviewer wants to know*—that is, what qualification is obviously important for this job, and how you can demonstrate that you have that qualification. Don't hesitate to ask for clarification if you don't understand the question.

It is totally acceptable to take a few moments to think about an answer. You undoubtedly have many experiences to draw from. However, if the question asks for an example you simply don't have—for example, "Tell me about a time when you had to fire a friend," and this has never happened to you—say so rather than trying to make up a story.

Many job-search experts recommend using the STAR approach when answering a behavioral question. It helps you organize your response and goes like this:

1. **S and T:** Choose and describe a **S**ituation or **T**ask that enables you to best demonstrate you have the qualification.
2. **A:** Explain the **A**ctions you took in dealing with the situation. Give enough detail to show your skills, but take care not to ramble or give unnecessary information.
3. **R:** Describe the **R**esults. Explain what happened, what you learned, and how the results made a difference. Give numbers and percentages when possible.

It's a good idea to write your examples out in the form of stories so you'll have the details in mind if you need them. Some questions may ask you to describe failures and how you've handled them, so it's a good idea to think of some examples. Reflect on what you learned from experiences that didn't turn out as you hoped they would.

Although you need to have examples in mind and practice telling your "stories," do not try to memorize what to say. You need to think about what you are saying during the interview and not give a canned response that may not exactly apply or sound sincere.

Prescription for Success: 14-3 Answering Behavioral Interview Questions

1. Think of five behavioral questions you might be asked in an interview.
2. Choose a specific job and facility (real or imaginary) and prepare an appropriate response for each question.
3. Say your answers aloud.
4. Continue to practice the exercise aloud until you can answer the questions smoothly, but without sounding "canned" or phony. You may not be asked these same questions, but this exercise will give you practice thinking quickly and creating targeted answers.

Situational Questions

Situational questions present situations and problems you might encounter on the job. You are asked to explain how you would respond and/or handle the problem. (See Box 14-1 for examples.) As with behavioral questions, you need to do some advance planning to be prepared to answer them:

- Learn as much as possible about the organization and the specific job. If possible, read the mission statement and goals of the organization.

BOX 14-1   Examples of Situational Questions

What would you do?
- You see a coworker who does not have the authority to administer medications taking some from a locked cabinet.
- You disagree with your supervisor about how to handle a problem.
- You hear a coworker discussing confidential patient information with her friend, who is not involved in the patient's care.
- You aren't sure how to prioritize your work, and no one is available to discuss it with you.
- You are working with an angry patient who insists on seeing the physician—who is not available—immediately.
- You have a problem to solve. What steps would you take?
- You offer ideas at staff meetings, but no one seems to take them seriously.
- Many of the patients you are working with are crabby people in pain.
- You are frequently asked to change tasks as priorities shift at the facility where you work.

- Recall your own values and mission statement. These may provide guidelines in answering questions that don't have easy answers but can be based on your sense of right and wrong.
- Review your personal inventory of skills and qualifications.

Prescription for Success: 14-4 Answering Situational Interview Questions

1. Think of five situational questions you might be asked in an interview.
2. Choose a specific job and facility (real or imaginary) and prepare an appropriate response for each question.
3. Say your answers aloud.
4. Continue to practice the exercise aloud until you can answer the questions smoothly, but without sounding "canned" or phony. You may not be asked these same questions, but this exercise will give you practice thinking quickly and creating targeted answers.

Occupation-Specific Questions

Questions in this category explore your specific knowledge, skill mastery, willingness to learn new procedures, and the general content of your training. The type of question will vary, as in the following examples:

- Describe how to perform a specific procedure.
- Explain how to operate certain equipment.
- Describe appropriate action to take in a given situation that directly relates to this job.
- Suggest how to solve a health care problem.

- Explain how you plan to keep your skills updated.
- What do you know about...? (a theory, new procedure, etc.)
- Why do you want to work in pediatrics (dermatology, children's dentistry, etc.)?

Some employers give practical skill tests or ask you to physically demonstrate your knowledge. Examples of these tests include a keyboarding speed test, filing or record-keeping exercise, spelling test, calculation of drug dosages, or demonstration of a procedure. If you are asked to perform a practical test that is appropriate for your level of training, do so willingly. Use the request to show that you have confidence in your abilities and can handle stress. If the task is something you have not been trained to do but is required for the job, tell the interviewer you would welcome the opportunity to learn.

Prescription for Success: 14-5 Answering Occupation-Specific Interview Questions

1. Think of five questions that apply to your field.
2. Prepare an appropriate response for each question.
3. Say your answers aloud.
4. Continue to practice the exercise aloud until you can answer the questions smoothly, and with confidence, but without sounding "canned" or phony.

Work Preference Questions

You may be asked about your job preferences. Review your answers to Prescription for Success 1-8, "What Do I Want?" In addition, be prepared to answer questions such as the following:

- Do you want full-time or part-time work?
- What hours you are able to work?
- What length of shift you prefer?
- What days and time of day can you work?

Remember to be realistic when applying for jobs. Don't waste employers' time—or your own—interviewing for jobs with conditions you already know are impossible for you to meet.

Prescription for Success: 14-6 Answering Questions About Your Work Preference

1. Think of five questions an employer in your occupational area might ask.
2. Prepare an appropriate response for each question.

Personality Tests

In today's employment world, you may be asked to take a personality test as part of the interviewing process. Personality assessment tests are increasingly being used, especially in larger organizations. These tests consist of answering a series of questions on paper or on the computer that measure such qualities as persistence and whether a person is an extrovert or introvert (highly social or more private). Some studies claim that better matches are found when applicants take these tests. This is because certain jobs require specific characteristics, and these are more reliably determined by tests than by interviews. Another claim is that individuals hired tend to be happier with their jobs because of this matching process.

The best advice for taking a personality test is to answer the questions honestly. It is also recommended that you take a deep breath and relax before starting the test. It is said that it is impossible to study for a personality test; however, one psychologist suggests that the "most important thing is to know who you are and to be in touch with your own core values, your own strengths, your own limitations."[2] Another suggestion is that you take a few personality tests (available online) to become comfortable with the process. One website that offers a number of interactive tests is http://personality-testing.info.

Personality tests contain a variety of questions to assess each trait. If you answer as you think you should or if you randomly select answers, this can show up negatively. If you do not "pass" such a test for the particular position you are applying for, it is very possible you would not have enjoyed either the work or the setting. This has been one of the reported benefits of personality assessments: lower turnover among employees who, with traditional hiring methods, end up deciding the job just isn't for them.

Computerized Job Interviews

Yes, believe it or not, some employers are conducting interviews with the help of a computer. The advantage for the employer, in addition to saving time, is that every applicant is asked a prepared set of questions, often as many as 100. Most interview programs consist of answers to be checked. This enables the comparison of "apples with apples" when deciding who to interview in person. The advantage for you, the applicant, is you may have a little more time to think about your answers and can, through the type of questions asked, learn a little about the organization before coming face-to-face with a human interviewer.

Answer the questions carefully and honestly. Computers are able to detect inconsistencies in your answers. Studies have shown that people are more likely to "tell" a computer information they would not reveal to another person.[3] If you are ever faced with a computerized interview, take care not to give unnecessary information that may harm your chance of getting hired. Also, be aware that most computer-assisted interviews must be completed in a certain length of time, so be sure you know how much time you have and keep track of it as you move through the questions.

Other uses of the computer in the hiring process include scenarios in which applicants explain what they would do in a given situation, skill tests, integrity tests, and personality tests. Some organizations administer computerized interviews and tests on their own computers at their facility; others make them available on the Internet and give applicants a password to gain access to testing websites.

Group Interviews

Some organizations are using group interviews in which several job applicants are interviewed at the same time. You may or may not know in advance if you will be participating in a group interview. If it comes as a surprise, do not show annoyance, shock, or surprise. Be gracious and if the interviewer does not begin the interview immediately, introduce yourself to the other candidates.

The same principles of preparation and conduct for individual interviews apply to group interviews. These include punctuality, appearance, positive body language, and having knowledge of the employer and the job. In addition to saving time by screening several candidates at the same time, group interviews tell the employer something about the applicants' interpersonal skills, self-confidence when presenting themselves in a group, teamwork, and presentation skills.

There are a number of ways you can present yourself as a strong candidate:

- During discussions, address the other candidates by name.
- Listen carefully to both the interviewer(s) and the other candidates.
- Do not repeat the same answer or information given by another candidate.
- Speak up when you have something to contribute, but do not interrupt or talk over others.
- Follow up on what others have said, when appropriate.
- Give praise, as appropriate, to other candidates.

Another type of interview (called a panel interview) involves one job applicant and several interviewers. If you encounter this type of interview, it may seem nerve-wracking, so try to stay calm. Acknowledge each person on the panel before the interview starts and note their name and position. It is recommended that you direct your answers to the person who asks the question. This will help you stay focused.

If you know you will be attending a panel interview, take special care with your appearance, body language, and presentation skills. With more than one person listening to and observing you, it is more likely that even small errors (such as mismatched socks or a limp handshake) will be noticed.

Telephone Interviews

A telephone interview is used by some organizations to reduce the number of applicants who are interviewed face-to-face. You may also be asked to do a phone interview if you live some distance from the employer or are relocating to a new area.

Preparation is just as important for a phone interview as for one that takes place in person. Have your resume and a description of the job you are applying for handy during the interview so that you can answer questions appropriately. (This is a good reason for keeping a job-search record as discussed in Chapter 12.) As with any job interview, prepare in advance by learning as much about the employer and the job as possible.

Your goals when participating in a phone interview are to show your enthusiasm and qualifications for the job in question and be invited to an in-person interview. Here are some suggestions to increase your chances of achieving these goals:

- Eliminate background noise, such as the television.
- Turn off call waiting, if you have that feature.
- Have a glass of water handy.
- Sit up straight and smile—it will come across in your voice.
- Address the interviewer with his title, not first name.
- Concentrate fully on the interview; do not multitask.
- Speak clearly and at a moderate speed.
- Be enthusiastic, but polite.
- Do not interrupt.
- Give complete answers, but don't talk too long.
- Take notes if you can do it without losing track of the conversation. If not, write up your notes immediately following the interview.
- Remember to say "thank you" before hanging up.
- Send a thank you note as you would for an in-person interview.

Practice: Your Key to Success

"Successful interviews usually depend on good preparation."
—John D. Drake

Of course, you cannot anticipate the exact questions that interviewers will ask. What you can do is prepare yourself to answer a variety of questions. There are some things you can practice to improve your interviewing skills:

- Listening carefully
- Asking for clarification when necessary
- Thinking through your "inventory" of capabilities and characteristics that apply when answering questions
- Thinking of examples to back up your answers
- Projecting self-confidence

Preparation means practice—actually answering questions, aloud, under conditions as close to those of an actual interview as possible. The best way to practice is to role-play with someone who acts as the interviewer. This can be an instructor, classmate, mentor, networking contact, friend, or family member. Many schools require mock (pretend) interviews as part of professional development classes. Take advantage of these opportunities, and do your best to conduct yourself as if you were at a real interview. Videotaping or having an observer take notes can be helpful, even if it's a little nerve-wracking. It's better to make a few mistakes now so you can avoid them at interviews.

If you believe that you might be asked to demonstrate skills or react to a scenario, include them in your practice sessions. The career services personnel at your school may be familiar with the interviewing practices of facilities in your area and can give you additional information about what to expect and how to best prepare.

The goal of interview rehearsals is not to memorize answers you can repeat. It is to develop a level of comfort about the interviewing process and have facts fresh in your mind so you can call on them as needed and respond to questions intelligently and confidently.

Be Prepared: What to Take Along

Having everything you might need at the interview will help you feel organized and confident. It also demonstrates to employers that you are organized and think ahead, valuable qualities for health care professionals. Although your own list will be different, here are some suggestions for what to take along:

- Extra copies of your resume
- Your portfolio
- Copies of licenses, certifications, and other documentation
- Proof of immunizations and results of health tests
- Reference sheet
- Any documentation of skills and experience not included in your portfolio (or if you have chosen not to create a portfolio)
- Pens
- Small notepad
- Your list of questions (discussed later in this chapter)
- All information needed to fill out an application (see Chapter 13)
- Appointment calendar, planner, electronic organizer, or phones
- Anything you have been requested to bring
- For your eyes only: extra pantyhose, breath mints, other "emergency supplies"

A small case or large handbag is a convenient way to carry your papers and supplies. It can be inexpensive, but it should be a conservative color, in good repair, and neatly organized so you can quickly find what you need.

First Impressions: Make Them Count!

"The way in which we think of ourselves has everything to do with how our world sees us."

—Arlene Raven

Just 30 seconds! That's how long you have to make a lasting impression. The average person forms a strong opinion of another in less than one minute. This is why so much emphasis is placed on professional appearance both during the job search and later, on the job. Although it is possible to eventually reverse a negative first impression, it's a lot easier to make a good one in the first place. Employers are basing their opinions on this first meeting.

Appearance

In Chapter 2, we discussed the messages that dress and grooming communicate. When you are applying for a job in health care, appropriate appearance lets the interviewer know that you:

- Understand the impact of your appearance on others (patients, other professionals)
- Know what is appropriate for the job
- Apply the principles of good hygiene
- Respect both yourself and the interviewer
- Take the interview seriously

There is no universal agreement about the proper clothing to wear when applying for health care jobs. Some schools encourage their students to wear a clean, pressed uniform. Other schools advise them to wear neat, everyday clothing that is not too casual. It is important to pay attention to the professional advice of the staff at your school. The best choices for clothing are generally conservative colors and simple styles. Figure 14-1 shows examples of professional appearance for interviews.

There are a few don'ts that always apply. Never wear jeans or clothing that is revealing or intended for sports and outdoor

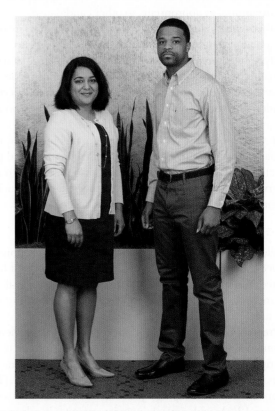

FIGURE 14-1 Your appearance makes an impression—make it a good one! These two job candidates are not dressed formally—in suits, for example—but their clothing is appropriate for a job interview. *Describe, in detail, why their appearance is appropriate.* (From Birchenall J, Streight E: *Mosby's textbook for the home care aide*, ed 3, 2013, Mosby.)

activities. Don't wear a hat or sunglasses during the interview. If you're not sure about what to wear, ask your instructor or someone in your school's career services department for help. If extra money for interview clothes is a problem, ask if your school has a clothes-lending program. Many cities have thrift shops that sell nice clothes at reasonable prices. Some even have staff who specialize in helping people dress for job interviews.

You may arrive at an interview and discover that most people at the facility are dressed very casually. Don't worry. It is far better to be overdressed in this situation than underdressed. You can adjust your style later, after you get the job.

There are some additional guidelines that apply to all health care job applicants:

- Be squeaky clean. Take a bath or shower, wash your hair, scrub your fingernails, and use a deodorant or antiperspirant.
- Save the fashion trends for later. Hair and nails should be natural colors, tattoos covered up, and visible rings and studs from piercings removed. Limit earrings to one set. Women should apply makeup lightly for a natural, not painted, look.
- Show that you know what is acceptable for the health care professional. Avoid long fingernails, free-flowing hair, and dangling accessories that can be grabbed by patients or caught in machinery. Wear closed-toe shoes. Strive to be odor free. For example, don't smoke on the way to the interview. Even the fragrances in perfumes and other personal products, intended to be pleasant, should not be worn because many patients find them disagreeable or have allergic reactions.
- Men who wear facial hair should groom it neatly.

> **Prescription for Success: 14-8**
> **Planning the Look**
>
> 1. Select an appropriate outfit for interviewing, including shoes. Make sure everything is clean, pressed, and ready to go on short notice.
> 2. If in doubt, ask your instructor, mentor, or career services staff for advice about what to wear to interviews.

Punctuality

Your appearance may be perfect, but if you arrive late for an interview, it may not matter. Being late is a sure way to make a poor impression. Time management is an essential health care job skill, and you will have failed your first opportunity to demonstrate that you have mastered it. In addition, arriving late is a sign of rudeness and inconsideration for the interviewer's time. Making a few advance preparations will help to ensure that this doesn't happen to you:

- Write down the date and exact time of the appointment.
- Verify the address and ask for directions, if necessary.
- If the office is in a large building or complex, get additional instructions about how to find it.
- Inquire about parking, bus stops, or subway stops.

- If you are unsure of the location and it is not too far away, go there a couple of days before the interview to be sure you can find it.
- Allow extra time to arrive, and plan to be there about 10 minutes before the appointed time.
- If there is an emergency that can't be avoided (a flat tire or unexpected snow storm), call as soon as possible to offer an explanation and reschedule the interview.

Courtesy

Many job applicants don't realize that the interview actually starts before they sit down with the person asking the questions. That's right. From the first contact you made to inquire about a job opening or set the appointment, you have been making an impression. If you arrive for the interview and are rude to the receptionist, you may have already failed in your bid for the job. You cannot know what information is shared with the hiring authority. (Keep in mind, too, that these may be your future coworkers!)

Learn the name of the person who will be conducting the interview. Be sure you have the correct spelling (for the thank-you note, discussed in Chapter 15) and pronunciation. When you are introduced, the following actions express both courtesy and self-confidence:

- Make and maintain eye contact.
- Give a healthy (not limp or hesitant) handshake.
- Express how glad you are to meet him or her and how much you appreciate the opportunity to be interviewed.
- Don't sit down until you are offered a chair or the other person is seated.

> **Prescription for Success: 14-9**
> **Practice Until It Comes Naturally**
>
> 1. In front of a mirror, practice your smile and posture.
> 2. With a partner, practice your handshake.
> 3. Rehearse the meeting until you feel comfortable with these actions: approach, smile, handshake, sitting down, maintaining positive posture.

Courtesy During the Interview

Maintaining eye contact (without staring, of course) while the other person is speaking indicates that you are interested in what he or she is saying. When you are speaking, it is natural to look away occasionally. Most of the time, however, you should look at the listener. This is a sign of openness and sincerity. (Review the guidelines for respectful communication in Chapter 10.) The following is a summary of behaviors to definitely avoid (even if the interviewer engages in them):

- Interrupting
- Cursing
- Using poor grammar (such as the word "ain't") or slang
- Gossiping, such as commenting on the weaknesses of other facilities, professionals, or your previous employer

- Telling off-color jokes
- Putting yourself down
- Chewing gum
- Appearing to snoop by looking at papers or other materials on the interviewer's desk, shelves, and so on
- Discussing personal problems
- Answering your phone (turn it off)

You don't want to come across as stiff or stuffy, but you do want to come across as professional. Try to be at ease and act natural while maintaining your best "company manners."

Trouble Ahead? 14-1

Abrianna has about had it with the job search. She graduated from her medical assisting program over two months ago and she still isn't employed. She knows it's not her fault. After all, the career services people at her school just aren't giving her good leads. She's tried to tell them that the employers they've sent her to are not really interested in hiring a recent graduate, but they just keep encouraging her to keep the appointments.

As she told her friend Janice, "Last Thursday was a waste of time. I went to an interview, but how was I supposed to act enthusiastic about a job in a little office working with an older doctor. It didn't look like it would be a fun place to work. So I answered his questions, but I really couldn't pretend I was interested."

"So what did he say when you finished the interview?" asked Janice.

"He thanked me for coming in and said goodbye," answered Abrianna.

"That was all?" asked Janice.

"Yeah, imagine that," said Abrianna. "After I went to the trouble of getting dressed up and going in. Even if I didn't want the job, he could have said he would call me back or something."

Abrianna believes that she has bad luck with interviews. Sometimes she arrives late because "the office was hard to find and they didn't give her good directions." Other times, career services called her at the last minute and she didn't have time to get her clothes ready, her car gassed up, or her resume copied. As she told Janice, "What is that school thinking? That I'm just waiting around for them to call me about an interview?"

Yesterday, Mr. Craig called from her school. "Abrianna, I'd like you to come in so we can talk about your job search and the interviews you've been on."

Abrianna responded, "That sounds like a good idea because I need to talk to *you* about these employers you've sent me to. What a waste of time."

Mr. Craig sighed. "Can you be here at 2:00?"

Abrianna arrived at Mr. Craig's office at 2:15. He looked at his watch. "Abrianna, our appointment was at 2:00. I want to help you, but this is one of the problems I'm hearing from the employers you've had interviews with."

"The babysitter arrived late and I had to stop and get gas," explained Abrianna.

"Abrianna, arriving late is not acceptable on the job," said Mr. Craig.

"Work is different. I can be on time. And even if I can't—you know, some kind of little emergency—there are coworkers who can cover for a few minutes. It won't kill them," said Abrianna.

"I must say that's a very unprofessional attitude, Abrianna. And it's not the only thing. You've had such a hard time becoming employed that I called a few of the employers who have interviewed you to see if there was something keeping you from receiving an offer," he said.

Abrianna was surprised but couldn't imagine any of them would have anything really negative to say about her.

Mr. Craig told her, "You seem to have a problem showing interest in the employers or their needs—or even showing respect for them. One employer told me you actually answered your cell phone during the interview! That is simply not done. It shows little regard for the employer and a lack of interest on your part in the interview or —"

"Well!" interrupted Abrianna. "That was an important call from a friend. I didn't think employers expected me to put my life on hold during an interview."

"The fact is, they want your full attention—just like they want it when you are working for them. The interview is like a test: are you the kind of person they want as an employee? And unfortunately, the behaviors you're demonstrating to me and to them are not going to get you employed."

Questions for Thought and Reflection

1. How is Abrianna's attitude affecting her job search?
2. What mistakes is she making at interviews?
3. How does she regard other people?
4. What advice would you give her?

Apply Your Communication Skills

A successful job interview depends on the effective use of communication. An interview is essentially a conversation between two people who are trying to determine whether they fit each other's employment needs. As a job applicant, you must take responsibility for making sure that you understand the employer's needs, questions, and comments. At the same time, you have to express yourself clearly so that the interviewer understands you.

Active Listening

Understanding begins by listening actively. The importance of carefully listening to the interviewer cannot be overemphasized. So many times we become so caught up in thinking about what we're going to say next that we fail to fully hear, let alone actively listen, to the other person. This is especially true in an interview when we are nervous and worried about whether we will say the right thing. But this is the very situation in which we can most benefit from listening carefully so we can base what we say on what we hear.

TABLE 14-2

Examples of Mirroring at the Job Interview

If the Interviewer Is	It Is Best to
Very business-like. Direct and to the point.	Answer questions concisely, quickly getting to the point. Avoid long introductions, wordiness, and unnecessary detail.
Warm and friendly. Conversational tone.	Reflect the interviewer's warmth without becoming too casual. Include human interest and details, when appropriate, in your answers.
Seemingly unhurried. Spends time describing the job in detail.	Include details to support your answers and fully explain yourself (without giving unnecessary or unrelated information).

Recall from Chapter 7 that active listening consists of paying attention, focusing on the speaker's words, and thinking about the meaning of what is said. This takes practice. When you participate in the mock interviews suggested earlier, do not look at the questions the person role-playing the interviewer is going to ask. Instead, focus on listening carefully to the questions and then formulating an appropriate response. Pausing to think and compose a good answer will be appreciated by interviewers. You are more likely to be evaluated on the quality of your answer, not on how quickly you gave it.

Mirroring

An effective communication technique for interviews is known as **mirroring**. This means you observe the communication style of the interviewer and then match it as closely as possible. This does not mean mimicking or appearing to make fun of the other person. It does mean adapting a style that will be most comfortable for the interviewer and help to build trust. Table 14-2 provides examples of mirroring.

Feedback

Whatever the style of the interviewer, use feedback when necessary to ensure that you understand the message. Feedback, as you recall from Chapter 10, is a communication technique used to check your understanding of the speaker's intended message. It is not necessary—or even desirable—to repeat everything the speaker says. It is annoying to speakers to have everything they say repeated, and you don't want to sound like a parrot. Using feedback unnecessarily will use up time better spent learning about the job and presenting your qualifications. Used when needed, however, feedback can help you understand the other person so you can respond appropriately and intelligently.

Q&A with a Health Care Professional

Rick Baird

Rick Baird is the former Chief Human Resources Officer at Bend Memorial Clinic in Bend, Oregon. Rick shares some interview tips for applicants.

Q What advice would you give applicants who are interviewing for a job at your clinic—or at any health care facility?

A First, I would say they should use sound common sense. I might add here that common sense is not always so common! What I mean is that applicants need to think about the impression they are giving the employer. If applicants are not at their best when they come in for an interview, what is the employer going to expect from them once they are on the job?

Q Can you be more specific?

A Sure. Good candidates for jobs in health care are friendly, concerned, and respectful. They show this in the way they interact with the interviewer. For example, they are on time, showing they respect the other person's schedule. Health care today is a high customer service environment, and we are looking for employees who take their work seriously. After all, we aren't selling shoes. Health *matters*, and that's what we're taking care of.

Q You mention appearance. Have the standards changed in today's health care facilities?

A To some degree, the answer is "yes." Social values drive business values, and, as we all know, styles and trends have changed. What we're looking for is "reasonable standards." For example, piercings and tattoos used to be job-blockers. But now they're more accepted if they aren't excessive or too outlandish.

Related to appearance is language. Communication and the impressions given to patients are really important, so inappropriate language is really not okay. Anything off-color or offensive—that kind of thing.

Q What kinds of questions should interviewees be prepared for?

A Patients today are considered to be *customers*, so I'm interested in knowing what an applicant can do, that will help us make our patients satisfied with our service. What will they do to make our patients feel important? Those are questions I would ask. The bottom line is that I'm looking for people who want to help make this place better. And I want to know how they're going to do it.

We sometimes give behavioral interviews. This means we give applicants scenarios of typical work situations and ask how they would handle them. What we are looking for is caring and respect for others—their general approach to work. Sometimes we require a demonstration of a skill related to the job.

Organization

When speaking, do your best to present your ideas in an organized manner so they are easy for the listener to follow. This can be difficult when you are nervous, so take your time to think before you speak. Recall the STAR technique described earlier in this chapter. Sometimes we are uncomfortable with silence and feel that we have to talk to avoid it. But taking a few moments to consider what you are going to say will result in better answers. Saying something meaningful after a pause is more important than simply responding quickly.

> **Prescription for Success: 14-10 Apply Your Communication Skills**
>
> Apply your communication skills at every opportunity: active listening, mirroring, and feedback. These are not just interviewing skills. Making an effort to use them consistently will benefit every aspect of your relationships with others.

Nonverbal Communication: It Can Make You or Break You

"The most important thing in communication is hearing what isn't said."
—Peter Drucker

You can speak smoothly and answer questions correctly and yet fail in your communication efforts. What has gone wrong? Your actions have betrayed you. That's right: what you do communicates as much as—or even more than—what you say. As we discussed in Chapter 10, our movements, posture, gestures, and facial expressions tend to reveal our true feelings. You can enthusiastically claim that you would love the challenge of working in a fast-paced, think-on-your-feet clinical environment. But if your face and body language reflect fear, anxiety, or subtle expressions of "yuck!," your verbal message will not ring true. Remember that more than half of the meaning of our messages is communicated nonverbally. This is why videotaping yourself is very helpful when practicing interviewing skills. You can observe your nonverbal language and catch inappropriate facial expressions and other behaviors that might betray your words.

The point is not to suggest that you should try to mask your true feelings and put on an act to impress interviewers. Rather, the purpose of this discussion is to encourage you to be aware of how important your actions are and what they say about you. If there are aspects of a job you know you

can't or don't want to perform, this is the time to find out. Keep in mind that one of your goals in an interview is to learn about the job and the organization so you can decide whether this is the place for you.

Developing a positive attitude about the interviewing process and having confidence in your own abilities will help ensure that your body language communicates appropriate positive messages. At the same time, developing the body language of a positive, confident person will help you become that person. Table 14-3 provides a number of ways to communicate self-confidence and, at the same time, respect for the other person. Figure 14-2 shows an example of body language that sends a positive message.

> **Prescription for Success: 14-11 Tune In to Nonverbal Messages**
>
> 1. Observe the behavior of other people throughout the day. Can you find examples that communicate cooperativeness? Self-confidence? Respect for others?
> 2. Describe some of the behaviors you observe that communicate positive messages.

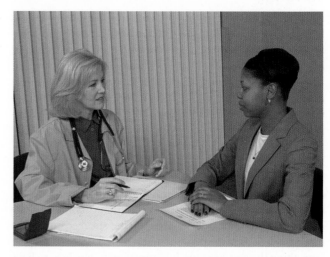

FIGURE 14-2 Your body language says as much—or more—about you than your words. *How is this interviewee's body language expressing her interest in what the interviewer is saying? Describe how her appearance is appropriate for a healthcare job interview.* (From Bonewit-West K, Hunt S, Applegate E: *Today's medical assistant: Clinical and administrative procedures,* ed 2, St Louis, 2013, Saunders.)

TABLE 14-3
Positive Body Language

What You Do	The Message You Send
Stand up straight, with your head held up and shoulders back	"I am a candidate worthy of your consideration."
Maintain eye contact	"I am sincere in what I am saying."
Avoid nervous actions such as jiggling a leg or fidgeting with your hands	"I want to be here."
Lean forward slightly toward the other person	"I am interested in what you are saying."

Using Your Portfolio Wisely

Portfolios are gaining popularity among job seekers, including those in the health care field. They can be a very effective way to support your claims of competence by providing evidence of your accomplishments and qualifications.

Not all employers are familiar with portfolios. Announcing at the beginning of interviews that you have brought one and asking interviewers if they would like to see it is not the most effective way of using it to your advantage. Remember that one of your main goals at the interview is to show how you meet the employer's needs. You won't know enough about these needs until you spend a little time listening. Then you may be able to use your portfolio constructively. The following interviewer questions and statements might be answered with material in your portfolio:

1. Asks a question about your skills and abilities
   "Can you…?"
   "Have you had experience…?"
2. States what skills are needed or provides a job description
   "This job requires…"
   "We need someone who can use medical terminology correctly and chart accurately."
3. Shares a problem or concern
   "One of our problems has been with ensuring accurate documentation…"
   "We have difficulties with…"
4. Isn't familiar with the contents of your training program
   "Did your program include…?"
   "What skills did you learn…?"
5. Asks for verification of licenses, certifications, and so on
   "Have you passed the _____ exam?"
   "Are you a certified medical assistant?"
   "Are you licensed in this state?"

It isn't necessary—or even a good idea—to try to back up everything you say with your portfolio. In fact, if overused, a portfolio loses its effectiveness. And many questions are better answered with an oral explanation and/or example.

Become very familiar with your portfolio's contents so you can find items quickly. If necessary, create an easy-to-read table of contents. Frantically flipping through pages to find something will make you look (and feel) unprepared and disorganized. You will also waste valuable time, a limited resource in most interviews.

At the end of the interview, you can use your portfolio to give a brief summary presentation if you are given an opportunity. For example, the interviewer might say, "Tell me why I should hire you," or ask, "What else should I know about you?" Use this presentation to quickly review your qualifications or to point out those you haven't already mentioned.

You may attend interviews where you don't use your portfolio at all. This is okay. It is always better—both during the job search and on the job—to be over-prepared. This prevents you from missing opportunities when they do present themselves.

Handling Sticky Interview Situations

In spite of your best efforts, some interviews can be a little rocky. Remember, not every employer is skilled at interviewing. Table 14-4 contains difficult situations and suggestions for handling them gracefully. Keep in mind that the questions reveal something about the interviewer and possibly about the organization, so consider them when deciding if this is a place you want to work.

Dealing with Illegal Questions

It is illegal for employers to **discriminate** against an applicant on the basis of any of the following factors:

- Age (as long as the applicant is old enough to work legally)
- Arrests (without a conviction or being proven guilty)
- Ethnic background
- Financial status
- Marital status and children
- Physical condition (as long as the applicant can perform the job tasks)
- Race
- Religion
- Sexual orientation

Questions that require the applicant to reveal information about these factors are illegal. They are sometimes asked anyway. Some employers are ignorant of the laws. Or the interview becomes friendly and conversational, and personal information is shared. ("Oh, I went to Grady High School, too. What year did you graduate?") Employers may take the chance that applicants won't know the questions are illegal. And a few will ask because they know that most applicants will not take the time to report them for discrimination. It may not be obvious from the questions that answering them will, in fact, reveal information that cannot

TABLE 14-4
Handling Difficult Interview Situations

If the Interviewer	What You Can Do
Keeps you waiting a long time	If you are interested in the job, do not show annoyance or anger. It is best not to schedule interviews when you have a very limited amount of time. Remember, this person may be overworked, and that's exactly why there is a potential position for you! Keep in mind that health care work does not always proceed at our convenience. A patient with an emergency, for example, will certainly have priority over an interviewee.
Allows constant interruptions with phone calls and/or people coming in	Again, do not show that you are irritated. This person may be very busy, disorganized, or simply having a difficult day. (This could be another good sign that this employer really needs your help.)
Does most of the talking and doesn't give you an opportunity to say much about yourself	Listen carefully, and try to determine how your qualifications relate to what you are hearing. Being a good listener in itself may be the most important quality you can demonstrate.
Seems to simply make conversation. Doesn't discuss the job or ask you questions	Try to move the discussion to the job by asking questions: "Can you tell me about what you are looking for in a candidate?" "What are the principal duties that this person would perform?" It is possible that this is a test to see your reaction, so take care to be courteous.
Tries to engage you in gossip about school, etc.	Say you don't really know about the person or other professionals, facilities, or situation and cannot comment. Ask a question about the job to redirect the conversation.
Allows long periods of silence	This may be a test to see how you react under pressure. Don't feel that you have to speak, and do your best to remain comfortable. (Say to yourself, "This is just a test, and I'm doing fine.") If it goes on too long, you can ask: "Is there something you'd like me to tell you more about? Discuss further?"
Doesn't seem to understand your training or qualifications	Explain as clearly as possible. Use your portfolio, as appropriate, to illustrate your skills.
Makes inappropriate comments about your appearance, gender, ethnicity, etc.	Depending on the nature of the comment and your interpretation of the situation, it may be best to excuse yourself from the interview. For example, comments of a sexual nature or racial slurs should not be tolerated. You should discuss this situation with your instructor or career services department for advice on how to proceed.
Is very friendly, chatty, and complimentary about you	Why in the world, you ask, is this a problem? It may not be. But be careful not to get so comfortable that you share personal problems and other information that may disqualify you for the job.

be considered when hiring. Take a look at the following examples:

QUESTION	WHAT IT CAN REVEAL
What part of town do you live in?	Financial status
Do you own your home?	Financial status
Where are your parents from?	Ethnic background
Which holidays do you celebrate?	Religion
When did you graduate from high school?	Age

Illegal questions put you in a difficult situation, and there are no easy formulas for handling them. In deciding what to do, you need to ask yourself the following questions:

- Is the subject of the question of concern to me?
- Do I find the question offensive?
- Does the interviewer appear to be unaware that the question is illegal?
- What is my overall impression of the interviewer and the facility?

- Would I want to work here?
- How badly do I want this particular job?
- If this person is to be my immediate supervisor, is the question an indication that this is a person I don't really want to work with?
- What do I think the interviewer's real concern is? Is it valid?

Based on your answers, there are several ways you can respond to the interviewer.

1. Answer honestly.
2. Ask the interviewer to explain how the question relates to the job requirements.
3. Respond to the interviewer's apparent concern rather than to the question.
4. Ignore the question and talk about something else.
5. Refuse to answer.
6. Inform the interviewer that the question is illegal.
7. Excuse yourself from the interview and leave.
8. State that you plan to report the incident to the Civil Rights Commission or Equal Employment Opportunity Commission.

Employers do have the right—as well as the responsibility—to make sure that applicants can both physically and legally

TABLE 14-5
Addressing Employer Concerns

Question	Possible Concern	Possible Responses
Do you have young children?	Your attendance and dependability	Explain your childcare arrangements, good attendance in school and on other jobs, and your understanding of the importance of good attendance.
Where do you live?	Reliable transportation and punctuality	Describe your transportation and previous good attendance.
Which religious holidays are you unable to work?	Scheduling problems	Explain that you are a team player and understand that all workdays must be covered. You are willing to cover when coworkers have a holiday you do not observe.

TABLE 14-6
Point Out the Positives

The Problem	The Bright Side
You're very young, with little work experience.	You are energetic, eager to learn, "trainable," and looking for long-term employment. ("One of the advantages of being young is….")
You have a criminal record.*	You have learned from your mistakes and are eager to have an opportunity to serve others.
You're over age 40.	You are experienced, have good work habits, and are patient.
You've had many jobs, none for very long.	You have a variety of experiences, are flexible, can adjust to the working environment, and have now found a career to which you want to dedicate your efforts.

*Note: Some states do not allow individuals who have been convicted of specific crimes to work in certain health care occupations. In some cases, these individuals are not even allowed to take certification exams.

perform the job requirements. Sometimes there is only a small difference in wording between a legal and an illegal question, as in the following examples[4]:

ILLEGAL	LEGAL
How old are you?	Are you over 18?
Where were you born?	Do you have the legal right to work in the United States?
What is your maiden name?	Would your work records be listed under another name?
Have you ever been arrested?	Have you ever been convicted of a crime?

Are you beginning to understand how employers can get confused and ask illegal questions? It is possible to be an excellent dentist or physical therapist but not an expert in the details of employment law. However you choose to respond to questions you believe are illegal, it is best to remain calm and courteous. You may decide you don't want to work there, but conduct yourself professionally at all times.

Many employment experts recommend that you respond to the employer's concerns rather than the questions. This requires that you determine what the concerns are. Table 14-5 shows some examples.

One recommended strategy for handling common employer concerns is to bring them up before the interviewer does. This gives you the opportunity to present them in a positive light.

Employers may be uncomfortable addressing certain issues and will simply drop you from the "possible hire" list. By taking the initiative, you gain the opportunity to defend your position and stay on the list. Table 14-6 contains suggestions for showing the employer the positive aspects of various employment "problems."

Personal Reflection

1. Is there anything you think employers might see as an obstacle to hiring you?
2. How can you turn the obstacle into a positive characteristic?

Stay Focused on the Positive

"Employers are hiring based on attitude: "Give me a 'C' student with an 'A' attitude."

—Melva Duran

Interviews are a time to do your best to stay positive. They are not the place to bring up problems or what you believe you can't do or don't want to do. Be positive and future-oriented, and prepared to emphasize the following:

* What you can do
* How you can help
* Ways you can apply what you've learned

As mentioned before, you should never criticize a previous employer, instructor, or anyone else. Potential employers realize they may someday be your previous employer and don't want to be the subject of your comments to others in the profession. It is also possible that the interviewer is a friend of the person you are criticizing!

Keep in mind that every interview is a sales presentation. A sales presentation is not the time to point out the product's faults. You want to emphasize the positive aspects of your skills and character, not your weaknesses. However, if you sincerely feel that you are not qualified for a job (and this is an important consideration in health care), you should never pretend that you are. Lacking needed skills is not a negative reflection on you as a person. It simply means that this job is not appropriate for you. Other jobs will be. In fact, there may be many reasons why jobs and applicants do not match. After all, that's the whole purpose of job interviews—for you and the employer to make that determination.

Discussion of personal problems should always be avoided. You are there to help solve the employer's problems, not find solutions to your own. Employers are looking for independent problem solvers. Bringing your own problems to the interview will not give them a good impression of your capabilities in this area. (There are exceptions. For example, if you are responsible for a disabled family member and need some consideration regarding your work schedule, it would be appropriate to mention this at the interview.)

Focusing on your own needs is negatively received by employers. Giving the impression that you are more concerned with what you can get from the job than what you can give is a sure way to get nothing at all. The following questions send the message "What's in it for me?" and should be avoided until you know you are actually being considered for the job:

- How much does the job pay?
- What are the other benefits?
- How many paid holidays will I get?
- Is Friday a casual day?
- Can I leave early if I finish my work?
- When will I get a raise?

It is acceptable to inquire about the work schedule, duties, and other expectations. The time to negotiate specific conditions, including your salary, is after you have been offered the job. (This is discussed in Chapter 15.)

Case Study 14-1

Jessica was really excited when she received the phone call yesterday from Blaine Clinic asking her to come in for an interview. This clinic had a reputation as a great place to work and she had dropped her resume off there last week. She had learned through doing research on the clinic that it had several specialties and there were advancement opportunities for employees who worked hard and showed promise.

She was surprised, then, by what happened at her interview. After arriving a few minutes early for her 10:30 appointment, it was almost 11:00 before she could see Dr. Spader, the director of the department that was looking to hire an administrative medical assistant. And she had no sooner introduced herself and sat down, when the phone rang. Dr. Spader took the call and was brief, but this was to be how the interview went. Not only did the phone ring a number of times, there were interruptions when staff members knocked on the door. Some even came in without knocking.

Jessica could see that Dr. Spader was stressed. He looked harried and apologized many times for the interruptions. Jessica tried her best to stay calm and answer his questions in ways that presented her as a good candidate for the job. Sometimes she lost her train of thought when an interruption occurred, but she would smile, take a breath, and continue. Dr. Spader seemed to understand that this was difficult for her.

That evening, Jessica thought about the interview and the clinic. It looked very busy with patients and personnel coming and going, especially in the department where she interviewed. She was still interested in working there, in spite of the interview that had seemed to go so wrong. She spent some time thinking about Dr. Spader and how stressed and apologetic he was. She didn't know whether to be annoyed or sympathetic and decided to think it over for a day or two.

The next day she remembered what she had learned in her job search class: focus on the employer's *needs*. Dr. Spader certainly had some needs. Obviously, there were problems in the department resulting in his not having the time to interview job candidates in a quiet environment. Jessica decided she really had nothing to lose and decided to write a thank you letter that included her observations—and how she could help. She had always been an organized person and mentioned this in her letter. Of course, she didn't say the department was disorganized, but worded her letter carefully, mentioning how busy Dr. Spader was and how she would like to help with the obviously heavy workload, using her organizational skills in the department. She included a couple of specific suggestions based on what she saw and heard.

Questions for Thought and Reflection

1. What do you think of Jessica's strategy in writing a thank-you–plus letter? (See Chapter 15 for thank-you notes.)
2. Do you think Jessica got the job? Why or why not?
3. How would you have handled the situation?

Sarah is a classmate of Jessica and graduated at the same time. She did well in the administrative medical assistant program and prides herself on being punctual and organized. Like Jessica, she is pleased to receive an appointment to interview with Dr. Spader at Blaine Clinic. And like Jessica, her interview is sprinkled with phone calls and staff interruptions. She finds it difficult to concentrate. She finally tells Dr. Spader that in spite of his apologies, she believes he is inconsiderate.

Sarah tells him, "I took the time to come in for an interview. As a recent graduate, I'm still a little nervous about interviewing and I expect to have your attention."

The situation doesn't improve, however, and by the time Sarah leaves, she is truly annoyed. "What a madhouse," she tells her boyfriend, Mike. "They could really use my organizational skills. Maybe Dr. Spader heard enough of what I said about myself to realize what a good employee I'd be."

"You're kidding, right?" asked Mike incredulously. "Why would you want to work in a place like that? Wouldn't it drive you crazy?"

"Probably. But that's only one department. The clinic has a good reputation and they do pay well. I'm thinking if I just got my foot in the door, I could get to know people in the other departments and get a transfer as soon as possible," explained Sarah.

"That's my girl," said Mike. "Always thinking ahead. Are you going to drop him a note and thank him for the so-called interview?"

"That would be a waste of time. He'd probably just lose it!" she laughed.

Questions for Thought and Reflection

1. How did Sarah's reaction to Dr. Spader differ from that of Jessica?
2. What do you think of Sarah's reasons for wanting the job?
3. Do you think Sarah got the job? Why or why not?

It's Your Interview Too

Interviews are not only for the benefit of employers. You have the right, and the responsibility, to evaluate the opportunities presented by the jobs you are applying for. This may seem to contradict what we discussed in the previous section, but it doesn't. In fact, well-stated questions about the job communicate motivation and interest.

When you are in class, it is generally true that "there are no stupid questions." However, at a job interview, the quality of your questions does count. There is a difference between questions that should be avoided and ones that demonstrate that you:

- Have a sincere interest in the job
- Want to understand the employer's needs
- Understand the nature of health care work
- Have thought about your career goal
- Want information that will enable you to do your best

What you ask will depend on the job, the interviewer, and how much you already know about the job and the organization. It is a good idea to prepare in advance a list of general questions, along with a few that are specific to the job and the facility. This will help you remember what you want to ask. As we pointed out earlier, it is easy to forget when we feel under pressure, as may happen in the interview situation. Not everyone is skilled at "thinking in the seat," especially when it feels like the hot seat!

Here are a few suggested questions to get you started:

1. How could I best contribute to the success of this facility?
2. What are the most important qualities needed to succeed in this position?
3. What is the mission of this organization or facility?
4. What are the major problems faced by this organization or facility?
5. How is the organization structured? Who would I be reporting to?
6. What values are most important?
7. I want to continue learning and updating my skills. What opportunities would I have to do this?
8. How will I be evaluated and learn what I need to improve?
9. Are there opportunities for advancement for employees who work hard and perform well?

It is perfectly acceptable to ask questions throughout the interview where they fit in. This will be more natural and lead to a smoother interview than asking a long list at the end. You don't have to wait until you are invited to ask them.

> **Prescription for Success: 14-14 What Do You Want to Know?**
>
> Make up at least five questions you might ask at an interview. The purpose of your questions should be to help you find out whether the job and organization are a match for your work preferences and qualifications.

In addition to asking questions, observe the facility and the people who work there. Does this "feel" like a place you would want to work? Is it clean? Organized? Does it appear that safety precautions are followed? What is the pace? Are the people who work there courteous and helpful? How do they interact with patients and with each other? If your interview is with the person who would be your supervisor, do you think you would get along? Do you believe you would fit in?

It may not be possible for you to see anything other than the interviewer's office. In fact, at a large facility your first interview may take place in the personnel office. You won't see the area where you would work. If this is the case, you will want to ask for a tour if you are offered a job.

Leaving Graciously

The end of the interview provides you an opportunity to make a final impression, so make it a good one. It is important to be sensitive to any signals the interviewer gives that it is time to wrap up. Failure to do so shows a lack of consideration for his or her time, and this is definitely not the parting message you want to leave. Some interviewers will make it obvious the interview is almost over by doing the following:

1. Telling you directly
2. Asking whether you have any "final" questions
3. Telling you that everything has been covered

Less obvious signs include looking at his or her watch, clock, appointment book, or papers on the desk; pushing his or her chair back; or saying that the interviewer has "taken enough of your time." Show respect for the interviewer's time by moving along with the final steps of the interview:

1. Ask any final questions (limit these to a couple of the most important ones that haven't been answered).
2. Make a brief wrap-up statement.
3. Thank the interviewer for his or her time.
4. Inquire about what comes next.

If you are interested in the job, say so in the wrap-up statement. Tell the interviewer why you believe you can make a contribution; what impressed you about the organization; why you believe your qualifications fit the position; and so on. Express your enthusiasm about working there and state that you hope you are chosen for the position.

Whether you want the job or not, always thank the interviewer for his or her time. This applies even if the interview did not go well. Health care professionals and personnel staff are extremely busy. Let them know how much you appreciate being given the opportunity to present your qualifications.

Finally, if you aren't told about the next step in the application process, don't hesitate to ask. Inquire about when the hiring decision will be made. Find out if there is anything more you need to do or send to the employer. If asked, give the interviewer your reference sheet. Be sure to get the interviewer's last name and correct title. An easy way to do this is to ask for his or her business card. And be sure that he or she has your telephone number and any other information needed to contact you. Then smile, give a firm handshake, and leave as confidently as you entered, regardless of how you believe the interview went.

> **Prescription for Success: 14-15**
> **Wrapping It Up**
> 1. Create several short summaries that express your interest in various jobs and statements about why you should be hired.
> 2. Practice your statements aloud, along with a "thank you" and questions about follow up. (Note: The purpose of this exercise is not to prepare a canned summary but to practice giving a good summary.)

Some Final Thoughts

"You wouldn't be nervous if you didn't care."

—Robert Lock

You may be feeling a little—maybe very—overwhelmed at this point. "How can I remember all this and act natural and maintain eye contact and give good examples and…?" It is a lot, and that's why it is so important to spend time learning about the interviewing process, preparing, and practicing. Take every opportunity to role-play. Make your practice sessions as realistic as possible. Figure 14-3 contains a summary list of positive interview behaviors.

When you inventoried your skills, were you surprised at how much you can do now that you would never have attempted before you started your educational program? You learned these skills by studying and practicing them—over and over. If you have been working on developing these skills, this is your chance to use them for job success. You are almost certainly more qualified for the job search than you realize. And using your skills to get a job will reinforce your ability to use them once you are on the job.

A final note: It's okay to be nervous. It can even be a good thing, because it means you are not taking this experience for granted. Interviewers know you are nervous, and it tells them that this job is important to you and that you care about the outcome. This is a positive message to communicate.

> **Personal Reflection**
> 1. What is my biggest concern about interviewing?
> 2. What can I do to best prepare for interviewing?

At the Interview: How To Show You've Got What It Takes	
Employers want to hire someone who is:	**How to show that you are that someone:**
Qualified to perform the job	1. Be familiar with and able to document all your skills. 2. Create a portfolio that contains evidence of your qualifications.
Reliable	1. Arrive on time to the interview. 2. Send any requested follow-up materials.
Trustworthy	1. Have a good handshake. 2. Maintain appropriate eye contact. 3. Include only accurate information on your resume and job application. 4. Do not lie during your interview. 5. Avoid saying anything negative about a previous employer. 6. Do not engage in any type of gossip.
Professional	1. Dress appropriately. 2. Be clean and well-groomed. 3. Bring needed materials to interview.
Motivated and willing to learn	1. Know something about the facility and why you want to work there. 2. Ask questions about the job. 3. Inquire about learning opportunities on the job. 4. Have a plan for professional development.
A good communicator and able to work well with others	1. Show consideration for everyone at the interview site. 2. Introduce yourself. 3. Behave courteously. 4. Listen actively throughout the interview. 5. Use feedback appropriately to check your understanding of the speaker's message. 6. Answer all questions completely but concisely. 7. Speak clearly and with proper expression.
Likable	1. Smile. 2. Be enthusiastic. 3. Have a sense of humor. 4. Show interest in job. 5. Express interest in employer's needs. 6. Be comfortable with yourself. 7. Show respect for interviewer. 8. Avoid showing impatience, annoyance.
A problem-solver	1. Describe examples of problems solved in the past. 2. Be prepared and willing to participate in any problem-solving exercises given. 3. Suggest specific ways you can help the employer.

FIGURE 14-3 A job interview is a sales opportunity for you to present yourself as the ideal candidate. *Study this list and consider how the behaviors described will help sell you to the employer.*

Summary of Key Ideas

- An interview is a sales opportunity, so consider the customer's—the employer's—needs.
- Advance preparation is the key to a successful interview.
- Practice will help you present your qualifications effectively.
- First impressions are critical.
- It's natural to be nervous at a job interview.

Positive Self-Talk for This Chapter

- I am well prepared for interviews.
- I present myself and my qualifications effectively.
- I answer questions clearly and confidently.
- I make a positive impression.

Internet Activities

For active links to the websites needed to complete these activities, visit http://evolve.elsevier.com/Haroun/career/.

1. The Monster website has a section with links to helpful articles on interviewing. Choose two articles to read. Create a list of the 10 tips you find most useful.
2. Quintessential Careers has links to dozens of websites dealing with job interviews. Browse sites of interest, and summarize what you learn.
3. The *Riley Guide* contains links to advice from job-search professionals about handling improper questions at an interview ("Handling Questionable Questions"). After reading the advice offered, describe how you would handle a question whose answer would reveal your age.

To Learn More

About.com

http://jobsearch.about.com/cs/interviews/a/aceinterview.htm
Read about all aspects of interviewing, including behavioral interviews, proper interview conduct, and suggestions for dress.

Quintessential Careers

www.quintcareers.com/intvres.html
Gain access to dozens of articles and links to websites with information about interviewing, including examples of questions.

The Riley Guide

http://www.rileyguide.com/interview.html
Get information and links to dozens of articles about all types of interviews and how to prepare for them.

References

1. Hansen K: Behavioral interviewing strategies for job-seekers. Available at: www.quintcareers.com/behavioral_interviewing.html.
2. Miller D: Personality tests on the job. Available at: http://www.theladders.com/career-advice/personality-tests-job-search.
3. Chang L, Krosnick JA: Comparing oral interviewing with self-administered computerized questionnaires: An experiment, *Public Opin Quart* 74:154–167, 2010. Available at http://web.stanford.edu/dept/communication/faculty/krosnick/docs/2010/2010_poq_chang_comparing.pdf.
4. Lock RD: *Job search: career planning guide, Book II*, ed 3, Pacific Grove, Calif, 1996, Brooks/Cole.

CHAPTER 15

After the Interview

OBJECTIVES

1. Learn from every interview you attend.
2. Write appropriate thank-you letters to employers following every interview and keep your references informed.
3. Explain when and how to call and inquire about hiring decisions.
4. Develop criteria for determining whether to accept a job offer.
5. Know how to discuss salary requirements and what information you should consider before accepting an offer, including the work schedule.
6. Understand benefits and calculate the total value of the compensation package.
7. Accept or turn down job offers properly and know what to expect once you are hired.
8. Describe how to deal with and learn from the experience if you are not selected for a job.

KEY TERMS AND CONCEPTS

Benefits Items of value provided by employers in addition to salary. They include insurance, tuition reimbursement, paid days off, and a uniform allowance.

Compensation The payment an employer gives for work done. It includes wages and other benefits.

401(k) Retirement Plan A retirement plan offered by some employers. It gives you an opportunity to save and invest for your retirement.

Reward Yourself

Attending an interview is a success, whether or not you are hired for a particular job. You have qualifications that were worthy of the interviewer's time, you prepared well, and you met the challenge of presenting yourself one-on-one to a potential employer. Take a moment to reward yourself for completing this important step.

Maximize the Interview Experience

"Nothing is a waste of time if you use the experience wisely."
—Auguste Rodin

Making the most of every interview means that you view each one as an experience that provides opportunities to improve your presentation skills and to learn more about the health care world. This knowledge can help you in future interviews and work-related situations such as performance evaluations. When you leave the interviewer's office, your reaction may be "Whew! That's over!" and the last thing you want to do is spend more time thinking about it. This is especially true if you feel the interview didn't go well. But this is precisely when you need to spend some time thinking about and evaluating the experience and your performance. Using an interview evaluation sheet will help you focus on the important factors that determine the success of an interview and create a plan for improvement. Make copies of the questions listed in Prescription for Success 15-1, and keep a record of your interviews in your job-search notebook.

Prescription for Success: 15-1 How Did I Do? Postinterview Self-Evaluation

Record the following information to evaluate your interview:

☐ Name of organization
☐ Interviewer's name
☐ Job title
☐ Date of interview
☐ Did I arrive on time?
  • If not, what can I do to make sure I'm not late for future interviews?
☐ Did I...
  • display good nonverbal communication skills?
  • smile?
  • maintain good eye contact?
  • wait to be seated?
  • shake hands properly?
☐ If not, what do I need to improve?
☐ Did I...
  • present my qualifications effectively?
  • use examples to support my skills and qualities?
  • use my portfolio effectively?
  • accurately answer questions that tested my knowledge?
  • perform hands-on skills correctly?

☐ If not, how can I improve my presentation skills?
☐ Are there subjects and skills I need to review?
☐ Did I...
  • prepare properly to answer the interviewer's questions?
  • understand the meaning of the questions?
  • compose my thoughts and organize good responses?
  • prepare properly for the types of questions that were asked?
☐ If not, what steps can I take to prepare to handle interview questions more effectively?
☐ Did I...
  • ask good questions?
  • think of them as the interview progressed?
  • fit them in appropriately?
  • have appropriate questions prepared in advance?
☐ If not, how can I be better prepared to ask what I need to know?
☐ What things seemed to make a positive impression on the interviewer?
☐ What things seemed to make a negative impression?
☐ What would I do differently if I could do it over?
☐ What things, on the part of the interviewer, made a positive impression on me?
☐ What things, on the part of the interviewer, made a negative impression on me?
☐ What did I learn from this experience?
☐ What questions, or kinds of questions, did the interviewer ask?

(Adapted from Drake JD: *The perfect interview: how to get the job you really want,* ed 2, New York, 1997, AMACOM.)

You might want to discuss your self-evaluation with someone you trust. Sometimes we are too hard on ourselves and need a second point of view to help us see the real situation. Review the interview with your instructor, career services staff, or mentor. You may have friends and family members who can provide insight and support. Create an improvement plan and practice so you'll feel more confident at the next interview.

When seeking help or discussing interviews with others, it is best not to make negative remarks about the interviewer or the facility. This serves no purpose, unless you are seeking advice about whether to accept a job you have doubts about. A friend may have a friend who works there, and your words, said "in confidence," may be passed along to the wrong party.

You may believe you will receive a job offer. You very well might. But don't cancel or turn down other interviews until you are formally hired. You may have done a superb job and the facility plans to hire you. Then the next day, your soon-to-be supervisor is informed of a facility-wide hiring freeze. You don't want to be left out in the cold with no other options. You may even find something better before they make the offer. Stay actively involved in the search until you have a job.

Thank-You Letter

Whether the interview went like a dream or a nightmare, send a thank-you note. This courtesy is something many job seekers don't do. Yet it is a simple action that can set you apart from the others. Suppose the employer interviewed nine people in two days, in addition to carrying on a normal workload. Tired? Very likely. Able to remember each candidate clearly and recall who said what? Maybe. But why take the chance of being lost in the crowd? Some employers even report that they won't hire a candidate who fails to follow up with a thank-you note. One survey reported that 22 percent of hiring managers are less likely to hire a job candidate who doesn't send a thank-you note after an interview. They believe not doing so demonstrates a lack of interest.[1]

If you know for sure that you don't want the job, send a thank-you note anyway. Keep it simple, say something positive about the interview, and express your appreciation for the time taken to meet with you. Do not say that you are not interested in the job. Figure 15-1 is an example of this kind of note.

Why, you might ask, would you write if you don't want to work there? There are at least three good reasons:

1. The employer may know someone else who is hiring. Impressed by your follow-up, he or she recommends you.
2. An opening for a job that you do want becomes available at this facility. You are remembered for your thoughtfulness.
3. At this time, when courtesy and consideration for others are declining, it is the right thing to do.

1642 Windhill Way
San Antonio, TX 78220
October 13, 2014

Nancy Henderson, Office Manager
Craigmore Pediatric Clinic
4979 Coffee Road
San Antonio, TX 78229

Dear Ms. Henderson:

Thank you so much for the time you spent with me yesterday. You have a busy schedule, and I appreciate the time you took to describe the opening for a medical assistant at Craigmore Pediatric. The Clinic enjoys a good reputation in San Antonio for the services it provides children in the community, and it was a pleasure to learn more about it.

Sincerely,

Karen Gonzalez
Karen Gonzalez

FIGURE 15-1 A simple thank-you note not only says "thank you," but also acknowledges the interviewer. In this letter, Karen expresses appreciation for her time. She also includes a sincere compliment about the clinic.

Although e-mail is becoming a major method of communication, it is highly recommend that you mail your note. It can be either handwritten or typed. (If typed, review Figure 13-7, which shows the proper format for a business letter.)

Some hiring managers see e-mailed letters as appropriate, but they can be lost in the numerous messages that some employers receive daily. Avoid texting a thank-you as only a small percentage of hiring managers view this method as appropriate.[1] At the same time, for some jobs, such as administrative positions, e-mailing a thank-you note may be acceptable because it demonstrates computer proficiency. Take the same care you would with a written letter: include a salutation, write complete sentences, use correct grammar, spell all words correctly, and use a proper closing. Career experts recommend that if you do decide to send a thank-you e-mail, you also follow up with a written letter.

Thank-you notes should be sent no later than the day after the interview. Consider keeping a box of cards in the car and writing the note immediately after you leave the interview. Interviewers will be impressed when they receive your note the next day.

Prescription for Success: 15-2 Thank You

1. Imagine a job for which you interviewed and that you will probably not accept if offered.
2. Write an appropriate thank-you note.

Thank-You–Plus Letter

If you want the job (see the next section for how-tos on making that decision), then take the time to write a thank-you–plus letter. The "plus" refers to a paragraph or two in which you do at least one of the following:

- Briefly summarize your qualifications as they relate to the job as it was discussed in the interview.
- Point out specifically how you can make a positive contribution—again, based on details you learned.

Let the employer know you want the job and hope to be the candidate selected. Include your full name and telephone number. Figure 15-2 shows an example of a thank-you–plus letter.

Prescription for Success: 15-3
Thank-You–Plus

1. Imagine that you have interviewed for a job you would most likely accept if offered.
2. Write a thank-you–plus letter, including a description of what you can contribute.

Alert Your References

If you left a reference sheet with the interviewer, call your references as soon as possible to tell them they may receive a call. Of course, they already know that you have given their names out as references. (You did ask them, right?) Give them the job title, nature of the work, and type of facility. Add anything you learned about the type of candidate the employer is seeking. This gives your references an opportunity to stress those features that best support your bid for the job. Help them to help you by keeping them informed.

When to Call Back

Following up after an interview is a kind of balancing act: you don't want to be considered a pest by calling too soon and too frequently. On the other hand, you took the time to attend the interview and have a right to be informed when the hiring decision is made. And a follow-up call tells the employer that you are both motivated and interested in the job.

The best strategy is to wait until the day after you were told a decision would be made. Call and identify yourself and inquire about the decision. If none has been made, ask when you might expect to hear. Use your best telephone manners. This is still part of the interview, and courtesy counts. Never express impatience about a delay. You want to show interest, but you don't want to pressure the employer for a decision he or she is not ready to make. Sometimes the interviewer is deciding between two candidates and the decision may be influenced by your follow-up.

Is This the Job for You?

Jobs are usually not offered on the spot during the first interview. If this does happen to you, it is a good idea to ask when a decision is needed and say that you are very interested (if you are) but need a little time to make a decision. There are exceptions, of course. You may have performed your externship at this facility and know for sure that this is the place for you. In this case, the interview may be a formality and it makes sense to accept the position immediately.

Interviewers will usually give you a time range during which a hiring decision will be made. You, too, need to make a decision: if this position is offered, will you accept it? Many factors will influence your decision. In Chapter 12, we discussed how the job market is affected by various economic and governmental conditions. When the unemployment rate is high, you probably can't be as choosy about the job you take. In fact, you may have only a few choices, because there will be more candidates competing for a limited number of positions. When the unemployment rate is low, you can be more selective. And your location and specific occupation will influence the number of opportunities available to you. Some parts of the country are highly desirable places to live, and competition is more intense. And some occupations may be in either high or low demand, depending on current health care trends. Box 15-1 contains questions to help you select an appropriate job.

Although you should consider these questions carefully, remember that the job that is "exactly what you want" probably doesn't exist. Finding the right job for you is a matter of finding a close match on the most important elements. You are starting a new career, and there are certain factors that will contribute to your long-term success. Working with someone who is interested in teaching you, for example, may

1642 Windhill Way
San Antonio, TX 78220
October 13, 2014

Nancy Henderson, Office Manager
Craigmore Pediatric Clinic
4979 Coffee Road
San Antonio, TX 78229

Dear Ms. Henderson:

Thank you so much for the time you spent with me yesterday. You have a busy schedule, and I appreciate the time you took to describe the opening for a medical assistant at Craigmore Pediatric. The Clinic enjoys a good reputation in San Antonio for the services it provides children in the community, and it was a pleasure to learn more about it.

After visiting your facility and meeting the health professionals who work there, I sincerely believe I could make a positive contribution to your facility. My ability to communicate in both English and Spanish would allow me to work with patients from various cultural backgrounds. My previous experience working in a day care facility gave me a love for and understanding of children that enables me to work effectively with them. Finally, my organizational skills and knowledge of current insurance requirements would be of benefit in helping to develop the new billing system you described.

I am interested in this position and enthusiastic about working at Craigmore Pediatric. Please let me know if you need anything further from me. I can be reached at (210) 123-4567. I look forward to hearing from you.

Sincerely,

Karen Gonzalez

Karen Gonzalez

FIGURE 15-2 A thank-you–plus letter not only expresses appreciation for the interview, but uses what the applicant learns in the interview to explain how he or she might contribute to the employer. In this case, Karen mentions several of her qualifications and how they apply to the job. This is much more effective than saying, "I know I can do a good job."

be a better choice than choosing a slightly higher-paying position that offers no opportunities for acquiring new skills. Many health care facilities make it a practice to promote from within. If there is a facility where you want to work, consider taking a job that gets you in the door.

Discussing Salary: When and How

Most career experts recommend that you do not discuss salary with a potential employer until you have been offered the job. In many cases, this won't be an issue because the salaries are predetermined and not negotiable. Some occupations, such as nursing, have labor unions, and the employer cannot change agreed-on salaries for specific positions.

Doing your research before you attend an interview may provide you with this information. If a range of salary is given for a position, the amount offered to you will most likely depend on the experience you bring to the job. Recent graduates tend to start at the low end of a range, earning more as they gain experience.

Here are some questions to guide your thinking about the specific job and facility in which you would be working:

1. Do the job duties match my skills and interests?
2. How closely do the job and facility match my work preferences?
3. Does the facility appear to follow safe and ethical practices?
4. Do I agree with the mission and values of the organization?
5. Can I make a positive contribution?
6. Who are the clients or patients? Can I work with them effectively?
7. How well do I think I would fit in?
8. Are there opportunities to learn?
9. Will there be opportunities for advancement?
10. Can I commit to the required schedule?
11. Is the management style compatible with my work style?
12. How did the facility "feel"?

Considering an Offer

A job offer may be extended in a telephone call, at a second or even third interview, or in a letter. Even if you feel quite sure that this is the right job, you still need to be sure that you have all the information needed to make a final decision. It is essential that you understand the following:

- The exact duties you will be required to perform. If you haven't seen a written job description, ask for it now. If there is no written description, ask for a detailed oral explanation if this wasn't done in the interview.

- Start date. Be sure you are clear about the exact date and time you are to report for work.
- The days and hours you will work. Ask about the likelihood of required overtime and any change of hours or days that might take place in the future.
- Your salary. Earnings are expressed in various ways: hourly, weekly, biweekly, monthly, or annual rates. If you are quoted a rate that you aren't familiar with, you might want to convert it to one you know. For example, if you are accustomed to thinking in terms of amount per hour but are given a monthly salary, you may want to calculate the hourly equivalent (Figure 15-3).
- Orientation and/or training given. This is especially important for recent graduates. Learning the customs, protocols, and practices of the facility can make a big difference in your success. Letting the employer know that you are interested in learning as much as possible about the facility and the job communicates the message that you are motivated and interested in being prepared to do your best.

You may have received all this information in the interview(s). Don't hesitate, however, to ask about anything you don't fully understand. It is far better to take the time now rather than to discover later that the job or working conditions were not what you expected. If you didn't have an opportunity to see any more than the interviewer's office, be sure to ask for a complete tour of the facility before deciding whether to accept the job.

Understanding Work Schedules

Health care facilities operate on a variety of schedules. Some, such as hospitals and emergency services, are staffed 24 hours a day, seven days a week. In addition to a regular, 40-hour

---

Calculating How Much You Will Earn

Basic Facts: Based on a 40-hour week: 1 year = 12 months = 52 weeks = 2080 work hours

If you are paid every 2 weeks, you will receive 26 paychecks per year.

Conversions Based on Annual Salary of $29,000.00

Monthly = $29,000/12 = $2416.66
Biweekly = $29,000/26 = $1115.38
Weekly = $29,000/52 = $557.69
Hourly = $29,000/2080 = $13.94

Conversions Based on Hourly Rate of $14.00

Weekly = $14 x 40 = $560.00
Biweekly = $14 x 80 = $1120.00
Monthly = $14 x 2080/12 = $2426.66
Annually = $14 x 2080 = $29,120.00

FIGURE 15-3 You may have been paid in different ways in the past. Take some time to learn how much the jobs offered to you pay in terms you are familiar with.

per week work schedule, there are others that are common in health care:

- Part-time: Continual, regularly scheduled employment for less than 40 hours a week.
- Per-diem: Very short-term temporary employment to fill in for an absent employee.
- Flextime: Scheduling arrangement that permits variations in the employee's starting and departure times. The number of hours worked in a week does not change. Employment may be either part-time or full-time.
- Casual work hours: Work done on an irregular basis. Worker is employed as needed by the employer and if the worker wants or is able to work when called.

Understanding Benefits

Benefits can represent a significant portion of your **compensation**. Health insurance, for example, can cost hundreds of dollars per month for a family of four. If full family coverage is offered by the employer, this may be worth thousands of dollars each year. Find out if you must pay part of the cost of the premiums and what type of coverage is provided. Health insurance for individuals (or families) is often more expensive than the group rates available through an employer. Health insurance is becoming an increasingly important benefit to consider when choosing where to work. There are other types of insurance, too, that can add value to the benefits package, including dental, vision, life, and disability.

If you are planning to continue your education, tuition benefits might be important to you. Some employers cover all or part of educational expenses if the studies are related to your work and you receive a grade of C or better. Time off to take classes and workshops is an additional advantage. This benefit is especially helpful for health care professionals who are required to earn continuing education units on a regular basis. Related professional expenses that some employers cover are the dues for professional organizations and required uniforms.

Other benefits to consider when calculating your overall compensation include the number of paid vacation, holiday, and personal days offered and whether there is a retirement plan such as a **401(k) retirement plan**. With this plan, you choose an amount to be deducted from your earnings each pay period. You pay no taxes on this money until you withdraw it anytime after you reach age $59\frac{1}{2}$. The money is invested, often in mutual funds. Some employers match a certain percentage of the money you save, which is like giving you an additional, tax-free salary.

When considering the compensation offered by an employer, think in terms of the total package. One job may offer a higher hourly rate but require you to pay part of your health insurance premium. You may end up financially ahead by accepting the lower salary. On the other hand, if you are included on your spouse's group insurance plan, this might not be significant. Salary alone should not be the determining factor when deciding whether a job "pays enough."

Accepting an Offer

When you accept a job, express your appreciation and enthusiasm. In addition to responding orally, write a letter of acceptance. The letter should include a summary of what you understand to be the terms of employment. Figure 15-4 provides a sample letter.

When speaking with the employer, inquire about any necessary follow-up activities. It is also a good idea to disclose any future commitments or other factors that will affect your work. For example, if your son is scheduled for surgery next month and you know you will need to take a couple of days off to take care of him, let the employer know this during the hiring process. It is a sign of integrity to make important disclosures before the hiring is completed. There may be little risk of losing the job by revealing reasonable, unavoidable future commitments. If the employer does refuse to accommodate you, it is better to learn now that this job lacks flexibility regarding family needs. You may want to reconsider your acceptance. (Be aware, however, that employers cannot grant repeated requests for days off because of family responsibilities. Their first responsibility must be to the patients they serve.)

You may want this job but need to negotiate some conditions. For example, suppose the work hours are 8:00 AM to 5:00 PM. You have a 3-year-old child who cannot be left at day care before 7:45 AM, and it takes at least 25 minutes to drive to work. It is better to ask if you can work from 8:30 AM to 5:30 PM than to take the position and arrive late every day. Many problems on the job can be avoided by discussing them openly in advance. (Again, you must also consider the employer's needs. Accommodations like this are not always possible if they disrupt the facility's schedule and patient flow.) And sometimes, having a "Plan B" will save the day—in this case, having someone reliable who can take your child to day care.

> **Prescription for Success: 15-4 I'll Take It!**
> Write a letter of acceptance for a job in your field.

What to Expect

Once you are hired, employers can ask questions that were unacceptable during the hiring process. Information that cannot be used to make hiring decisions is often necessary to complete personnel requirements. Examples include the following:

1. Provide proof of your age (to ensure you are of legal age to work).
2. Provide verification that you can legally work in the United States.
3. Identify your race (for affirmative action statistics, if applicable in your state).
4. Supply a photograph (for identification).
5. State your marital status and number and ages of your children (for insurance benefits).
6. Give the name and address of a relative (for notification in case of emergency).
7. Provide your Social Security number (for tax purposes).

1642 Windhill Way
San Antonio, TX 78220
October 13, 2014

Nancy Henderson, Office Manager
Craigmore Pediatric Clinic
4979 Coffee Road
San Antonio, TX 78229

Dear Ms. Henderson:

I was very pleased to receive your telephone call this morning advising me that I have been chosen to fill the medical assistant position at Craigmore Pediatric. This letter confirms my response to accept your offer. I am very excited about joining your organization and look forward to reporting for work at 9:00 a.m. on October 20, 2014.

Thank you for placing your confidence in me. I will do my best to merit your support.

Sincerely,

Karen Gonzalez

Karen Gonzalez

FIGURE 15-4 Send a letter of acceptance to formalize the agreement between you and the employer. Include what you understand to be the details: start date and time; anything else the employer has requested of you before beginning to work.

There may be mandatory health tests and immunizations. In addition, some employers require drug tests and background checks for all employees.

If you are asked to sign an employment contract (may also be called an employment agreement), read it carefully first. As with all other employment issues, ask about anything you don't understand. Also, be sure to ask for a copy of anything you sign. See Figure 15-5 to see a sample agreement.

Turning Down a Job Offer

After careful consideration, you may decide not to accept a job offer. It is not necessary to explain your reasons to the employer. Do express your appreciation and thanks for the opportunity, and do send a thank-you note. In addition to being an expression of courtesy, this leaves a positive impression on the employer. You may want to work at this facility in the future. Figure 15-6 is a sample refusal letter.

Prescription for Success: 15-5 No, Thank You

Write a sample refusal letter.

EMPLOYMENT AGREEMENT

(Complete form in duplicate: one copy for the employer; one copy for the employee.)

EMPLOYEE'S NAME   Debbie Quigley, CDA

Date ____11/08/xx____   Full time/Part time ____full time____

JOB TITLE   Chairside assistant to Dr. Hernandey
See attached list for details of duties and responsibilities:

PRACTICE WORK SCHEDULE
(Your hours will be scheduled within these times.)

Usual days per week: S _____   M __√__   T __√__   W __1/2__   Th __√__   F __√__   S __1/2__

Usual working hours: ____8:30____ to ____5:30____ ; lunch ___1 hr___ ; breaks _____ .

Work schedules are posted: ___two weeks in advance; assigned hours may vary___

SALARY AND BENEFITS

Pay days: ___every other Friday___   Starting rate: ___$ XX. per hour___

Basis for increases: ___review at 6 months, then annually___

Vacation days: ____5____ ; Sick days: ____5____ ; Personal time: ____2____ .

Additional benefits: group insurance is available

                                    retirement plan after 3 years

TERMINATION

For each new employee, the first ____6____ weeks are a provisional period of employment.
During this time, the new employee may leave or be dismissed without notice.

After this period, the employee is expected to give ____2____ weeks notice.

If dismissed, the employee will receive ____2____ weeks notice or the equivalent in severance pay.

In the event of fraud, theft, illegal drug use, or unprofessional conduct, the employee may be dismissed without notice or severance pay.

Debbie Quigley, CDA   _J. Hernandey, DDS_
Employee's signature   Employer's signature

FIGURE 15-5 If you are given an employment agreement, read it over carefully and fill it out accurately because it can serve as a legally binding document. Be sure to ask questions about anything you don't understand. (From Bird D, Robinson D: _Modern dental assisting,_ ed 11, St Louis, 2015, Saunders.)

If You Don't Get the Job

"Failure is a delay, but not a defeat. It is a temporary detour, not a dead-end street."

—William Arthur Ward

It can be difficult when you are not selected for a job you really want. There are many reasons why applicants don't get hired. Some you can't change and must simply accept, such as the following:

- There was another applicant with more experience or skills that more closely met the employer's current needs.
- An employee in the organization decided to apply for the job.
- The employer believed that someone else was a better "match" for the organization in terms of work style, preferences, and so on.
- Budget cuts or other unexpected events prevented anyone from being hired at this time.

On the other hand, you may have lost this opportunity for reasons you can change. How do you know? First, do an honest

1642 Windhill Way
San Antonio, TX 78220
October 13, 2014

Nancy Henderson, Office Manager
Craigmore Pediatric Clinic
4979 Coffee Road
San Antonio, TX 78229

Dear Ms. Henderson:

Thank you so much for your telephone call this morning advising me that I have been chosen to fill the medical assistant position at Craigmore Pediatric. I told you I would give you a response within one day. After much careful consideration, I have decided to decline the offer at this time.

This was not an easy decision to make, and I hope it does not exclude me from future consideration at Craigmore Pediatric. I am sincerely grateful for your time and consideration.

Sincerely,

Karen Gonzalez

Karen Gonzalez

FIGURE 15-6 Even if you tell the employer by phone that you won't be accepting the job, follow up with a letter. Writing a letter of refusal is both courteous—the right thing to do—and a smart career strategy.

review of your postinterview evaluation, school record, and resume. Are you presenting yourself in the best possible way? Second, look over the list in Box 15-2. Health care employers and career services personnel name these as major reasons why job applicants fail to get hired. Do you recognize anything that might apply to you?

You must be honest with yourself and commit to improving your attitude and/or job-search skills. If necessary, seek advice from your instructor, career services personnel, or mentor. Work on creating a winning attitude that will help you develop the interviewing skills it takes to get hired. Seek support from friends and family members if you are feeling down. They can help you keep your perspective and boost your self-confidence if it's a little low.

Although you may not feel enthusiastic about writing a note to an employer who chooses another applicant, consider this: you may have come in a close second. The next opening may be yours! So take a few moments and demonstrate your high level of professionalism by thanking the employer and letting him or her know that you are still interested in working for the organization (Figure 15-7).

Prescription for Success: 15-6 Thank You, Anyway

Write a follow-up letter for a position that you wanted but for which you weren't chosen.

BOX 15-2 Why Job Applicants Fail to Get Hired

1. Failure to sell themselves by clearly presenting their skills and qualifications
2. Too much interest in what's in it for them rather than what they can give
3. Unprofessional behavior or lack of courtesy
4. Lack of enthusiasm and interest in the job
5. Poor appearance
6. Poor communication skills
7. Unrealistic job expectations
8. Negative or critical attitude
9. Arrived late, brought children or the person who provided transportation, or other demonstrations of poor organizational skills
10. Fail to follow up by sending a thank-you note

If you don't get hired after attending an interview that you think went well, ask for assistance from an instructor or career services personnel. You may be able to get good feedback. Or perhaps this person can call the employer on your behalf to find out how you might improve your presentation or to see if you appeared to lack needed skills. Employers are sometimes more willing to share reasons with school personnel so they can better assist their students. Be willing to listen to any constructive criticism offered and to make any needed changes.

Personal Reflection

1. If you don't get a job you want, what can you learn from this experience?

1642 Windhill Way
San Antonio, TX 78220
October 13, 2014

Nancy Henderson, Office Manager
Craigmore Pediatric Clinic
4979 Coffee Road
San Antonio, TX 78229

Dear Ms. Henderson:

Thank you for letting me know that you have chosen another candidate for the medical assistant position at Craigmore Pediatric. I am still very interested in working at Craigmore and hope you will consider me for future openings. I believe I can make a real contribution.

I am sincerely grateful for your time and consideration. I was treated professionally by everyone at Craigmore and have great respect for your organization.

Sincerely,

Karen Gonzalez

Karen Gonzalez

FIGURE 15-7 If you are not offered a job—even one you have already decided you don't want—write a letter acknowledging the employer's decision. Don't hesitate to let him or her know if you are still interested in the position.

Follow-up Counts!

Nick had recently completed his degree in respiratory therapy. He enjoyed his studies, and now hoped to become employed soon so he could increase his contribution to the family budget. His wife, Cindy, had worked overtime while he was in school and he really wanted her to be able to cut back on her hours. He appreciated how she had been willing to step up when he decided to return to school.

Nick had done well in school, although he wasn't able to earn the highest grades as he had hoped and he had to be absent a couple of times when one of his children was ill and had to stay home from school. But he was dedicated and enthusiastic and sincerely interested in helping patients. He empathized with people who had lung and breathing disorders. He could imagine how frightening it would be to have to struggle for a breath.

There was only one hospital, St. Frances, and an associated pulmonary clinic in Nick's city, so he knew that jobs were limited in his field and there would be competition for the few openings that came up. He spent time practicing his interviewing skills. His school offered a lot of advice and he attended a workshop in which the students did mock interviews with the school administrators. He had Cindy role play so he could get more practice at home. Nick also remembered what one of his instructors had said about listening to employers to learn about their needs—what they were looking for in an employee.

It took a few weeks, but Nick finally was called for an interview at St. Frances where he had dropped off his resume shortly after he had passed the exam to obtain his registered respiratory therapist (RRT) credential. He was nervous, but tried to focus on Dr. Foster's questions and what he said about the respiratory therapy department at the hospital. Nick explained that he became interested in respiratory therapy after his uncle died of lung cancer. He wanted to combine his interest in helping others with his ability to work with technology and complex equipment. Dr. Foster mentioned that the job was fast paced and that the hospital depended heavily on employees being dependable and always on time.

Nick left the interview feeling he had done his best, especially considering that he had little experience interviewing for jobs. When he got home, he and Cindy discussed how it had gone and how he might do better at future interviews. That night, Nick wrote a letter to Dr. Foster thanking him for the interview. He included a paragraph about why he wanted to work at the hospital: the orientation program that Dr. Foster had told him about at the interview; the opportunity to work with the latest equipment; and the chance to learn from the more experienced therapists. Nick decided to add one more paragraph about how he enjoyed working with older patients. Dr. Foster had told him that many of the patients were elderly and Nick thought it was important for the doctor to know that he was interested in contributing to their welfare. He knew that some of his classmates preferred working with younger patients—preferably children, in some cases—so he thought this might be a plus for him.

Nick heard back from St. Frances a week later and it was not good news. The job had gone to a therapist who had previously worked for the hospital and just returned to town. Dr. Foster felt that it would be better to hire someone who was experienced and knew the protocols. Nick was disappointed, but sent a note saying he understood but to please keep him in mind for the future.

Several weeks passed and Nick was starting to look for employment in nearby locations. He and Cindy thought that perhaps they should move to a larger city where there might be more opportunities. So it was a great relief when Nick received a call from St. Frances to come in and meet once again with Dr. Foster. There was an unexpected opening in the pulmonary clinic and after another meeting with the physician, Nick was hired. When he expressed his appreciation for the opportunity, Dr. Foster told him, "Nick, you interviewed well and demonstrated the qualifications we need. But what sealed the deal was your follow-up. You showed your interest by sending me a thank-you letter. Not only that, but when you didn't get the job you responded graciously. I could tell you would be the kind of person we would want to work with."

Questions for Thought and Reflection

1. In what ways did Nick interview well?
2. What do you think would have happened if Nick hadn't followed up his first interview with a thank-you note?
3. What did taking these follow-up actions tell Dr. Foster about Nick?
4. How does the old phrase, "Actions speak louder than words" apply to this situation?

Trouble Ahead? 15-1

Alex was feeling pretty proud of himself. He had recently earned his certificate in medical assisting. Working hard, he had done well in school and was eager to let local employers know what he had to offer. He was confident he'd land a good job soon.

Like Nick, Alex lived in a fairly small city with around 75,000 people, but there were two fairly good-sized clinics that employed a number of medical assistants. Alex contacted the human resource department at each and submitted his resume—which he believed was pretty impressive. On it had he noted his top grades, good attendance, and positive externship evaluation. When he was contacted by the largest facility for an interview, he was quite confident he'd be hired. As he told his friend, Adam, "I know I'll be a great MA. They'll be glad to have me on staff."

At the interview, Alex focused on pointing out his many qualifications: recent training, top grades, expertise in lab skills—and on and on. When the interview drew to a close, he believed he'd done well and asked the interviewer when he would hear about the job.

"We'll give you a call within the next week," responded Shirley Rose, the human resource director.

Ten days later Alex hadn't heard back from the clinic and decided to give them a call. He was totally surprised when he was told they had hired someone else.

"What can they be thinking," he asked himself. He decided to talk it over with career services at his school. He explained to Mr. Acosta that he knew he had done well at the interview and that he believed himself to be an excellent candidate.

"Well, Alex," asked Mr. Acosta, "what did you learn about the employer at the interview?"

"What do you mean?" asked Alex. "I know about the employer. What would I need to learn? I was there to sell myself—let them know what a good candidate I am."

"I see. So let me ask you another question: what did you do to follow up after the interview?"

"Oh, I called them after they didn't call me back. I waited ten days and thought they had lost my number or something," responded Alex.

"That's all you did?" asked Mr. Acosta.

"Well, yeah. What else would there be?" asked Alex.

"I'm referring to a thank-you note—showing your appreciation for the interview, for the time they spent with you."

"You know, Mr. Acosta, that really sounds like a waste of time. They need an employee. I was there for the interview—and on time. They talked with me. I told them about myself. What do these people expect? Why would I need to send a note?"

Questions for Thought and Reflection

1. Alex thought his interview went well. What do you think?
2. Why do you think Alex didn't get the job?
3. How will his attitude affect his ability to get a job?
4. Why is a thank-you letter always appropriate, even if you believe you interviewed well?

Summary of Key Ideas

- Make it a point to learn something from every interview you attend.
- Write thank-you notes to everyone who interviews you.
- Consider all aspects of a job when deciding whether it is the one for you.
- Learn to accept defeat gracefully.

Positive Self-Talk for This Chapter

- I am performing better at each interview I attend.
- I am a considerate person and follow up all interviews with a thank-you note.
- I can gracefully handle being either selected or rejected for a job.

Internet Activity

ⓔ For active links to the websites needed to complete these activities, visit http://evolve.elsevier.com/Haroun/career/.

1. Use the search phrase "job interview follow-up" and write a summary of suggestions for increasing your chance of being hired.

To Learn More

About.com

"Job Interview Follow-Up"
http://jobsearch.about.com/od/interviewsnetworking/a/intfollowup.htm

Purdue Online Writing Lab (OWL)

"Follow-Up & Thank You Letter Overview"
https://owl.english.purdue.edu/engagement/34/43/135/

Quintessential Careers

"Job Interview Follow-Up Do's and Don'ts"
www.quintcareers.com/interview_follow-up-dos-donts.html
"Job Interview and Thank You Letters"
www.quintcareers.com/sample_thank-you_letters.html

Reference

1. Quast L: Want that job? Send a thank-you note after your interview, *The Seattle Times*, 2014. Available at http://jobs.seattletimes.com/careercenter/work-life-blog/want-that-job-then-send-a-thank-you-note-after-your-interview.

CHAPTER 16

Success on the Job

OBJECTIVES

1. Know how to shift your focus now that you are a new health care professional.
2. Make a good impression when starting a job.
3. Apply your study skills to learning a new job and create a personal workplace guide for quick and easy reference.
4. Develop your workplace competencies to increase your value as a health care professional and be sure to maintain a positive relationship with your supervisor.
5. List five acts (laws) and one regulatory agency that protect the rights of employees.
6. Develop effective ways to deal with difficult situations at work.
7. Know when to use a grievance procedure.

KEY TERMS AND CONCEPTS

Approval Agency An organization that sets standards for health care facilities.

Blood-Borne Pathogens Microorganisms (germs) that cause disease and are transmitted from one person to another by means of the blood.

Burnout A state of physical and emotional exhaustion related to conditions on the job.

Charting Recording patient data in written or computerized form to document all aspects of diagnosis and care.

Code of Ethics Standards of conduct created by professional organizations to guide the conduct of members of the profession.

Coding Numbers (codes) that correspond to specific diagnoses and health care procedures. The three major sets of codes are (1) Current Procedural Terminology (CPT), (2) the Health Common Procedure Coding System (HCPCS), and (3) the International Classification of Diseases, Tenth Revision, Clinical Modification (ICD-10-CM).

Compliance Reports Reports submitted to approval agencies to demonstrate that their standards are being followed.

Courtesy More than saying "please" and "thank you," courtesy means treating others with kindness, consideration, and respect.

Cross-Training Learning to perform tasks in addition to those traditionally assigned to a given occupation.

Employee Manual A written document that contains policies, rules, and guidelines for employees.

Grievances In the workplace, circumstances believed to be unjust and/or harmful to an employee and grounds for filing a formal complaint.

Integrity Conducting oneself honestly, sincerely, and in a manner guided by high moral principles.

Morale Group feelings of confidence, enthusiasm, and willingness to work hard to achieve goals.

Reasoning Organizing facts so they make sense and/or help you draw correct conclusions.

Scope of Practice Duties you are legally allowed to perform in a specific occupation. They are established and monitored by governmental or professional regulatory bodies.

Standard Precautions Specific practices and procedures to prevent the spread of infection.

Toxic Poisonous.

Work Ethic A belief in the importance and benefit of work.

Hit the Ground Running

You have achieved a major goal when you start your first job in health care. Enjoy the satisfaction of your success. At the same time, be aware that how you perform during the first months on the job will influence your future career success.

The first few weeks at work can be busy and stressful. There will be a lot to learn and many adjustments to make. Sometimes it may seem as if getting through each day is a major accomplishment. Be patient with yourself. Do your best, but remember that it takes time to learn a new job and to develop a level of comfort. There are three actions you can take to help you get a good start:

1. Shift your focus.
2. Make a good first impression.
3. Learn all you can about the job.

Action 1: Shift Your Focus

As a student, your main career-related concern was getting through school: mastering new material, learning new skills, completing assignments, and performing well in tests and evaluations. Your principal responsibility was to yourself, perhaps to a family and a job, and to your personal progress. As a health care professional, you must now shift your attention to the goals and needs of others: your employer, patients, and coworkers. You are now accountable to people who are depending on what you do and how well you do it.

Important components of professionalism in health care are the ability to understand and the willingness to attend to the needs of others. Being a professional includes possessing the ability to determine what is most appropriate and necessary to provide high-quality service. This is true whether you work in direct patient care or in services that support the health care delivery system, such as medical billing (Figure 16-1).

Demonstrate Empathy

Empathy, discussed in Chapter 10, means trying to see the world through the eyes of others. Health care is a people business, and understanding the feelings and experiences of others—patients, supervisors, and coworkers—is essential. To be empathetic requires caring about the other person. Patients who have experienced an illness or injury sometimes feel as if they have lost control of their lives. The empathy shown by caregivers and other support personnel can be a critical component of their recovery. Empathy is also important in relationships with supervisors and coworkers. Mutual understanding promotes effective working relationships.

Each of us interprets a given set of circumstances differently. This interpretation is shaped by factors such as cultural background, education, religious beliefs, and previous experiences, which lead us to make certain assumptions about the world. Difficulties and misunderstandings can arise because most of us take our assumptions for granted and don't see them as only *one* possibility out of many. Our view makes

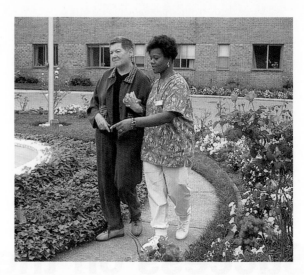

FIGURE 16-1 Being a successful health care professional means dedicating yourself to meeting the needs of others. By helping this patient take a walk outside, which he couldn't do alone, this professional is improving his quality of life. *What opportunities do you envision for helping others in your future career?* (From Sorrentino S, Remmert L: *Mosby's textbook for nursing assistants*, ed 8, St Louis, 2012, Mosby.)

sense to us and provides us with a basis for dealing with life. We believe our way to be the right way, and it may not occur to us to question it. But the fact is, what is obvious to us is not necessarily obvious to others.

It takes awareness and effort to see beyond our own assumptions, but that's what is necessary to be empathetic. Let's review the following suggestions from Chapter 10 for developing empathy:

• Listen carefully to what the other person is saying. You must know his or her view before you can begin to understand, and you can't know unless you listen.

• Don't judge what you hear. You are gathering information to help you understand the other person, not to decide if he or she is right or wrong.

• Ask questions or give feedback to ensure that you have received the other person's message as it was intended.

An important point to keep in mind is that it's not necessary to agree with the beliefs of others. You must simply be aware of them and how they influence their perceptions and actions. In some cases, providing the appropriate care requires you to try to persuade others to change their ideas that may be harmful to their health. For example, many patients demand to be given antibiotics for colds and flu. They don't understand that these common illnesses are caused by viruses that cannot be killed by antibiotics. Overprescribing these drugs has caused many bacteria (which antibiotics are intended to treat) to mutate and become resistant. In cases like this, being empathetic does not mean accepting the beliefs of the patients. It does mean respecting the individuals and understanding that what they want is relief from their symptoms. Through this understanding, you increase your chances of convincing them that they can benefit from your knowledge.

Empathy for Your Supervisor

Brian was happy to be hired by the pharmacy at St. George Hospital after graduating from his pharmacy technician program. This was the major hospital in his city and offered many opportunities for him to learn and for possible advancement. It was the largest hospital in the region, serving not only the city, but also the surrounding rural areas. St. George had a cancer treatment center, so that, in addition to the type of prescriptions filled in a typical drug store, this pharmacy had a special department that prepared chemotherapeutic drugs and other intravenous medications. These were based on the individualized dose requirements for each patient. Brian was especially interested in learning about new advances in cancer treatments.

As a new graduate, Brian tried to develop good relationships with his coworkers and his supervisor, Dr. Sutter. He found most of his coworkers willing to help him learn the protocols and fit in with the daily routines. A couple of them even invited him to join them for a beer after work. Dr. Sutter, however, was another matter. She was moody, and he had difficulty communicating with her. When he tried to ask her a question, she seemed either distant or in a hurry and not interested in spending time with him.

Brian was disappointed that he couldn't establish a better relationship with his boss. After a few weeks on the job, he went on a weekend fishing trip with his dad and one of his dad's friends, Mr. Morrison. They headed out on Friday evening after work, setting up camp after arriving at Gem Lake two hours from the city. Brian had experienced a tense week, having been reprimanded by Dr. Sutter for an error he made while documenting a prescription. He knew that accuracy was critical, but he wished that she would help him learn, rather than yell at him so that everyone in the immediate area could hear. He'd been really embarrassed.

The woods and sound of the lake lapping the shore were soothing and he felt himself relaxing. After a dinner of beans heated up on the camp stove and hot dogs cooked over the campfire, he felt at ease. The after-dinner conversation was about the morning plans for fishing then shifted to talk about work. Brian's father asked him how things were going at the pharmacy.

Brian felt comfortable confiding, so he shared his struggles with Dr. Sutter.

"I don't really understand what her problem is. I try to do my best. Everyone does. We all understand how important our work is—and the consequences if we goof up. But she's just difficult to work with."

His father asked, "You say difficult. In what way?"

"She just seems unhappy and grumpy. Nothing we do is good enough," Brian answered.

"Have you tried talking to her about this?" asked his father.

"That's just it. Talking with Dr. Sutter just seems to annoy her more."

Mr. Morrison leaned forward. "Did you say your boss is Dr. Sutter? The pharmacist?"

"That's right. I work at St. George. Do you know her?"

"I used to work with her husband, Phil," said Mr. Morrison. "But he had to quit a few months ago. He was diagnosed with cancer and the last I heard, didn't have long to live. I think he's home but they have hospice come in every day. Poor guy. He's only 53."

"Oh my gosh!" exclaimed Brian. "I didn't know anything about that."

"Yeah," said Mr. Morrison. "It's really a sad situation. His wife came with him to a few of the company functions. They seemed real devoted to each other."

Questions for Thought and Reflection

1. Do you think that knowing what he learned from Mr. Morrison will change Brian's opinion of Dr. Sutter?
2. How do you think this knowledge will affect his relationship with her?
3. Do you think he will be better able to handle the way she works with the employees? Why or why not?

Action 2: Make a Good First Impression

Each time you meet someone new or perform a task for the first time, you have an opportunity to make a first impression. The saying "You have only one chance to make a good first impression" is worth thinking about. Why is it so important? Because people tend to make judgments about others very quickly and often on the basis of very little information. In the employment setting, information from first contacts may be used by others to form opinions about the level of your professionalism and competence, as well as about the quality of the entire facility. You represent the organization for which you work.

As a recent graduate, you may not be 100% confident of your abilities. You may feel a little anxious about your performance. Keep in mind that no one expects you to know everything. However, there are two key factors under your control that influence first impressions: appearance and courtesy.

Most people are strongly influenced by visual impressions. If you look as though you know what you're doing, you are likely to be perceived that way. In Chapter 2, we discussed the appropriate appearance for a health care professional. To review quickly, we said that the desired manner of dressing and grooming is as follows:

1. Conservative—out of consideration for patients
2. Clean—for the safety and consideration of others
3. Safe—for the benefit of self and others
4. Healthy—to provide a good example of wellness

The discussion about appearance in Chapter 14 applies to the workplace as well as to the interview. You will probably find there are variations in the dress and grooming considered appropriate. Some facilities are more formal than others, and what is appropriate in one is unacceptable in another. Follow the directions you receive during your interview or orientation. Read the written dress code. And remember, for a new employee it is better to be more rather than less conservative.

Much more than simply using good manners, **courtesy** refers to being considerate and helpful. It means respecting the feelings of others and showing appreciation for the help you receive when you are new on the job. An important way to show respect and courtesy is to learn and use people's names. You are establishing relationships with coworkers, and courtesy will go a long way toward providing a good foundation for these important relationships.

Personal Reflection

1. Describe a time when someone made a negative impression on you when you first met. Did your impression change after you got to know the person? Why and how? Did it take a long time to change? How does this relate to the first impressions you make at a new job?

Action 3: Learn All You Can About Your Job

The first few weeks at a new job can seem overwhelming. Your educational program provided you with occupational knowledge and skills. But there will be a lot more to learn when you start your first job—any new job, in fact—because each facility has its own policies, rules, and procedures. Add to this the need to know the proper operation of equipment, the location of supplies, and the correct way to fill out forms, and you have a full course to master: Job 101.

The good news is you have what it takes to pass this course with flying colors. If you approach it with a "can do" attitude and apply the same skills that helped you succeed in school, you can learn and master your job systematically, and effectively. Chapter 1 pointed out that "school skills" have valuable applications on the job. Let's see how you can use some of them now to succeed in your new environment.

Using Your Note-Taking Skills

Your supervisor and coworkers will be important sources of useful information. Just as you took notes in class, you can profit from taking notes on the job. These notes can serve as both learning aids and reference materials. Some note-taking situations will be formal, such as structured orientation sessions and employee training programs. Informal situations in which note-taking is useful include receiving explanations and demonstrations from your supervisor and fellow employees. You can gain a lot from taking notes, including the following:

- It allows you to concentrate on what is being presented.
- It reinforces what you hear, through the act of writing it down.
- It creates a record of information to study later.

- It enables you to put together a reference so you won't have to ask the same questions again.
- It demonstrates to your employer and coworkers that you care about your work and are detail-oriented.

Taking and using notes involves three different ways of learning: listening, writing, and reading. This variety will reinforce your learning and help you master the new information you need for your job.

Remember that a key factor in effective note-taking is careful listening. This applies, of course, to all communication, whether you are taking notes or not. Take full advantage of learning opportunities in the workplace by clearing your mind of other thoughts, focusing on what the speaker is saying, and asking questions to clarify anything you don't understand.

As you did in class, use an organizing scheme when taking notes: write down the key ideas, the steps in a procedure, and/or important facts. Spend a few minutes after work editing your notes, if necessary, and reviewing the important points. Taking a few minutes each day to review them and "rehearse" your job duties will give you confidence and make your time on the job more productive. You might want to review the section on note-taking in Chapter 7.

Asking Questions

The potentially negative consequences of workplace errors make the ability to ask appropriate questions an essential professional skill. This applies to all types of health care employment situations, such as the following:

- Direct patient care in which the physical safety of both you and the patient is at risk
- Use of equipment, chemicals, and other materials that can be hazardous if handled incorrectly
- Administrative responsibilities in which errors can jeopardize the facility's standing with a regulatory agency
- Coding and billing tasks in which errors can cause the rejection of payment by insurance companies, Medicare, or other agencies

Knowing when to ask questions is important. Whenever possible, use your resources, observe, and think through situations to find the answer for yourself. If you cannot find the answer, there isn't time to do research, or the situation is urgent, don't hesitate to ask an appropriate person—someone who has the training and experience to know the answer or where to find it. In situations that are not urgent, choose a convenient time for the other person. It is also important not to ask questions about patients in the presence of anyone else, including other patients. Remember that the patient's right to privacy is protected by law. Patient confidentiality is discussed in more detail later in this chapter (Figure 16-2).

Creating a Workplace Reference Guide

When starting a new job, it can be helpful to create a workplace reference guide. If you started a personal reference guide, as recommended in Chapter 9, you can add an on-the-job section. What should you include? The following are some items you might find useful:

- Materials given to you during orientation or training sessions

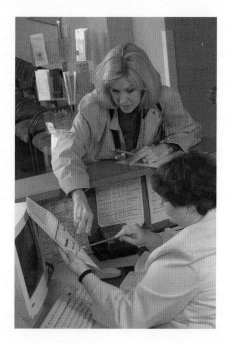

FIGURE 16-2 The ability to ask good questions is an important job skill. Never hesitate to ask questions of your instructors or future supervisors when necessary. *Why is essential that when you ask questions about a patient, you do so in a location where you cannot be overheard by other people?* (From Bonewit-West K, Hunt S, Applegate E: *Today's medical assistant: clinical and administrative procedures*, ed 2, St Louis, 2013, Saunders.)

- Notes taken during training sessions
- The name and telephone number of the person to contact if you must be absent
- Schedules: holidays, vacations, meetings, and weekly schedules if they vary
- Facility staff directories and important phone numbers
- Maps and floor plans if you work in a large facility
- Notes from meetings attended
- Printed instructions and other how-to information
- Instructions about what to do in case of an emergency
- Procedures to follow during inclement weather
- Organizational charts and chains of command (who supervises whom)

You can organize your guide in several ways. If you work mostly at a desk or in one location, a standard-sized three-ring binder is a convenient place to store information. For jobs that involve moving around, such as in a hospital, a pocket-sized reference system you can carry with you works well. For example, you can write important information on index cards, punch a hole in the corner of each card, and hook the cards together with a metal ring. Or carry a small notebook. You might want to record notes on a smart phone or other electronic device. Having everything in one place will be a big help when things get busy and you want to find something quickly.

Using Your Reading Skills

Reading is not limited to classroom-based learning. Printed materials are the source of important job-related information.

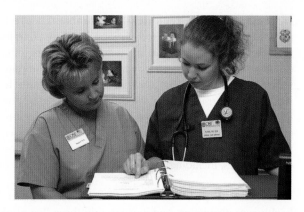

FIGURE 16-3 Health care has become increasingly complex. Policy and procedure manuals contain important information for employees. *What are possible safety and legal consequences when health care workers don't know and don't follow facility policies?* (From Sorrentino S, Remmert L: *Mosby's textbook for nursing assistants*, ed 8, St Louis, 2012, Mosby.)

The following examples highlight a few of the most common ones:

- **Employee manuals.** These contain policies and rules regarding employee conduct, holidays and vacations, the grievance procedure (discussed later in this chapter), and other topics related to the employer–employee relationship. Unfortunately, many people don't take the time to study the employee manual. Although it may not be very exciting reading, it contains facts to help prevent problems and misunderstandings that cause the kind of excitement you don't want to happen on the job. If you don't receive an employee manual your first day on the job, request one.

- **Policy and procedure handbooks.** Facilities create manuals to provide standard instructions for routinely performed tasks. Although it may not be necessary for you to read the entire manual, you should study the sections that apply to your job. Pay special attention to the procedures to follow in emergency situations. Knowing where to find this information quickly when it is needed has the potential to save lives. It is your responsibility to read and study workplace manuals and handbooks. You may not be tested on them, but you cannot use the defense that you "didn't know" if the information was in a manual you should have read (Figure 16-3).

- **Regulatory and approval agency standards.** Health care facilities are regulated by a variety of government and private agencies. Following the standards and rules set by these agencies is critical in determining the success—even the survival—of a facility. For example, reimbursement for Medicare patients requires the strict observance of certain guidelines. It is important that you know and understand all the requirements that affect your job. Important regulatory agencies include the Occupational Safety and Health Administration (OSHA), which oversees worker safety; the Clinical Laboratory Improvement Amendments (CLIA), which regulates all laboratory testing on humans; and The Joint Commission, which evaluates the quality and safety of care for more than 15,000 health care organizations.

- **Instructions and technical manuals.** The techniques and equipment for today's jobs are more complex than ever. Being able to read and follow instructions (often called *documentation*, especially when applied to computer software) is an important job skill. Examples include instructions for using equipment, performing laboratory tests, mailing special packages, and using computer programs. The proper use of equipment and supplies is essential in health care because their misuse can result in serious consequences, including injury to the professional and/or patient.
- **Professional publications.** These include general health care newsletters and journals and those that apply to your specialty. They help you keep up-to-date in your field, which is essential in health care. (See the section entitled "Continue to Learn," later in this chapter.)

When reading technical material, apply the following techniques for effective reading, suggested in Chapter 7:

1. Preview the material quickly.
2. Ask yourself questions about the material and look for the answers as you read each section.
3. Mark anything you don't understand.
4. Periodically review the material.

Remember that repetition over time is the best way to learn. You can see the power of repetition in action by observing experienced professionals at work. Their self-confidence and ability to perform duties smoothly and effectively develop over time.

Using Your Observation Skills

There are important things you need to know about the workplace that you may not be told. They are not written down anywhere and may not even be discussed. Everyone simply takes them for granted. These are the factors that make up the organizational culture, discussed in Chapter 10. Recall that this culture consists of the customs and expectations of an organization and includes the following:

- **Level of formality:** Does Dr. Patricia Abrams want the staff to call her "Dr. Abrams" or "Dr. Pat"?
- **Amount of at-work socializing among employees:** Does everyone go out to lunch to celebrate birthdays and holidays, or do individuals who have become friends at work plan these events on their own time?
- **Organizational values:** What are the most valued employee characteristics?
- **Management styles:** Are employees closely supervised or given lots of freedom?
- **Methods of communication:** Does your supervisor prefer all requests in writing?
- **Daily customs:** Who goes to lunch first?

You can learn the organizational culture and discover how to fit in as a new employee by observing carefully and asking questions. "Knowing the ropes" can influence your job performance. It usually takes time to understand the organizational culture, but it is well worth the effort.

You may notice that some of the procedures and methods used at your workplace are different from those you learned in school. As we discussed in Chapter 9, there is often a variety of correct ways to perform a given procedure. Some experienced professionals develop preferences or acceptable (in terms of safety and effectiveness) shortcuts. Your facility may have specific reasons for using a different method. Use the method that is most comfortable for you *and* meets the facility's requirements. Never suggest that another employee is wrong because he or she is not doing something the way you learned it in school. The only exception is if you believe a law or safety measure is being violated. Under these circumstances, it is usually best to speak first with your coworker. Then, if necessary, speak with your supervisor. And never feel pressured, because you are new, to perform a task in a way you know to be unsafe.

Prescription for Success: 16-1
Applying Your Study Skills

Think of three "study skills" not discussed in the previous sections that might help you succeed in your job.

Developing Your Workplace Competencies

In Chapter 1, we introduced lists of competencies that employers value in their employees, including items from the SCANS report and standards from the National Consortium for Health Science Education. What better way to learn about achieving success on the job than going directly to the source of information—the employers themselves? The following sections discuss a number of these competencies and how you can apply them to your job in health care.

Believe in Your Self-Worth

"Positive feelings about oneself are essential to enhancing the life force in self and others."

—Mattie Collins

Believing in your self-worth means that you value yourself and your actions. You consider both to be important and deserving of respect. You recognize that you and your work can truly make a difference. These beliefs provide the foundation for all other career competencies, because they generate the self-confidence necessary to ask questions, learn new skills, and build positive relationships with others.

Prescription for Success: 16-2
Recognize Your Value

1. List five things you like about yourself.
2. List five accomplishments that give you pride.
3. List five things you believe will make you a good employee.

Demonstrate Integrity and Honesty

Integrity means having sound moral principles and being sincere and honest. Let's look at some examples of workplace behavior that demonstrate integrity.

- **Admit when you make a mistake.** Covering up errors in the health care environment can have serious consequences. For example, if lab results are reported for the wrong patient, a false diagnosis can cause ineffective—or even harmful—treatment to be prescribed (Figure 16-4).
- **Practice ethical behavior.** This means conforming to established standards for moral and correct behavior. In addition to ethical standards that apply to society as a whole, each health care profession has a **Code of Ethics** that serves as a guide for proper conduct. Box 16-1 contains a Code of Ethics developed for medical assistants by the American Association of Medical Assistants (AAMA). (**Note:** The American Medical Technologists organization also has a code for medical assistants.) You should become familiar with the code for your profession.
- **Develop a strong work ethic.** This means taking a positive approach to work. It means that you take your work seriously, are responsible, and give each task you perform your best effort.
- **Be loyal to your employer.** As long as you are being paid by an employer, it is your obligation to demonstrate loyalty. Examples of ways to show loyalty include the following:
  - Dedicating your time on the job exclusively to work. Personal tasks and telephone calls should be limited to the lunch hour or break time.
  - Not using your employer's computer to send personal e-mails or to surf the Internet at any time. This is becoming a growing problem for employers. Remember, anything that occurs online can be traced back to you.
  - Never taking anything that belongs to the employer. Even small items, such as pens, add up when every employee thinks, "This is so small it won't make any difference." Taking something, however small or inexpensive, is theft. Don't contribute to the rising cost of health care by increasing your employer's expenses.
  - Not speaking badly about your employer. Speaking badly serves no purpose other than to lower employee **morale.** If overheard by patients, it can create doubts in their minds about the quality of care they are receiving. Seek solutions by discussing legitimate concerns directly with your supervisor.
  - Not complaining about your job, working conditions, and so on. Again, this does nothing to resolve the problem. Seek positive solutions through action or by speaking with someone who has the power to address the issue.

> **Prescription for Success: 16-3**
> **The Code as Your Guide**
>
> 1. If you don't already have one, obtain a copy of the Code of Ethics for your profession.
> 2. Read the Code and describe how it addresses the following issues:
>   - A. Integrity
>   - B. Human dignity
>   - C. Loyalty
>   - D. Honesty and sincerity
>   - E. Responsibility to patients
>   - F. Lifelong learning
>   - G. Community service

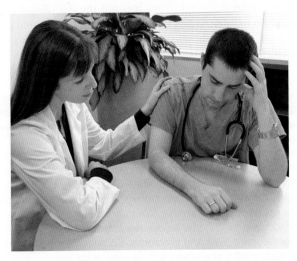

FIGURE 16-4 Everyone can make a mistake. Seek help if you misunderstood instructions, didn't realize that you were performing a procedure incorrectly, or made some other type of error. *How can you use mistakes as opportunities to learn?* (From Yoder-Wise PS: *Leading and managing in nursing*, ed 6, St Louis, 2015, Mosby.)

> **BOX 16-1** **American Association of Medical Assistants Code of Ethics**
>
> The Code of Ethics of the American Association of Medical Assistants (AAMA) shall set forth principles of ethical and moral conduct as they relate to the medical profession and the particular practice of medical assisting.
>
> Members of AAMA dedicated to the conscientious pursuit of their profession, and thus desiring to merit the high regard of the entire medical profession and the respect of the general public which they serve, do pledge themselves to strive always to:
> A. Render service with full respect for the dignity of humanity
> B. Respect confidential information obtained through employment unless legally authorized or required by responsible performance of duty to divulge such information
> C. Uphold the honor and high principles of the profession and accept its disciplines
> D. Seek to continually improve the knowledge and skills of medical assistants for the benefit of patients and professional colleagues
> E. Participate in additional service activities aimed toward improving the health and well-being of the community
>
> Copyright by the American Association of Medical Assistants Inc.

Respect Confidentiality

As a health care professional, you have an ethical and legal responsibility to respect patient confidentiality. As mentioned in Chapters 1 and 10, this includes both oral and written communications. You must be willing to monitor your work habits and conversation to make sure this important patient right is constantly guarded. Confidentiality must be safeguarded for both the patient's sake and yours. Serious or habitual disregard of this principle can be a cause for dismissal of health care personnel, as well as fines and disciplinary action against the facility.

The necessity to maintain patient confidentiality has increased as a result of federal legislation, known as HIPAA, passed in 1996. These letters stand for the Health Insurance Portability and Accountability Act. The following are a few of the major provisions of this act:

1. Make it easier for employees to maintain health insurance coverage when they change jobs
2. Adopt national standards for electronic health care transactions
3. Protect the privacy of every patient's health information

All health care facilities have developed policies and procedures to ensure that medical privacy is maintained. It is essential that you learn and follow these policies strictly to prevent problems for yourself and for your employer. The following suggestions, although not comprehensive, can help you avoid unintentional "leaks" of private information during a busy workday:

- Never discuss patient issues with anyone other than health care professionals who are directly involved in the care of the patient, and confine discussion to matters pertaining to this care.
- Limit allowable discussion to locations where you won't be overheard.
- When speaking with patients about personal matters, do so in a voice that they, but not anyone else, can hear.
- Take care when speaking to and about patients on the telephone so that others cannot overhear you.

- Leave patient-related matters at the workplace. Although it is natural to want to share your work with family and friends, any reference to patients and "interesting cases" is illegal.
- Do not share any information about particular situations at your workplace on social media, such as Facebook.
- Clear computer screens containing patient records when you leave the computer.
- Don't leave paperwork or files containing patient information on reception counters or other areas where unauthorized individuals can see them.
- Do not discuss any information with anyone, even a patient's spouse or relative, without the written permission of the patient.

Prescription for Success: 16-4 Focus on Confidentiality

1. Does the Code of Ethics for your profession include a statement about patient confidentiality?
2. List at least five techniques you can use in your work to guard patient confidentiality.

In addition to patient confidentiality, health care professionals have an obligation to protect the privacy of the facility where they work. Engaging in conversation about problems at work is a common employee activity. But airing what you consider to be the facility's "dirty laundry" does nothing to help the situation. In fact, it can have the opposite effect by damaging its reputation and undermining patient confidence. Problems must be addressed at the source if positive changes are to be made.

A final note regarding privacy is to respect your own. This means that personal problems don't belong at work and should not be discussed there. It is not the responsibility of coworkers to listen to and spend time advising you about personal affairs. Remember that your focus should be on work activities.

Trouble Ahead? 16-1

Whitney works as a home health aide for the Remain-At-Home agency. She hopes to be a nurse someday, but decides to take the shorter aide training program and do this work to see how she likes working in health care. Nursing school is expensive and she wants to save money for the tuition. She also hopes to build her self-confidence. She's doesn't have a strong sense of self and has a difficult time making friends, feeling she has little to offer.

As an aide, Whitney works with three clients each week under the supervision of Carol Stuart, RN. Whitney tries to be friendly and discovers that she likes visiting with her clients. Two of them are without family in the area and as a result, are quite lonely. They enjoy talking with Whitney while she is in their homes checking on their condition, doing

the laundry, preparing meals, and other tasks as needed. Having few people to visit them, they share their problems with Whitney: their worry about an alcoholic son, their concern about a sister in another state who has just suffered a stroke. Or they may tell her stories of happier times when their spouses were still alive. Whitney admits she is an advice-column junkie; she enjoys reading and hearing about other people's lives and problems. So taking an interest in the elderly folks she works with is natural for her.

In addition to hearing about their past and current lives, Whitney is aware of their physical condition because she takes them to their doctors' appointments, and assists them with exercises, bathing, and grooming. And being in their homes nearly every day, she knows about their personal habits. Mrs. Greene, she discovers, is somewhat of a hoarder. Her back bedrooms are stacked with books, papers, and mementos of her life. Mrs. Watson seems addicted to soap operas, even getting "involved" in the lives of the characters.

When Whitney spends time with others outside of work, including a few of the other aides that work for the agency, she enjoys sharing her experiences on the job. She giggles as she tells about Mrs. Watson crying over the problems of Carrie, a character on her favorite TV show. She tells about the old-fashioned dresses she found in Mrs. Greene's closet. "She must have had quite a social life," Whitney suggests.

A few weeks after she has started her job with Remain-At-Home, Whitney is asked to stop by the agency to meet with Carol, her supervising nurse.

Carol starts the conversation with a compliment, telling Whitney how her clients enjoy having her help them. "But Whitney," continues Carol. "I have real concerns about what goes on when you are not in their homes."

Whitney is puzzled and asks Carol what she means.

"It's what you are sharing with others—personal information about the clients," explains Carol.

"But they tell me these things. I don't think they care if a few other people know—they'd probably tell this stuff themselves," responds Whitney.

"No, Whitney. That's not an excuse. We have a duty to maintain confidentiality. You simply can't reveal anything about the people you work with."

Whitney doesn't say anything, but thinks to herself. What is she going to talk about if she can't share her experiences at work?

Questions for Thought and Reflection

1. Why do you think Whitney enjoys sharing what she knows about the people she works with? Do you think it is related to her lack of self-confidence?
2. What could be the consequences for the home health agency if Whitney continues to share confidential information about her clients?
3. Do you think Whitney realizes the seriousness of sharing information about the clients?

Be Responsible

Employees who are responsible and can be depended on to do what is expected—and then some—are worth their weight in gold. Today's health care environment puts many demands on employers. For example, they must provide high-quality services for patients, meet administrative deadlines, comply with a variety of regulations, and control operating costs. This is why it is essential that your employers can depend on you. Acting responsibly means that your actions include the following:

- **Complete all tasks.** This includes returning equipment and supplies to their proper places for the next person who needs them.
- **Strive for accuracy.** Examples of the many health care tasks in which accuracy is critical include patient **charting**, medical **coding** and billing, filling out **compliance reports** and lab reports, preparing sterile fields, and providing patient education.
- **Help out when needed, even when it's not your job.** The unexpected must be anticipated in health care. Coworkers are sometimes absent, emergencies occur, and situations can quickly change from routine to urgent. A career in health care requires you to be willing to do what it takes to get the job done.
- **Be on time.** This includes arriving at work on time every day, returning promptly from lunch and breaks, and getting to meetings and appointments on time. One of the major complaints of patients is having to wait. They feel that their time is not respected. Sometimes this cannot be helped, but avoid being the cause yourself. Absences should occur only for real emergencies. Have backup plans for transportation, childcare, or any other condition that might interfere with your attendance.

- **Follow through with everything you are directed or have offered to do.** If you cannot perform a task or need assistance, let your supervisor know so the task can be reassigned or help recruited. Don't allow work to go undone because you couldn't get to it yourself.

Prescription for Success: 16-5
Consider the Consequences

A medical assistant who works in a busy pediatric office fails to autoclave the instruments as directed. As a result, the physician cannot perform minor elective surgery scheduled for a young patient. Discuss the possible impact on the following:

1. Patient
2. Parents
3. Physician
4. Medical assistant

Work Effectively with Others

Getting along with others is one of the most talked-about, yet taken-for-granted workplace skills. Failure to work well with others is a major cause of employee dismissal because it reduces the health care facility's capability to provide high-quality service. Applying the people skills discussed in Chapter 10 and earlier in this chapter will help you establish positive relationships with coworkers. How well you develop your people skills will greatly influence your future.

High-quality health care requires the cooperation of many specialized individuals. And new types of professionals, in response to medical advances and increasingly complex delivery systems, continue to join the team. Whatever your particular occupation, you will be working with a variety of people who will bring different personalities, work styles, personal goals, and skill levels to the job. Your challenge will be to work in harmony with them all because each one is equally important to successful care delivery.

Trouble Ahead? 16-2

Charlie's mother, Ellen, had a difficult life. Raised by an alcoholic mother, she sought comfort from her high-school boyfriend. Their relationship resulted in her becoming pregnant at 17. Believing she was in love, Ellen hoped she and the young father would get married and enjoy a life together. Her boyfriend, however, had other ideas. Believing himself too young to be responsible for a wife and child, he left the area, leaving Ellen to take care of herself.

Ellen chose to have the baby and after giving birth to Charlie, did her best to provide for him. Her sister watched him while she worked the evening shift at a local restaurant, the best time for receiving good tips from customers. She felt guilty about not having more for Charlie; she was especially worried about him not having a father. She tried to make up for what was missing by spoiling him at best she could. She made an effort to build his self-esteem by giving him lots of praise, telling him what a good boy he was regardless of his behavior. When he got into serious mischief, she passed it off as "just something boys will do." There was very little discipline and while Charlie never got into real trouble as a teen, he had an unnaturally high opinion of himself. Because he was a good football player, the other kids gave him a little slack.

Charlie had a number of pets growing up and decided to become a veterinary technician. He enrolled in a two-year program. His mother had saved for years so that Charlie could pursue his education and he appreciated her efforts. He worked hard and did well in school. After graduating, Charlie passed the Veterinary Technician National Examination and was hired at a local animal clinic.

Excited and enthusiastic, Charlie plunged into the work. He wanted to make a good impression and show what he could do. He believed his training had prepared him well and as usual, received encouragement from his mother who was proud of his achievements. It was perhaps because of her continual praise and belief in him that he never hesitated in pointing out what he thought to be errors on the part of his coworkers. As they performed a procedure, such as a lab test or administering anesthesia to an animal, he would inform them that he had been taught differently in class and that "due to his recent training," he was quite sure his way would be best. "That's probably not the most up-to-date way to do that," he would say. For a while his coworkers ignored him, but things got really tense one day when he made a "correction" in the presence of a cat's owner, Mrs. Grisham. She overheard a remark that she interpreted as meaning her beloved pet was not receiving appropriate care. She complained to the veterinarian, Dr. Link.

Dr. Link had heard some grumbling about Charlie, but disliking confrontation, he hadn't said anything to his new employee. But after being confronted by Mrs. Grisham, he knew he couldn't let the situation continue. Calling Charlie into his office, he told his new employee what he had been hearing.

"Charlie," he told him. "I've been told that you've been correcting your coworkers—even experienced employees who have been with the clinic for several years."

"That's true. And maybe the ones who have been around for a while are the ones who need some correcting," Charlie said.

"There are often a number of ways to perform a procedure. And you need to know that the staff here at the clinic attend workshops regularly to learn the latest techniques," explained Dr. Link.

"Well," responded Charlie. "That may be, but I really think I should share what I know. You should be glad to have someone with my recent training and good skills."

Questions for Thought and Reflection

1. How do you think Charlie's mother has contributed to his current behavior on the job?
2. What do you think of his attitude about having "the most recent training?" Does this mean he is always correct?
3. Do you think Charlie will become a successful employee at the clinic? Why or why not?
4. What advice would you give Charlie?

Working with Your Supervisor

How well you get along with your supervisor can make the difference between looking forward to each workday or dreading the thought of showing up (Figure 16-5). The nature of this relationship influences promotions, raises, and the quality of work assignments. Indeed, it is a critical factor in determining both job success and work-life quality. Make an effort to get to know this important person. Use the information in this section to avoid missing what can be a career-enhancing opportunity.

Just as instructors have their own teaching and classroom management styles, described in Chapter 10, supervisors are characterized by a variety of management styles. These are shaped by the supervisor's personality, beliefs about management, personal experiences, and the organizational culture in which they work. Table 16-1 contains examples of different management styles. Your supervisor may demonstrate more than one of the styles listed. Keep in mind that there is no one right way to manage in all situations. Each has advantages and disadvantages. Certain styles are more appropriate than others in specific situations and work settings. The following are a few examples:

- Being friendly with employees is not positive if it results in too much downtime spent socializing. There is also the danger that some employees will believe there is favoritism if the supervisor is more friendly—or perceived to be so—to some employees than to others.

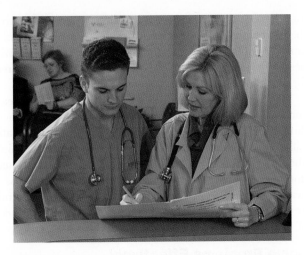

FIGURE 16-5 Make an effort to get along with and learn from your supervisor. *What are some ways you can make a favorable impression on your supervisor as you start a new job?* (From Proctor DB, Adams AP: *Kinn's the medical assistant: An applied learning approach*, ed 12, St Louis, 2014, Saunders.)

- There are brilliant people who seem to be very disorganized. They may have numerous projects going and don't feel they have the time to tidy up. Don't lose the chance to learn from them because you have judged them negatively for their disorderliness.
- Inviting employee input and encouraging creativity is beneficial in some work settings. But in others, such as the emergency room, it is not appropriate. Here, employees must work as directed. Procedures must be strictly followed. Lives depend on doing work the right way—and quickly.

Your work style may not match the management style of your supervisor. This is not uncommon. Mature employees see these differences as challenges rather than obstacles. A number of constructive ways to work effectively with your supervisor in spite of differences include the following:

1. Keep communication open. One of the worst things you can do is avoid someone with whom you disagree or have difficulty. Cutting off contact is likely to increase distance and decrease understanding.

TABLE 16-1
Common Management Styles

Management Style	Examples of Supervisor's Actions
Micromanages	Closely monitors your work. Frequently checks on you and wants regular progress reports.
Believes employees work best on their own	Doesn't appear to pay much attention to your work unless something goes wrong.
Likes a friendly work environment	Conversation is warm and friendly. Interested in your family and other aspects of your personal life. Birthdays and holidays are celebrated at the workplace.
Maintains a businesslike environment	Keeps most conversation work-related. Coworkers who become friends engage in social activities outside the workplace.
Disorganized or too busy to keep order	Loses reports you've turned in. Forgets scheduled meetings. Doesn't give you promised follow-up in a timely way. (Caution: Don't assume that because your supervisor is disorganized, he or she will tolerate *your* disorganization and accept actions such as completing assignments late.)
Values and practices order	Rarely misses deadlines and expects you to meet them, too, correctly and efficiently. Keeps lists, calendars, and orderly files.
Communicates directly	Lets you know how you are doing. Offers suggestions and criticism as needed. You know where you stand.
Communicates indirectly (or not at all)	Doesn't want to hurt your feelings. Avoids confrontations. May not tell you if you are doing something incorrectly or not to his or her liking. (Caution: May complain about you behind your back, thus depriving you of the opportunity to learn and resolve the problem.)
Believes it is the supervisor's responsibility to make most decisions	Employees are not consulted about policy changes, future plans, etc.
Believes that better decisions result when employees participate in making them	Employees are asked for their opinions. Some decisions are made as a group. (Caution: Group decision making can bog down the group and result in little being accomplished.)

2. Follow the chain of command. This means speaking with your supervisor before going to the next level with concerns and complaints. If you are having problems with your supervisor, talk with him or her first. It is all too common for employees to bad-mouth their supervisors and discuss problems with everyone except the one person who can actually do something to resolve them: the supervisor. In fact, complaining usually results in everything but resolution. It may actually create new problems: lowered morale among coworkers who hear your complaints, lost work time, a decrease in the quality of service to patients, and worsened relations with the supervisor who hears about the grumbling through the grapevine. Failure to follow the proper order can even result in dismissal.

3. Be empathetic. Your supervisor may have pressures and problems that explain his or her actions.

4. Ask questions to learn your supervisor's priorities and find out what is most important. If the following questions weren't answered in the job interview, ask them now:
   - What are your expectations of me?
   - What do you most value in an employee?
   - How can I best contribute to the success of the organization and/or facility?
   - How often would you like me to report to you?
   - What is the best time to report to you, ask questions, and receive progress reports about my work?

5. Let your supervisor know how you work best. This can be a positive conversation: "I really want to be able to do my best work for the radiology department. I find that when my work is constantly being checked, I get nervous and tend to make more errors. Could we work out another way to monitor my progress that still meets the needs of the department?"

6. Ask for clarification if you are unclear about your job duties or exactly what is expected of you.

7. Realize the bottom line is this: you must work with your supervisor, and this means adapting to his or her style. Do your best to make the situation positive. Focus on learning as much as possible from both the supervisor and the situation.

Prescription for Success: 16-6
Management Styles

1. What types of supervisors have you worked for in the past?
2. How did you get along?
3. Did you learn any strategies that you can apply at future jobs?

Think About What You Are Doing

Work in health care requires continual thinking. Nothing can be taken for granted. You must constantly pay attention to make sure that your actions make sense. Suppose that Mr. Cardenas, who doesn't understand English well, is scheduled for a lab test that requires him to follow certain procedures the day before. It wouldn't make sense for the medical assistant to give him a written instruction sheet in English. He will need directions in Spanish to ensure he is properly prepared for the test.

Health care professionals must keep their minds in gear, continually observing and thinking as they perform their duties. Your daily work can never be performed automatically. You must continually ask yourself questions, think about the significance of what you see, and use this information to determine the most appropriate action to take. As a health care professional, you cannot cruise along in neutral. Your work is too important, and the potential consequences of failing to be alert and thinking are too serious.

Solve Problems Effectively

The problem-solving method introduced in Chapter 9 is an essential workplace tool. To review it quickly, it consists of the following six steps:
1. Define the problem.
2. Gather information.
3. Brainstorm alternative solutions.
4. Consider possible results and consequences.
5. Choose a solution and act on it.
6. Evaluate the results and revise as needed.

Good problem-solving skills involve both **reasoning** and creativity. Start by examining what you believe to be the problem. Try to see it from different angles. Mentally walk around the problem, looking at it from all sides. Are you defining the problem in terms of the symptoms rather than the problem itself? (Recall the case of Kathy in Chapter 9. She believed her problem to be low grades in pharmacology when it turned out to be her lack of math skills.)

Use brainstorming to come up with possible solutions. Recall from Chapter 9 that this means thinking of as many ideas as possible, from the sensible to the crazy. Seeing new possibilities requires you to think creatively because problems are often solved by using an original approach.

Although creativity generates ideas, reasoning helps you to put the ideas together in ways that work. It also helps you test potential outcomes mentally. Use it to check "What would happen if..." scenarios for the possibilities you have brainstormed. Reasoning helps you ask the right questions, such as the following:
- Based on what I know, could this solution work? Why or why not?
- Do all the pieces fit together?
- Does it make sense?

Effective solutions are the result of using creativity to generate new ideas and applying reasoning to test them. Creativity is the artist and reasoning is the critic.

Before you approach your supervisor with a problem, think it through. Do your best to come up with solutions to suggest. This demonstrates your initiative and willingness to take an active part in the problem-solving process. With experience, you will better know when to ask questions and when to choose and implement solutions on your own.

Continue to Learn

To continue to learn is important in all fields today, but it is especially so in health care. This field is in a state of continual change brought about by medical discoveries, transformations in the delivery system and methods of payment, government regulations, and technological innovations. Outdated knowledge and skills can be useless. You've got to keep up to remain effective. There are many ways to do this, including the following:

- Attend the meetings and learning activities sponsored by your professional organization.
- Read journals and publications devoted to your field, as well as books and articles about the general field of health care.
- Take courses at local schools and colleges.
- Observe and ask questions at work.
- Check the websites of organizations, such as the American Heart Association and the American Cancer Society, that provide up-to-date information.
- Join newsgroups on the Internet, as described in Chapter 12.
- Use the Internet to explore topics of interest. (Be sure to check the reliability of Internet sources, as explained in Chapter 7.)
- Check the availability of resources at your workplace: library, reference books, journals, people with expertise and special interests.

Some employers pay for professional journal subscriptions, classes, and workshops, so ask about the policy where you work.

Case Study 16-2

Learning About the Job

Steve, like Charlie, is a recent veterinary tech graduate. Unlike Charlie, he is feeling overwhelmed by what he is expected to know at his new job. Steve worked hard in school, but working daily with people's pets, it seems like there's a lot he doesn't know—or that he feels unsure about. On weekends, he and some of his former classmates get together for a beer or to watch a game on someone's big screen. Charlie is in this group and it doesn't help Steve's confidence when he hears Charlie talk about how much more he knows than some of the people at the clinic where he works. Steve wonders to himself if there was something he missed at school. Why doesn't he feel as confident at Charlie?

After a month on the job with his self-doubts mounting, Steve considers turning in his resignation. When he mentions this at home, his wife suggests that he talk to his boss, Dr. Garcia. Steve is not sure this is a good idea. After all, if Dr. Garcia knows how he feels, he may have doubts about him and let him go. He won't even have to quit.

But Steve really enjoys working with the animals. And he did invest a lot of time and money in his education. So he decides to talk with Dr. Garcia. He is surprised to learn that his boss is quite understanding. He knows that students can't learn everything they will encounter on the job and appreciates that Steve is conscientious.

At the same time, he realizes that Steve needs help to acquire additional knowledge and improve his skills in order to feel more confident on the job.

Questions for Thought and Reflection

1. List five suggestions that Dr. Garcia could give Steve to help him learn more and increase his self-confidence.
2. What might Steve have done when he first started working for Dr. Garcia?
3. How can students best prepare to feel more confident when they start working at their first health care job?

Prescription for Success: 16-7
What's Available?

1. Does your professional organization have a local chapter?
2. What types of learning activities does it sponsor?
3. Name the journals that are available in your field. Where are they available?
   - By subscription?
   - As part of a professional membership?
   - In the library?
   - At your health care facility?
4. What types of continuing education classes are available in your occupational area?
5. Choose a topic of interest in health care, and conduct an Internet search for information.
   - What kind of information is available?
   - Who are the sponsors?
   - How reliable do you believe the information to be? Why?

Practice Cost Control

Cost control is a major concern in health care today. The United States spends more of its total income on health care than any other nation. How can you help control costs? There are a number of ways. They may seem insignificant, but if practiced by everyone, they can make a difference.

- Work carefully and thoughtfully so tasks don't have to be repeated by you or anyone else.
- Don't waste supplies. Use what is needed and no more.
- Learn how to use supplies correctly. For example, follow the instructions when using lab test kits.
- Take care of equipment. Follow the directions, use it carefully, practice preventive maintenance, and report any problems promptly.
- Never take supplies or use services for your personal use. A few pens tucked in your pocket or runs of personal documents through the copy machine can add up quickly.
- Use work time for work. Your salary is a major employer expense.

Manage Yourself

Managing your personal habits effectively enables you to serve others better. How does this work? We discussed the following major components of self-management in Chapter 3:

- Attitude
- Personal organization
- Time management
- Stress reduction techniques

Failure to maintain control in these areas can negatively affect your work in a number of ways, as shown in the following examples:

- Arriving late can disrupt the schedules of patients and co-workers.
- Running out of energy before the workday is over can delay the completion of important tasks.
- Repeatedly calling in sick because of stress-related illnesses forces coworkers to fill in for you, disrupts schedules, and/or leaves tasks undone.
- Failure to prioritize tasks can result in missing important deadlines.
- Feeling tired can reduce your ability to concentrate and complete work assignments accurately.

As you can see, your personal habits are no longer just personal—they affect other people, too. Efficient use of time, for example, is especially critical in today's busy offices and clinics. The inability to maintain schedules and complete tasks in a timely way can be a serious liability on the job. By choosing a career in health care, you have made a commitment to serve others, and you owe it to your profession to make your best efforts. And this requires good self-management.

This does not mean, however, that your life should be entirely devoted to work. In fact, just the opposite is true. You need to take time out to attend to your own needs. The key is to achieve a balance between your needs and those of others in your life: patients, employer, coworkers, family members, and friends. If you continually ignore your own needs, you can deplete your physical, mental, and emotional resources. The result will be that you have nothing left to give others.

Maintaining this balance between self, family, and work requires prioritizing and practicing good organizational and time-management skills. There will always be more to do than there is time and energy to do it. We all must make choices, and these should be based on our values. Your mission statement, described in Chapter 3, should guide these choices. For example, if spending time with your children is important to you, and you have only two free hours in the evening, you might choose to play games with the children instead of watching television. If your weekends are filled with housework and errands, you might look for ways your children can help with the chores and then plan a fun activity together as a family.

Prescription for Success: 16-8 Are You Ready?

1. What are your backup plans for transportation, child-care, and/or any personal responsibilities that could interfere with your job?
2. What organizational strategies have you developed to help balance your professional and personal life?
3. Do any of your self-management skills need improvement? If so, what can you do to improve them?

At the workplace, self-management means the ability to work without constant supervision. Supervisors don't have the time to continually monitor their employees. You can increase your value as an employee by identifying what needs to be done and following through on tasks. Working without being reminded will help you achieve a reputation as a dependable and responsible employee. In the event you complete your work and have some extra time, look for something else to do or ask for an additional assignment. There is no such thing as "free time" on the job, and you owe it to your employer to stay busy and productive.

It is more likely you will experience the opposite problem: too much to do in too little time. In this case, learn to prioritize tasks according to the needs of your employer so the essential ones always get completed. If you are unsure about priorities, ask your supervisor for direction.

Adapt to Changing Conditions

Change is to be expected in health care environments. Adapting to change—and doing so willingly and agreeably—is an essential job skill. We have mentioned the continuing changes in health care. Other factors that require flexibility include responding to patient emergencies and ensuring that all responsibilities are covered when other employees are absent. Here are a few everyday examples that demonstrate the need for flexibility:

- A dental assistant learning to assist the dentist with new laser equipment that has replaced traditional drills
- A medical insurance biller keeping informed and using revised reporting methods required for Medicare reimbursement
- An emergency medical technician agreeing to change her work schedule to cover for a fellow worker who is ill
- The members of a clinic's staff learning to work with a new supervisor and under new policies that accompanied an ownership change
- A nurse developing relationships with new coworkers after the hospital reorganizes departments and staff to create a team approach to patient care
- A lab technician applying new OSHA requirements to the handling of chemicals and biological waste
- A medical assistant learning new medical office management software

Change can be viewed as an opportunity to learn and avoid boredom on the job—or as an inconvenience that requires you

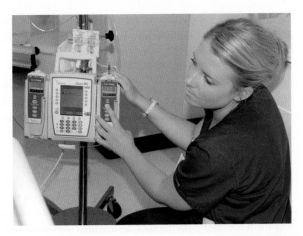

FIGURE 16-6 Health care is a particularly fast-changing field. This 21st century IV pump has many features that previous pumps lacked, presenting both challenges for nurses, and increased accuracy and safety for patients. *What kinds of changes do you anticipate for your career field?* (From Yoder-Wise PS: *Leading and managing in nursing*, ed 6, St Louis, 2015, Mosby.)

to "grin and bear it." The approach you choose will influence how much satisfaction you gain from your work. Be aware that the words "That's not my job," if heard by your employer, can be fatal in the workplace. (Exception: performing tasks you are not trained or legally allowed to perform.) See Figure 16-6.

Prescription for Success: 16-9 Knowing Ahead Gives You the Edge

Research your occupation to see how it has changed over the last 20 years. Sources of information include interviewing someone who has worked in the field for several years, your professional organization, the Internet, and your instructors.

1. Does your occupation require more training than it did in the past?
2. Describe any duties or responsibilities that have been added and/or deleted.
3. Have licensing or certification requirements been added or changed?
4. What changes are anticipated for the future?
5. How can you start preparing to be ready for these changes?

Be Willing to Cross-Train

Learning tasks that are usually—or used to be—performed by professionals outside your specific occupational area is known as **cross-training**. Job duties are not separated as distinctly by occupation as they once were. Certain tasks that were once performed only by nurses, for example, are now performed by other professionals. The movement toward the expansion of responsibilities has been encouraged by one

of the major goals driving health care today: increasing the quality of patient care while controlling costs.

Learning additional skills adds to your value as an employee. In some cases, it will even determine your success in securing the job you want. Having opportunities to learn new skills on the job should be viewed as a benefit, not an imposition. Take advantage of them. You are learning new skills that will enhance your career, and you're being paid at the same time!

One word of caution: check the **scope of practice** for your professional level. Some skills require you to be licensed or certified before you can legally perform them. Be sure that you know and stay within your legal limits.

Prescription for Success: 16-10 Scope of Practice

1. Does your profession have a published scope of practice?
2. Who defines the occupational roles for your career?
3. Who determines the duties you can perform?
4. What are these duties?
5. What are you prohibited from doing?

Serve as a Role Model for Wellness

Personal habits are now recognized as having a major impact on health. In a dual effort to help people live healthier lives and avoid the expense of preventable medical problems, health care providers are placing more emphasis on promoting wellness. This is in contrast to the traditional focus on treating disease and injury. A growing number of patients want to take a more active role in the management of their health. Part of your work may involve teaching patients, as appropriate for your profession, about the practice of preventive and good wellness habits.

As a health care professional, you can encourage this positive trend by promoting the benefits of healthy living. Serve as an example of healthy lifestyle choices. Are you a good "advertisement" for the industry you represent? This applies to your life in the community outside the health care facility, too.

Avoid Burnout

Burnout is a work-related condition in which a person experiences physical and emotional exhaustion. People experiencing burnout often have a feeling of hopelessness. They believe their efforts have no purpose.

Burnout is a growing problem among health care professionals because of the responsibilities of working with people who are ill, heavy workloads, and the increasing emphasis on efficiency and cost control. Signs of burnout include extreme fatigue, irritability, frequent illnesses, and a feeling of discouragement. Several conditions can lead to burnout, including the following:

- Continual job stress caused by factors such as constantly changing schedules, lack of feedback about work performance, and lack of recognition for accomplishments

- More tasks assigned than can be accomplished during work hours
- Long work hours and inadequate time for rest
- A feeling of never getting caught up on tasks
- Continual pressure to meet tight deadlines and complete demanding assignments

Consistent use of good self-management techniques provides protection against burnout. Box 16-2 contains a list of suggestions for avoiding burnout.

Your Legal Rights

It may seem, as an employee, that there is an endless list of "shoulds" and "must dos." In fact, there are safeguards to protect your rights on the job. These range from laws to prevent discrimination to agencies charged with ensuring your physical safety. You should be aware of the major employment laws described in the following sections. Ask your employer for information about company policies, and check the library and/or the Internet for further resources.

Family Medical Leave Act

The Family Medical Leave Act (FMLA) is an act of federal legislation that was passed in 1993 to make it easier for employees to take time off to attend to health and family matters. There are certain eligibility requirements that include the following:

- You must be a public employee or work for an employer who has at least 50 employees.

- You must have worked for at least 12 months and at least 1,250 hours during the 12 months immediately before the leave is to be taken.

The purpose of the leave must be (1) to take care of serious personal health problems or those of a spouse, parent, or child, or for the birth or adoption of a child; or (2) to take care of a family member who is in the Armed Forces and undergoing medical treatment or therapy or who is on temporary disability because of a serious injury or illness.

Employees who take leave under the Act must be given their previous job or the equivalent at the same pay on their return. The employer is not required to pay the employee during the leave, but benefits such as medical insurance must stay in effect.

Equal Pay Act

The Equal Pay Act was passed in 1963 as an amendment to the Fair Labor Standards Act, the federal regulation of wages, hours, and working conditions. Its purpose is to protect workers from pay discrimination based on gender. Although the act protects both men and women, it is women who have traditionally been prohibited from performing certain jobs and have been paid less than men for doing the same work. Therefore, most equal pay complaints are filed by women.

For a successful claim, the jobs in question must be proven to be equal. This means showing they are similar in skill, effort, and responsibility. Also, claims of unequal pay can only apply to employees working for the same employer in the same geographic location. In other words, a medical assistant can't file a claim because the physician at another office pays a higher wage to medical assistants. She could, however, file a claim if a male medical assistant in the same office is paid more for performing what is substantially the same work. The Equal Pay Act covers all categories of employees, including executives and managers.

Civil Rights Act of 1964

The Civil Rights Act is important legislation that was passed to protect the rights and opportunities of all Americans. Title VII of the Act prohibits the denial of employment opportunities on the basis of race, color, religion, sex, or national origin. Once hired, employees cannot be treated differently based on these factors.

Sexual harassment is classified as a form of discrimination and is therefore illegal under Title VII. It refers to unwelcome and unwanted sexual attention.

Sexual harassment can take many forms, ranging in severity from telling dirty jokes to rape. It does not prohibit mutually agreed-upon behavior between employees such as flirting and dating. (These behaviors are not recommended, however, because workplace romances that go sour can become workplace nightmares for the people involved.)

An important point to keep in mind is that the victim of sexual harassment does not have to be directly involved. Consider the example of two hospital employees who have become friends and regularly share jokes of a sexual nature. They find them amusing and stress-reducing. A third person, who works in the same department, finds them extremely offensive. She asks them to stop, but they consider her to be prissy and unreasonable. The third person may have a legitimate claim of sexual harassment.

Some people find any reference to sexual matters offensive, so it is best to play it safe by avoiding any speech or behavior that is sexual in nature. This is especially important when you are new on the job. It takes time to get to know people and the organizational culture. People respond differently, and it is best to avoid anything that might be misinterpreted. For example, remarks you intend as compliments, such as references to any part of the body, may be misinterpreted. You are in the beginning stages of establishing your reputation as a health care professional. Do everything possible to get a good start and avoid any behavior that might be interpreted as harassment.

At the same time, you need to know what to do if you are the victim. Most experts recommend that the first step of defense should be to speak directly with the harasser and request an immediate stop to the behavior you find objectionable. It is best not to let it go, hoping the problem will go away, because this can send the message that the person's actions are acceptable. As a result, the actions are likely to continue and may even get worse.

When speaking with the harasser, focus on the objectionable behavior. State exactly what you find unacceptable and tell him or her to stop. Keep a dated, written record of all events connected with the incident(s), including when you spoke to the harasser. If the behavior continues, report it to the appropriate person. This may be your supervisor or a specific person who has been appointed to deal with discrimination issues at your organization. Follow the proper procedures for filing a complaint. It is best to seek a resolution within the organization. If the problem is not resolved, however, a complaint can be filed with the Equal Employment Opportunity Commission. This must be done within 180 days of the incident.

Americans with Disabilities Act

The Americans with Disabilities Act (ADA) protects the right of disabled workers, who are qualified for the job, to secure and maintain employment. A disability can be either physical or mental. The Act requires employers to make "reasonable accommodations" for disabled employees who have the necessary qualifications to perform the job. A reasonable accommodation refers to both the financial impact on the employer and how the modifications affect the ability of the organization to function. Examples of reasonable accommodations are to provide a specially designed desk and chair for an employee with a back injury or an adaptive computer keyboard for an administrative worker who has the use of only one hand. Ramps, wheelchair access to work areas, and phone equipment for the hearing impaired are other examples of accommodations that might be considered reasonable under the Act.

Federal Age Discrimination Act

Passed in 1967, the Federal Age Discrimination Act protects applicants and employees over the age of 40 from discrimination in the workplace. Employers who have more than 20 employees are subject to this Act. The following actions are prohibited if they occur because of an employee's age:
- Refusal to hire
- Dismissal
- Layoff
- Denial of a promotion
- Limits placed on wages and other benefits

Complaints about possible age discrimination that are not resolved at the workplace can be filed with the Equal Employment Opportunity Commission.

Occupational Safety and Health Act

OSHA, passed in 1970, requires employers to provide safe workplaces. The Act is very comprehensive and contains a wide variety of provisions to protect workers by doing the following:
- Ensuring that equipment is safe and in good operating order.
- Keeping the environment free of **toxic** and potentially harmful wastes, chemicals, and other materials.
- Providing employees with training about the safe handling of chemicals, equipment, and other materials that are potentially hazardous when used improperly.
- Offering hepatitis B vaccines free of charge to employees who are at risk for contracting the disease. (Hepatitis B is a serious disease of the liver that can be transmitted through contact with the blood and other body fluids of an infected person.)
- Requiring **Standard Precautions to** be followed in the handling of blood and other body fluids. (Standard Precautions are specific practices and procedures to prevent the spread of infection.)
- Providing protective equipment, such as gloves and protective eyewear, to employees who are exposed to **bloodborne pathogens**.
- Disposing of medical waste properly.
- Having Material Safety Data Sheets (MSDSs) for all products used in the workplace. These sheets list every ingredient, as well as precautions and clean-up instructions in case of spills.

Although OSHA requirements are intended to protect workers, they also carry a burden of responsibility for employees. You will be required to follow certain OSHA policies and procedures on the job. It is essential that you become familiar with the ones that relate to your occupational duties because failure to comply can have serious consequences for both you and the facility where you work.

State and Local Employment Laws

In addition to federal laws, state and local entities enact employment laws. These cover many specific aspects of employment, such as the following:
- Pregnancy leave
- Minimum wage

- Jury duty leave
- Drug testing
- Overtime payment
- Holiday leave
- Number of hours worked

Focus on the Goal

In spite of your best efforts, difficulties may arise on the job. These can range from the annoying to the intolerable. The ability to handle them effectively is a major job and life skill. Some problems can be handled with your own resources. Others require the assistance of others to resolve.

In Chapter 2, we introduced Stephen Covey's advice to "Begin with the end in mind." Slightly modifying this sentence gives us words to keep in mind when we are faced with a serious problem at work: "Act with the end in mind." This means that you approach problems with the intention of finding solutions to enhance rather than jeopardize your career. Choose actions that are appropriate for the situation. Some situations must simply be tolerated. For example, patience may be required when working with people who have annoying habits. Actions such as refusing to work with them and/or complaining to others behind their backs may hurt you professionally. On the other hand, resigning from a workplace in which illegal actions are taking place—and not being corrected—may be the most appropriate action.

Dedicate your efforts to finding solutions to difficult situations. It's easy to wear yourself out by worrying or complaining about a problem, leaving you with little energy for actually dealing with it. Be clear about the resolutions you hope to achieve and look for ways to achieve them.

If you have a mentor, he or she may be a good source of advice for dealing with workplace issues. Talking them over with someone experienced in the field can help you gain perspective and see potential solutions that may not have occurred to you. Take care, however, to protect the confidentiality of the facility if your mentor does not work there.

The following are some examples of workplace problems that occur in health care settings:

1. *You are asked to perform duties that fall outside your scope of practice, tasks for which you were not trained, or tasks that are illegal.*

    Fortunately, this problem is rare. Unfortunately, when it does happen, it places the health care professional in a difficult situation. The best advice in these cases is "don't." Even if you are pressured by your supervisor or are assured that it is okay and "everyone does it," this is too big a risk to take. Once lost, your professional trustworthiness is very difficult to re-earn. Furthermore, illegal acts can result in fines and/or imprisonment.

2. *You find it difficult to get along with your supervisor.*

    Begin by taking an honest look at your own behavior to see whether there is something you are doing—or not doing—to contribute to the problem. Speak privately and frankly with your supervisor about how important your job is to you. Tell him or her that you want to have a good working relationship. Ask if there is anything you need to do to improve your performance.

Identify your supervisor's priorities and communication style. Use mirroring, the technique discussed in Chapter 14, to match your communication styles. Not all supervisors have good communication skills. Listen carefully, and use feedback to increase the quality of communication and the likelihood of mutual understanding.

Make an effort to find out what is important to your supervisor. Take a look at Table 16-1 to see descriptions of common management styles. Do your actions conflict with his or her management style? Does the management style conflict with your preferred way of working? Do you have different assumptions about the right way to do the work? This can lead to major misunderstandings in which each of you seems uncooperative and difficult to the other. We must become aware of the assumptions and expectations of the other person before we can attempt to get along with them.

When trying to communicate with your supervisor, keep in mind that your purpose is to promote mutual understanding and get the information needed to perform your job effectively. It is not to prove you are right or to tell your supervisor off, actions that will most likely make the situation worse. Look for ways to relieve your stress without venting your frustration at your supervisor.

3. *Low employee morale. Your coworkers are unhappy and complain a lot. You'd like to get along with everyone and be part of the group, but the conversation and atmosphere are getting you down.*

    This can be a tough situation because it's unlikely you can change the opinion of the group. And being a newcomer, you want to fit in, but not at the expense of joining in the complaint sessions. Complaints that are justified are resolved through action, not endless discussion that wastes time, drains energy, and generally leads nowhere. Apply your communication and problem-solving skills to try to find solutions. And do your best to avoid participating in complaint sessions. It's a negative note on which to start a new career.

4. *There's too much to do and you can't finish all your work.*

    Start by reviewing your work habits. Are you taking too much time to complete each task? Are there some tasks that you are still learning? Are you practicing good time management skills? You may be able to draw on the experience of your supervisor and/or coworkers to help you increase your efficiency. Talk with your supervisor about prioritizing your work. If you can't complete everything, which tasks are the most critical? What help is available? The time crunch is a growing problem in health care as professionals are being required to do more work in less time. Learning to maximize your efficiency will serve you well.

Work can be very satisfying in spite of problems like these. At best, problems provide opportunities for professional growth. Some situations, however, cannot be resolved or require compromises that you are not willing to make. You may choose to leave and seek employment elsewhere, a topic that is discussed in Chapter 17. In the meantime, it is critical that you do everything possible to maintain your professionalism and build a good reputation as a competent and cooperative employee.

Suppose you are newly hired and have been trying your best to complete what you understand to be your assignments. However, you only received a one-hour orientation for the job and are not completely clear about your duties, the policies at the facility, and exactly what you are expected to do. You haven't been able to locate all the supplies and resources you need and aren't sure how to operate the computer system. Your supervisor is always rushed. You now have 15 minutes to talk with him. What would you say?

Grievance Procedure

A grievance procedure is a written policy that gives employees a formalized, structured method to resolve workplace issues, or **grievances**, that they do not believe have been satisfactorily resolved by the supervisor. Common grievances concern fair treatment, discrimination, and disciplinary actions. For example, if an employee believes she did not receive a promotion because her supervisor unfairly favors another employee because they are friends, she should first speak with her supervisor. If she is dissatisfied with the explanation or believes that company policy regarding promotions was not followed, she can speak with her supervisor's manager. If, after seeking resolution by following the chain of command, she still believes she has been treated unfairly with respect to the promotion, she can file a grievance.

Organizations develop their own procedures, which consist of specific steps to take to file a grievance. This procedure is usually described in the employee handbook or in a policy and procedure manual. If you belong to a labor union, ask your representative how to file a grievance. It is important to follow the directions and meet any deadlines outlined in the policy. Grievances should be filed only when all of the following conditions are met:

1. You have made a sincere attempt to handle the issue, starting with speaking to your supervisor about the problem.
2. The issue is serious.
3. You are willing to follow a formal process.

Used appropriately, the grievance procedure can be an effective and fair means of resolving employee issues in an organization.

Seek Satisfaction in Your Work

Many of your waking hours are spent at the workplace. If you are to live a high-quality life, it makes sense for your work to be a source of satisfaction. This doesn't mean finding the "perfect job." In fact, it is unlikely such a thing exists. It does mean approaching work with a positive attitude and focusing on those aspects that give you the opportunity to do the following:

• Perform meaningful work
• Make a positive contribution to the well-being of others
• Work in an interesting environment
• Continue to learn

Satisfaction is self-perpetuating. This means that health care professionals who project a positive attitude and like their work are likely to create satisfaction in those who receive their services. Performance levels and efficiency are also raised, further increasing the professional's sense of satisfaction.

Q&A with a Health Care Professional

Bernie Stults, Registered Nurse

Bernie had 44 years of experience as a registered nurse in hospitals and clinics and now teaches clinical rotations for nursing assistant students. Bernie discusses tips for career success.

Q What advice would you give graduates who are starting their first job in health care?

A The basics are still very important for success on the job. Things like professional appearance. In the last 10 years or so, trends like tattoos have become a problem because some older patients find them objectionable. They don't understand they are just a fashion statement and no longer have the negative connotations they had years ago. Another style that's a problem is low-cut blouses and tops on female employees. These are seen just about everyplace these days, but they just aren't appropriate on the job in health care.

Q Along with appearance, what other recommendations would you offer?

A It's important to show an interest in the job. New employees should want to learn, and they can do this by asking questions—and then following up. By this I mean writing the information down and making an effort to learn and remember it. We had a new hire recently who would ask questions and then fail to pay attention. She ended up doing the work her way, which unfortunately wasn't always correct.

Q There are instances in which recent graduates believe their current training actually makes them more qualified than experienced health care workers. Have you run into this problem?

A Yes. This know-it-all attitude is a problem with quite a few graduates. What they don't realize is that much of their learning will be based on years of experience on the job. They need to do their best to perform efficiently and correctly while also being willing to learn.

Q What other advice do you consider essential for success in health care?

A In a few words: be prepared to meet the needs of others. And I don't just mean your patients. I used to work in the ER. When there was a seriously injured accident victim, for example, I was not only helping the patient, but dealing with the family members, friends, and working with other hospital personnel. There were lots of things to consider, and they all dealt with people. Regardless of the situation, good social skills are really a must.

A win-win situation is created in which everyone benefits.

To keep yourself on the right track, ask yourself the following questions as you work:

- Who is benefiting from the tasks I am performing now?
- What contributions am I making to the well-being of others?
- What can I learn today?
- Are there positive aspects of my work that I am overlooking?

◻ Prescription for Success: 16-12 Increasing Your Job Satisfaction

1. What were your reasons for choosing a career in health care?
2. In what ways do you think you will receive satisfaction from your work?
3. How will you measure your success and satisfaction at work?
4. What can you do to make your work fulfilling?

Summary of Key Ideas

- Your first job sets the groundwork for your future career success.
- Your study skills are also useful employment skills.
- Mastering workplace competencies leads to workplace success.
- Learning to work well with your supervisor is worth the effort.
- Employees have rights that are protected by law.

Positive Self-Talk for This Chapter

- I will be a confident and competent health care professional.
- I have the skills to handle various kinds of workplace problems.
- I work well with others.
- My health care career is off to a good start.
- My job will bring me great satisfaction.

Internet Activities

ⓔ For active links to the websites needed to complete these activities, visit http://evolve.elsevier.com/Haroun/career/.

1. Many specific OSHA regulations apply to workers in health care facilities. Explore the OSHA website and choose a topic related to your future career, such as blood-borne pathogens or needlestick prevention. Write a short report about the extent of the problem and OSHA's recommendations for the protection of workers.

2. Concern about medical privacy has increased significantly with the passage of HIPAA and the creation of federal privacy standards that took effect on April 14, 2003. The U.S. Department of Health and Human Services has created fact sheets on patient privacy that are available online. Read the fact sheets for consumers, and list the five provisions designed to protect patient health information.

3. Mind Tools has information on job success topics such as stress and time management, problem solving, and practical creativity. Choose a topic to explore, and write a plan for incorporating suggestions you find useful into your daily life.

To Learn More

About.com: Workplace Survival and Success

http://careerplanning.about.com/od/workplacesurvival/Workplace_Survival_and_Success.htm

This page contains links to dozens of short articles that include topics such as getting along with your boss and coworkers, office etiquette, and personal issues at work.

Covey S.R:. *The 7 habits of highly effective people,* New York, 1990, Fireside

This popular book lists seven principles that help individuals live effective lives. These can be applied for success in the workplace.

Flight M: *Law, liability, and ethics for medical office professionals,* ed 5, Clifton Park, NY, 2011, Cengage Delmar Learning

This book presents legal and ethical matters for health care professionals in an interesting and easy-to-read format. Actual cases are used as examples.

Mind Tools

www.mindtools.com

The "tools" include skills that contribute to workplace success including time management, problem solving, and stress management.

CHAPTER 17

Navigating Your Career

OBJECTIVES

1. List ways to gain maximum benefit from performance reviews.
2. Describe the continuing education requirements for your career, if applicable, and list ways to earn them.
3. Explain why it is important to maintain your professional network throughout your career.
4. Explain how to become a leader in your profession and how to increase your chances of earning a promotion.
5. List the characteristics of an effective supervisor.
6. Describe the proper actions to take when leaving a job voluntarily and how to use a decision matrix to choose the right job.
7. Explain how to survive and learn from the experience of being fired from a job.
8. List various ways to enrich your career.

KEY TERMS AND CONCEPTS

Decision Matrix A table you create to compare and rate alternatives when making an important decision.

Downsizing Reducing the number of employees.

Entrepreneur Someone who starts and operates a business.

Job Shadow To spend time with a professional during typical workdays to observe the kinds of tasks performed, the environment in which the work takes place, and so on.

Step-Up Programs Educational programs in which credits and/or experience earned for one occupational level can be applied for credit when studying for a higher level. Example: LPN/LVN to RN.

Staying on Course

"Only he who keeps his eye fixed on the far horizon will find his right road."

—Dag Hammarskjöld

You're on your way! You have launched your health care career and should be enjoying the results of your efforts. But maintaining a successful career is like traveling successfully by ship. Without plotting and paying attention to your course, you can end up drifting aimlessly. Even worse, inattention can result in collisions that can sink your ship.

Performance Reviews

Many people think that performance reviews (work evaluations) are the responsibility of supervisors only. In fact, *you* should be conducting your own regular self-evaluations to monitor your progress and keep yourself on course. Review your performance periodically using your job description and your employer's evaluation form as guides. Figure 17-1 is a sample evaluation form. Honest self-evaluations are like an internal quality control system, alerting you to when you need to make improvements and possibly get help from your supervisor.

Self-awareness empowers you to be proactive and in control. Rather than waiting for others to suggest needed improvements, you continually review your performance and set your own goals. At the same time, you should be documenting your achievements on the job.

Your supervisor is, of course, a valuable source of information and feedback about your progress. Take the initiative to maximize the value of your formal performance evaluations. More than one-sided progress reports, these meetings should be an opportunity for you to review your supervisor's expectations and determine whether you are meeting them. Take advantage of your meeting to ask questions such as the following:

1. Which tasks am I performing well?
2. Which tasks need improvement?
3. Do you have suggestions for improvements?
4. Can you recommend sources that might help me?
5. How can I increase my value to the team (department, facility)?

Don't hesitate to request information. If you are unsure about certain job duties, rules, policies, or procedures, use this opportunity to ask. If you receive a low rating in some area and don't understand why, ask for an explanation and examples that demonstrate how you do not meet the criteria or have performed poorly. In the case of low ratings, you can offer explanations, but don't make excuses. If you believe you have a good reason for performance on which you were rated poorly or believe there has been a misunderstanding, it is perfectly acceptable to give an explanation. For example, if it turns out you were given incorrect instructions about how to perform a procedure, let your supervisor know and ask for help.

In the spirit of developing a positive relationship and increasing your value to the facility, tell your supervisor how he or she can assist you. Examples include providing additional information about the job, explaining rules, giving you regular feedback about your work, or directing you to sources of additional training and information. Work with your supervisor to set professional goals for yourself. In some organizations, setting and reviewing goals are the main part of the performance review.

Withhold criticism and complaints during the review. This is not the appropriate time to present your list of complaints about the workplace. You will come across as defensive. Do not become angry. Use your energy to learn as much as possible in the current situation. Suggestions from your perspective can best be presented at another time.

Formal performance evaluations, when approached as opportunities rather than something to be endured, can be constructive experiences. Combine them with self-evaluations to help keep your career on course.

Case Study 17-1

Being Willing to Learn

Jason Handler owns a physical therapy agency that employs two other physical therapists and three assistants. He has built a good reputation with local physicians, especially orthopedic surgeons, for his work with patients who have had joint replacements. There are other physical therapists in town and creating these relationships has taken Jason several years of hard work.

Part of Jason's success is the result of hiring good employees. He emphasizes good customer service and looks for therapists and assistants who have a combination of good technical and people skills. Physical therapy is often uncomfortable for patients who have been injured or have recently undergone surgery, so encouraging them can be critical to their successful healing.

Empathy and the ability to communicate are essential skills.

Jason has worked with the career services director at nearby Sterling College for several years. The physical therapist assistant program has an excellent reputation for training highly qualified graduates. So when Ms. Waller recommends Sean Stuart, Jason agrees to interview him. The interview goes well and Sean agrees with Jason that customer service is indeed important.

Sean is hired to begin work under the supervision of Julie, one of the agency's therapists. After a couple of weeks, Sean is able to work without direct supervision. And this is when problems begin to surface. One morning Jason receives a call from Dr. Stewart who tells him that his knee-replacement

Wellness Plus Physicians Group
Employee Performance Review

Name: _____   Position: _____

Hire Date: _____   Date of Last
                                             Performance
Supervisor: _____   Evaluation: _____

Rating Scale: 1 = Excellent   2 = Very good   3 = Satisfactory   4 = Needs some improvement   5 = Needs much improvement

A. Quality of work performed   Comments:

    Rating   1   2   3   4   5

B. Use of judgment   Comments:

    Rating   1   2   3   4   5

C. Dependability   Comments:

    Rating   1   2   3   4   5

D. Cooperation with others   Comments:

    Rating   1   2   3   4   5

E. Appearance and hygiene   Comments:

    Rating   1   2   3   4   5

F. Attendance and punctuality   Comments:

    Rating   1   2   3   4   5

G. Time management   Comments:

    Rating   1   2   3   4   5

H. Proper use of equipment   Comments:
   and supplies

    Rating   1   2   3   4   5

I. Ability to work independently   Comments:

    Rating   1   2   3   4   5

(1)

FIGURE 17-1 **Sample performance review.** Note how many of the qualities evaluated are soft skills. *How can you use performance evaluations to monitor your own progress on the job?*

Continued

**Wellness Plus Physicians Group
Employee Performance Review**

Rating Scale: 1 = Excellent   2 = Very good   3 = Satisfactory   4 = Needs some improvement   5 = Needs much improvement

J. Communication skills   Comments:

   Rating   1   2   3   4   5

K. Willingness to take direction   Comments:
   and suggestions

   Rating   1   2   3   4   5

L. Ability to adapt to change   Comments:

   Rating   1   2   3   4   5

Employee's greatest strengths: _____
_____

Progress in meeting goals from last review: _____
_____

New goals for improvement: _____
_____

Plan for achieving goals: _____
_____

Overall evaluation of this employee: _____
_____

Reviewed by: _____

Date: _____

Employee signature _____

Date: _____
       (Signature does not necessarily
       mean agreement)

(2)

FIGURE 17-1, cont'd

patient, during a post-operative follow-up visit, reported that he was unhappy with his physical therapy.

"I'm surprised—and sorry to hear that," said Jason.

"Yes, I was too. My patients have always been happy with your agency. We've had good results working together in the past," said Dr. Stewart.

At this point, Jason isn't sure what to say, but he assures Dr. Stewart he'll look into the situation. After hanging up the phone, he checks the files and finds the record for Dr. Stewart's patient. Julie evaluated the patient and developed the treatment plan. The assistant who is working with the patient is Sean.

Jason looks into the situation to see if the dissatisfaction is limited to Dr. Stewart's patient or if there are other problems. He asks the therapists to speak confidentially with the patients who have worked with Sean to learn if they are happy with their treatment. After a few days, he receives reports from Julie, and Craig, the other therapist. He is concerned with what he hears, but glad he looked into the matter. Several of the patients feel that Sean lacks compassion, but were hesitant to speak up because they had been told that without physical therapy, they wouldn't recover from their surgery successfully. They assumed that pain was to be expected. Their doctors had sent them to Jason's agency and they didn't think to complain. A couple of the patients didn't want to say anything negative about their therapy, but it is evident from their body language and lack of enthusiasm that they aren't totally satisfied.

It's a few weeks early for Sean's 90-day evaluation as a new employee, but Jason knows he must take action now. He calls Sean into his office the day after receiving the reports from the therapists.

"Sean," starts Jason. "You've only been out of school a short time and I've been impressed with your knowledge of therapeutic modalities. But working with our patients requires more than that—much more, actually. Patients who come to us obviously have physical problems that need addressing. But they also bring psychological and emotional issues with them."

"Yes," Sean tells Jason. "Inspiring patients to do their best is something that was emphasized in our program at school."

"Well, Sean, I'm confused to hear you say that. Because what we're hearing from patients is that they feel you lack compassion—that you don't empathize with their condition."

"I want them to get better—to recover from surgery or whatever. That's my job, isn't it?" asks Sean. "I tell them they must do the exercises prescribed for them if they want to improve."

"This is true," says Jason. "But I think they want you to understand what they've been through and how difficult it is for them sometimes. They're in pain, they're worried about whether they'll ever get back to where they were. They may even be wondering if they should have had that knee replacement. Or they may be beating themselves up about having the accident that caused their injuries. It's really a hard time for them."

"You know," says Sean. "I guess I didn't really think about all this. I was so focused on helping them improve physically, I didn't realize all they're going through."

"Realizing this is a good start," says Jason. "What I'd like you to do are some exercises to increase your empathy and therapeutic communication skills. There's a really good workshop given at the hospital downtown every month. And I recommend that you take a look at the charts of the patients you work with and see what their situation is—learn more about them and what they are dealing with. Are you willing to do this?"

"I am," says Sean. "I really do want to help people. And I appreciate your helping me to do that. I guess you could have just fired me. So thanks, Jason."

Questions for Thought and Reflection

1. How did Sean misinterpret what it means to inspire patients to do their best?
2. What do you think about the way Jason handled the situation with Sean?
3. Why is empathy important when working with patients?
4. How can the way the health care provider communicates with patients influence their healing?
5. Do you think Sean will become a successful physical therapist assistant? Why or why not?

☐ Prescription for Success: 17-1
Make Reviews Work for You

Role-play the following situations with a classmate who takes the role of your supervisor.

1. Explain that you failed to follow certain safety procedures because you weren't told about them when you were hired.
2. Discuss three goals you want to achieve by your next formal evaluation.

Keeping Current

In Chapter 16 we discussed the importance of staying current in your field and how there will be continual changes and advances

in health care (Figure 17-2). In some professions, earning a certain number of continuing education units (CEUs) or participating in continuing professional education (CPE) is mandatory for renewing your license or certification. The required numbers are set by licensing boards, state regulatory agencies, and/or professional organizations. It is important for you to know exactly what is required for your profession. There are a variety of ways to earn these credits, including the following:

- Classes at local colleges and universities
- Workshops sponsored by your employer, another health care facility, or your professional organization
- Written assignments offered through correspondence courses or offered in your professional journal
- Distance education classes and workshops offered over the Internet

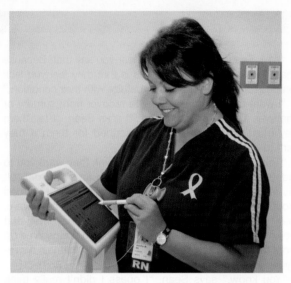

FIGURE 17-2 Computers are so common today it's hard to believe that many health care workers began their careers before computers were used. Advancements in technology have occurred at a fast rate, resulting today in hand-held computers, such as the one in the photo, that permit point-of-care documentation. *How can you be prepared to adapt to changes that will occur throughout your career?* (From Yoder-Wise PS: *Leading and managing in nursing*, ed 6, St Louis, 2015, Mosby.)

The agency or organization that requires the units, not the education provider, determines which units will be accepted. Before participating in any learning activity for credit, make sure it will be accepted by the appropriate agency, then request documentation showing that you attended and/or completed the work necessary to earn the credits. You may be required to submit proof along with your certification renewal application. Some employers provide training allowances and pay for classes to help their employees stay current.

An important source of learning throughout your career is your own experience. As you repeat the tasks of your profession, make decisions, and solve problems, you will gain confidence and the "knowing" that comes with practice.

Prescription for Success: 17-2
Getting Those Units

Identify ways you can earn the continuing education units (CEUs) necessary for your profession. Record the sponsor, requirements, units, and cost for each of the learning activities given below:

- Workshops
- College classes
- Distance learning
- Reading assignments
- Hands-on activities
- Professional conferences
- Other

Staying Connected

Once you are employed, maintain and expand your network. Stay in touch with your instructors, career services staff, classmates, mentors, and any professionals who assisted you during your training or job search. There are a number of reasons for staying connected. Other professionals can help you keep up-to-date in your field by sharing knowledge, ideas, and sources of information. If you want to change jobs in the future, they can be good sources of information. And networking is a two-way street: others may need your assistance. Finally, it's fun to have friends in the profession. Seeing them at meetings, workshops, and conferences adds to the enjoyment of having a career.

Becoming a Leader in Your Profession

Achieving excellence on the job is the first step toward becoming a leader in your profession. As you gain experience, there are other actions you can take to both enhance your career and increase your contributions to your employer, profession, and the general health care field.

- Participate actively in your professional organization. Join committees, run for office, give presentations, and attend the annual conference.
- Help new employees get started. Volunteer to orient, train, and act as a mentor.
- Become an externship supervisor at your facility. Help students acquire the on-site experience they need to complete their education.
- Teach seminars and workshops for your professional organization, facility, or local schools and colleges.
- Write articles for professional journals.
- Support legislation that promotes health care issues.
- Promote wellness and public access to health care.

Earning a Promotion

"Recognize opportunities and go through the door when it's open."
—Rick Baird

Earning a promotion is a satisfying reward for your hard work. Did you notice the use of the word "earning"? You must demonstrate that you have what it takes to be given more responsibility. If earning promotions is on your list of career goals, there are a number of ways to increase your chances, including the following:

- Be 100% dependable. Develop a reputation for being on time, being on task, and following through on all assigned duties.
- Demonstrate leadership skills. Help and encourage others, be a productive and cooperative team member, and develop excellent communication skills.
- Strive for excellence. Set high personal and professional standards. Continually develop your skills and acquire new ones.

- Increase your value to the organization. Take on additional responsibilities, and volunteer for committees and special projects. Look for ways to make positive contributions.
- Advertise your interest. Let your supervisor know you are interested in a promotion. Find out about the necessary qualifications, and develop a plan for acquiring any you don't have.

- Sell yourself. If you must apply for the new position formally, be prepared. Review your accomplishments and select examples of work that demonstrate why you are qualified for the new position. Don't assume that the interviewer—even if it is your own supervisor—is aware of all your qualifications.

Trouble Ahead? 17-1

Erin has worked in the billing department at Hallmark Hospital for 11 years. She enjoys working with numbers and is good with details, so this job has been a good fit for her. Erin especially likes the fact that she has a nine-to-five job. She sees the long hours that other staff members are sometimes required to work when there is an emergency, a nursing shortage, or other occurrences for which patient-care personnel are needed. As Erin tells her friend Jeanine at lunch one day, "I'm just not into work that much. I mean, I need to earn a living, but eight hours a day is enough. There's way more to life than work!"

At the same time, Erin prides herself on the quality of her work. She rarely makes errors. This is a good thing because she really doesn't like to "waste her time," as she puts it, having to explain to her supervisor or worse, to patients, about mistakes and how she will correct them. Because she believes her work to be among the best in her department, she is surprised—and upset—when Luann, an employee who has worked at the hospital for only four years, is promoted to supervisor, a job Erin had believed was rightfully hers as the employee with the most seniority.

"I really can't believe this!" she tells Jeanine the evening after the promotion is announced. "I nailed that interview with Mr. Hopkins. I've been around there longer than anyone and totally know what's going on in the department."

"Yeah," agrees Jeanine. "It seems like you've been there forever. I'm sure you know how to run that department."

"I wonder if Luann knows someone higher up—maybe she's friends with somebody who has some influence," Erin wonders out loud.

"Well," says Jeanine, "I guess it wouldn't hurt to check it out."

That night, Erin thinks about approaching Mr. Hopkins tomorrow. She knows she was the best candidate for the supervisory position and plans to point out to him what made her the best choice. The next day she goes to Mr. Hopkins' office, but is told he won't have time to see her until the next week. Erin lets his assistant know this is unacceptable, but it seems there isn't anything that can be done. Mr. Hopkins is busy with meetings and is preparing for a presentation he will be giving at a conference later in the week, so she will have to wait to see him.

The following Tuesday at her meeting with Mr. Hopkins, she lets him know how disappointed she is at not being promoted to supervisor of the billing department.

"After all," she points out to Mr. Hopkins, "I've been working in that department for 11 years. I know the systems inside and out. I'm definitely the most qualified."

"Erin," explains Mr. Hopkins. "Knowing the systems is not the only requirement for a supervisory position. What we need is someone who has people and leadership skills. Someone who can set positive goals for the department, inspire the employees to do their best, help them when they want to improve their skills—someone who will lead the department."

"Really, Mr. Hopkins," says Erin. "It seems to me that my setting an example of how best to do the work would be what you're looking for."

"I'm afraid that's not always the case," explains Mr. Hopkins. "In fact, from the impression you gave during your interview, you told me that you thought employees should 'buckle down and do their work' without a lot of supervision. I think you also told me that there were some people in the department that probably shouldn't be there."

"Well, yes," responds Erin. "If people can't pay attention to their work and do a good job, they should find something else to do."

"A supervisor's responsibility is to encourage employees—help them learn and realize their potential," explains Mr. Hopkins. "I also want to mention that your refusal to put in extra time was not in your favor. Sometimes it's necessary to put in a little extra time—this is especially true for supervisors at the hospital."

"That doesn't make sense to me. If people are efficient, they really shouldn't have to put in extra time," said Erin.

Questions for Thought and Reflection

1. Do you think Erin should have been promoted to the supervisory position? Why or why not?
2. How does Mr. Hopkins handle being confronted by Erin?
3. What would you have said to Erin if you were Mr. Hopkins?"
4. What is your opinion of Erin's attitude about her job?
5. What are five important characteristics of an effective supervisor?

Becoming the Supervisor

"The purpose of management is to maximize people's strengths and make their weaknesses irrelevant."

—Peter Drucker

Receiving a promotion is something you can be proud of. Enjoy the good feelings that come with having attained a significant accomplishment. At the same time, recognize and be willing to accept the increased responsibilities that are almost certainly included. If you are promoted to a supervisory position, you are now accountable not only for your own work, but for that of others as well. A special challenge occurs if former coworkers now report to you. This is sometimes an awkward situation, especially if you are friends outside the workplace. You may feel uncomfortable giving them directions and evaluating them. On the other hand, you can build on these positive relationships to develop a team that pulls together to accomplish group goals. Your priority now must be to ensure that the assigned work is completed satisfactorily. True friends will understand and support these efforts. Do take care that all employees are treated equally and fairly, regardless of previous relationships.

Being a successful supervisor may mean adding some new skills to the ones that helped you earn the new position. For example, building productive teams, organizing work schedules, and running effective meetings require skills that are different from those needed to be a good dental assistant, medical transcriptionist, or laboratory technician. The information in this section is only a brief introduction to supervision, intended to stimulate further study. If your future goals include becoming a supervisor, prepare ahead by acquiring the necessary knowledge by taking classes and/or self-study on topics such as personnel management, motivation, public speaking, budgeting, evaluation techniques, and long-range planning. Successful supervisors have good people skills. An important part of their job is to inspire others to do their best. There are many ways to accomplish this, including the following:

- Setting a positive tone for the group. Promoting the mission of the organization. Emphasizing the value of the work. Being enthusiastic and sharing your enthusiasm with others.

- Keeping the group focused on accomplishing worthy goals: delivering high-quality patient care, performing work accurately, and supporting the efforts of the organization.
- Giving continuous, appropriate feedback. Encouraging the employees' best efforts with public praise. Helping them improve by giving constructive criticism in private. Employees deserve the opportunity to make needed changes, and this is possible only if they know what the problems are.
- Recognizing and building on each employee's strengths and weakness, whenever possible, by assigning appropriate tasks.
- Clearly communicating your expectations. Assumptions are dangerous: what is obvious to you may be "as clear as mud" to others.
- Delegating appropriately. Too much and employees will resent you. Too little and you will find yourself worn out and/or unable to complete your work.

(See Figure 17-3.)

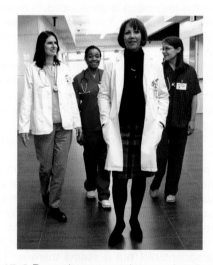

FIGURE 17-3 Becoming a supervisor requires the acquisition of new skills. In addition to being technically competent, good supervisors organize and inspire others to do their best. *Are you interested in becoming a supervisor in the future? What skills will you need to develop to be a successful supervisor?* (From Yoder-Wise PS: *Leading and managing in nursing,* ed 6, St Louis, 2015, Mosby.)

Rick Baird

Rick Baird, former Chief Human Resources Officer at Bend Memorial Clinic in Bend, Oregon, discusses how to succeed in the workplace and shares how his clinic evaluates employees.

Q How can health care employees increase their value to their employers?

A Customer service is the focus of today's health care environment—at least for our clinic. I want employees who will help make my business better. A major way they can do this is by increasing customer satisfaction—making patients feel important. Empathy is key to accomplishing this.

Showing appreciation for coworkers and being courteous with everyone may seem obvious but are sometimes overlooked. The ability to flourish in a social environment makes work satisfying and helps employees get ahead.

Q Do you have other suggestions for getting along with others?

A Yes. Demonstrate a positive, can-do attitude. Go with the flow. Be curious and seek out opportunities to learn. At the same time, be careful about not being a know-it-all. This can get you ostracized at work.

Q How do you measure employee performance?

A We do performance reviews annually. The ratings are based on objective performance standards written in concrete terms instead of them being very general. For example, we include the number of times a person was absent. We also have specific criteria that pertain to the job—for example, giving appropriate treatments to patients.

We always assign goals as part of performance reviews—two or three for each employee. We work with them to establish SMART goals.

Q What exactly are SMART goals?

A *S* stands for simple; *M* for measurable; *A* for attainable; *R* for reasonable; and *T* for time constrained—that is, it can be achieved in the time available.

At our clinic, we do focal reviews.

Q What are these?

A It means we do all employee reviews at the same time—during the month of October. This is instead of doing reviews based on each person's hire date. We plan in-house education and other activities to focus on self-improvement during the whole month.

Deciding to Leave a Job

Making the decision to leave a job should be done thoughtfully. It is important that you are clear about why you want to leave. Take time to review the situation carefully and identify the real problems. If you are unhappy at work, changing jobs may not be the answer. For example, if your own work habits are at the root of your dissatisfaction, working elsewhere will not necessarily be an improvement. Our personal baggage, consisting of our attitudes, habits, and abilities, goes along with us. Some people spend years jumping from one job to another, yet never find the right one. They fail to realize that the changes need to come from within themselves.

Review your current job by answering the following questions as honestly as possible:

1. How might I be contributing to my own dissatisfaction?
2. Do I have difficulty communicating effectively?
3. Does it take me longer than others to complete assigned tasks?
4. What can I do to improve my performance?
5. Have I asked for help?
6. Have I spoken with my supervisor about my dissatisfaction?
7. Do I need additional skills?
8. Are my expectations about work realistic?
9. Would requesting a transfer or promotion resolve the problem?
10. Do I have the experience and training for the job I really want?

You may discover that you can transform your current job into one that is more acceptable. Once you have identified the problems, you may be able to solve them by changing your attitude, developing a plan, seeking help, and applying your best efforts. On the other hand, some factors are simply out of your control. Your best efforts may not be enough to overcome poor management, disorganization, lack of adequate resources, and low integrity. An example is being repeatedly told to perform tasks beyond your level of training and experience or outside your scope of practice. Before making the decision to leave a job, consider filing a grievance, described in Chapter 16, if you feel you are being treated unfairly or illegally. When all efforts at resolution fail or if the facility is simply unable to accommodate your needs, finding employment elsewhere may be in your best professional interest.

Seeking New Opportunities

You may like your job but still feel the need to make a change. This can happen as you gain work experience, discover areas of particular interest, and/or want more opportunities for professional growth. Changes can be necessary steps on the road to achieving your long-term personal and career goals such as in the following situations:

- You are ready—and qualified—for more challenge and responsibility, but opportunities are limited because of the size or organizational structure of your place of employment.
- You want to spend more time working in a particular occupational area.
- You need assistance paying for additional training, but your employer's budget does not include funding for this purpose.
- You want to spend more time with your family, but the required work schedules do not permit this.
- Your duties are limited, and you want a chance to apply more of your training.
- You would like to work with a different patient population or health care specialty.

Sometimes opportunities simply present themselves. For example, a friend tells you about an opening in the clinic where she "just loves working." Or a facility with an excellent reputation in your field announces a promising position. You may find yourself in the position of having to make a choice between the known—your current job—and the unknown—a new job that may or may not be better.

Using a Decision Matrix

When you are faced with choosing among alternatives, a **decision matrix** helps you compare how they meet your requirements. The matrix is a table consisting of squares in which you record ratings and scores for each alternative. Here are the steps for putting together this handy tool:

Step 1: On a piece of paper, or on your computer, prepare an empty table using Table 17-1 as an example.

Step 2: List all the features of work that apply to the jobs you are considering. Review the list you created in Prescription for Success 12-2 and the examples in Table 17-1. Add any others that apply to you.

Step 3: Rate each feature with a number:
1 = Not important to me (no preference)
2 = Somewhat important to me
3 = Very important to me

TABLE 17-1
Sample Decision Matrix for Choosing a Job

Feature	Ratings (1, 2, 3)	Current Job	Proposed Job
Population served	2	1 2×1 = 2	2 2×2 = 4
Geographic location	1	2 1×2 = 2	1 1×1 = 1
Specialty	1	2 1×2 = 2	2 1×2 = 2
Independence given employees	3	1 3×1 = 3	2 3×2 = 6
Work pace	1	2 1×2 = 2	2 1×2 = 2
Variety of duties	2	1 2×1 = 2	2 2×2 = 4
Training opportunities	3	1 3×1 = 3	2 3×2 = 6
Reputation of facility	3	2 3×2 = 6	2 3×2 = 6
Opportunities for advancement	2	1 2×1 = 2	2 2×2 = 4
Challenge	2	1 2×1 = 2	2 2×2 = 4
Responsibility	2	1 2×1 = 2	2 2×2 = 4
Cooperativeness of coworkers	2	2 2×2 = 4	2 2×2 = 4
Work and mission align with your values	3	2 3×2 = 6	2 3×2 = 6
Orientation to health care (emphasis on wellness, acceptance of alternative therapies)	3	1 3×1 = 3	1 3×1 = 3
Pay	2	1 2×1 = 2	2 2×2 = 4
Benefits (insurance, vacation, etc.)	2	2 2×2 = 4	2 2×2 = 4
Work schedule	1	2 1×2 = 2	1 1×1 = 1
Contribution to society	2	2 2×2 = 4	2 2×2 = 4
Total Scores		**53**	**69**

Write the corresponding number next to each feature in the ratings column.

Step 4: Rank each job as you believe it will meet your needs:
1 = Unlikely or unknown
2 = Very likely

Write the numbers in the top right section of the corresponding squares.

Note: This may require some research to find out about the proposed job: good interview questions, talking with people who work at the facility, and reviewing the organization's website and published information.

Step 5: Multiply the number assigned to each feature (rating) by the ranking number for each job (1 or 2).

Step 6: Add the results of your calculations. The job with the highest score is most likely to meet your needs.

You can create a decision matrix that includes your list of features before you interview for a new job. This provides a method for planning questions to get the exact information you'll need to make an informed decision.

If going through this process seems like too much trouble, consider the trouble that can result from making poor career decisions. Where you spend the majority of your waking hours affects the quality of your life. Taking sufficient time to research, review, and properly manage your career will pay off. Using a decision matrix enables you to identify what matters most to you and to measure to what degree your professional needs are being met.

The decision matrix is also a useful tool for periodically reviewing your level of job satisfaction. Instead of comparing two or more jobs, rate the one you have every few months, and compare the results over time. How well does it continue to meet your needs? Have your preferences changed over time? Clearly identifying the sources of dissatisfaction makes it much easier to seek solutions, whether this means making changes in the job you have, or looking for another one. Saying "I'm bored here" is not very informative. Saying "I perform only three tasks over and over each day" is more useful information. You can request more assignments at your present job or look for a job that offers a wider variety of tasks.

Finally, using the matrix allows you to see whether your preferences align with your personal qualities and abilities. For example, if you rate "opportunities for advancement" as "very important" and "independence," "challenge," and "responsibility" as "not important," your goals are not realistic. Desires must be balanced with willingness to perform.

You can use a decision matrix in other areas of your life. Some examples include choosing the most practical car to buy, the most appropriate medical insurance plan for your family, the best school to attend for your advanced training, and the most desirable house to buy or rent. Try using a decision matrix the next time you must choose between alternatives. Use the left column to list the features most important to you. Then assign rating numbers and compare the alternatives.

Preparing to Change Jobs

Most employment experts recommend that you do not resign from a job until you have a firm offer for another one. It is generally believed that individuals are more employable if they are currently working. Perhaps more important, you are in a better position financially to look around and find a suitable position. This is especially true if the job market is tight and not many positions are available.

You may decide, however, that you need time to reenergize and reorganize. Difficulties at work can take all your attention and leave you with little energy to look for another job. In this case, plan to have at least six months of living expenses put aside. (Actually, it is good personal management always to have at least six months of living expenses available in case of an emergency, even if you aren't planning to leave your job.)

Develop a network of support among friends and family members. Even leaving a job voluntarily can be stressful. Call on people who endorse your decision and can offer encouragement during your job search and transition.

Long-term career success requires that you establish a stable work record. A pattern of frequent job changes can discourage employers from hiring you. They want employees to stay for a reasonable period of time because hiring and training expenses represent a substantial investment of time and money. On the other hand, remaining too long in a position that drains your enthusiasm and stifles your progress is not a sound career decision. Consider your mission, personal values, and long-term goals when deciding whether to change jobs.

Leaving on a Positive Note

Regardless of the circumstances, make your departure as gracious as possible. "It's a small world" certainly applies to employment, including health care. Employers meet at professional meetings, seminars, and country clubs. Even if you didn't like your last supervisor, he or she may play golf with someone you would love to work for. Here are some suggestions for keeping the relationship as positive as possible:

- Give sufficient notice. Two weeks is considered the minimum.
- Write a letter of resignation in which you thank the employer for the opportunities extended.
- It is not necessary to state the reason you are resigning, although in some cases it is appropriate.
- It's not a good idea to include complaints in the letter. See Figure 17-4 for a sample letter of resignation.
- Submit your resignation to your supervisor before discussing it with anyone else at work.

1642 Windhill Way
San Antonio, TX 78220
February 16, 2015

Nancy Henderson, Office Manager
Craigmore Pediatric Clinic
4979 Coffee Road
San Antonio, TX 78229

Dear Ms. Henderson:

I am writing this letter as my official resignation from Craigmore Pediatric Clinic effective March 16, 2010. I have accepted a position at Cooke Children's Hospital.

The decision to leave Craigmore was not an easy one to make. I have enjoyed my work over the past two years and feel very fortunate to have had the opportunity to begin my health care career here.

Please accept my sincere thanks for all your help. A constant source of encouragement, you are a true example of professionalism and caring. You always inspired me to aim for excellence in my work.

I wish you and Craigmore Pediatric continuing success in the future.

Sincerely,

Karen Gonzalez

Karen Gonzalez

FIGURE 17-4 Sample letter of resignation. Note the positive tone of the letter. *Why is it recommended that you don't include complaints or criticism in a letter of resignation?*

- Pursue job leads and attend interviews on your own time, not that of your current employer.
- Be willing to help train your replacement (Figure 17-5).
- Refrain from complaining and informing your employer and coworkers about everything you find wrong with the workplace.
- Put forth your best efforts through your last day. Finish all tasks and leave your work area, equipment, and files in order.

During your last days on the job, you may find it difficult to focus fully and maintain a positive attitude. Situations like these are true tests of professionalism. Doing your best and completing your obligations, under any circumstances, will help you build your reputation as a dependable health care professional. You are, in a sense, buying insurance for a successful future.

If you have enjoyed working with your supervisor, let him or her know. A thank-you note, separate from the letter of resignation, is a nice gesture. Express your appreciation for the supervisor's help. You may work with this person in the future. Add him or her to your network of contacts and stay in touch. Ask for a letter of recommendation for possible future use.

Take a little time to reflect on what you accomplished and learned on this job. Add anything that demonstrates this to your professional portfolio, along with your letter of recommendation.

Andrew has never been a happy person. Things just never seem to go his way—and it's always someone else's fault. When he didn't have the clothes or electronic devices he wanted as a kid, it was his dad's fault. His father just "didn't earn enough money," he told his friends. As a high school student, he had to drive an old car given to him by his grandmother after his grandfather died. Rather than appreciating having a car at all—many of his friends had to walk or take the bus—he grumbled about having to drive a "junker." His parents encouraged him to get a job during the summers, but he told them the jobs available were boring and besides, it would cut into his fun time. His parents knew they should encourage Andrew to look for a job, perhaps even insist, but he would argue and become so unpleasant, they just gave up.

Andrew did graduate from high school, although he had to take extra classes between his junior and senior year to ensure that he had enough credits. After all, he explained, his teachers did a poor job in the classroom and it wasn't his fault that he didn't pass all his classes.

A couple of months after Andrew graduated, his father suffered an accident at work and had to take time off to recover. It would take weeks before he was able to collect disability payments and in the meantime, the family had no income. Although Andrew resented the fact that he would have to make an effort to help out, he did get himself hired at a local grocery store stocking shelves and helping customers out to their cars with their groceries. It annoyed him how inconsiderate people were when they sometimes put items back in the wrong place on the shelves. And he was sure that many of the people he helped with their purchases could have taken care of themselves. But it was a paycheck, so he kept his complaints to a minimum.

Andrew's father eventually recovered enough to be given a desk job by his employer. And his mother had started a child day-care business in their home. Between the two of them, they again had enough income to get by. Andrew decided to quit his job at the grocery store and find something better. A friend of his was in school studying to be a laboratory technician and what he shared about his studies sounded interesting to Andrew. Maybe this was something he should look into.

He did enroll in a training program and in spite of his usual complaining about incompetent instructors, substandard equipment, and no one telling him what he needed to know about school rules (published in the school catalog), he managed to graduate. He even had to admit to himself that he found the subject interesting. He discovered that he enjoyed chemistry and biology and he liked working with the specialized equipment and computers.

Andrew lives in a large city and was able to get a job in a diagnostic laboratory that performed tests for many local physicians and small clinics that didn't have their own labs. He discovered that in the beginning, he would be doing basic tasks such as setting up equipment, sanitizing glassware, and preparing specimens. He believed these tasks to be beneath his training and complained about it to his coworkers. After a few days, they grew tired of his complaints and explained they had all started out this way—that he needed to get oriented to the lab before starting on performing tests and other more complex work.

However, even after Andrew was allowed to perform tests and oversee automated analyses, he was not happy. In his opinion, some of his coworkers were incompetent; his supervisor didn't give clear instructions, resulting in Andrew making mistakes; and in his opinion, the lab was disorganized. As in the past, Andrew blamed any problems he experienced on others. Finally, one day, a coworker who had had to work closely with Andrew told him, "Look, if you really don't like it here, why don't you just quit?"

Andrew was angry about this remark and decided to approach the lab's director, Dr. Ferragamo. Their conversation was not as Andrew had expected because rather than taking Andrew's side, the director told him that he had been receiving complaints about his negative behavior.

"Andrew," said Dr. Ferragamo. "The fact is that you are unpleasant to work with. For the lab to work efficiently we need to work as a team. And you just don't seem to want to be a contributing member of that team."

"Well," responded Andrew. "I just call it like it is. That's just being honest, isn't it? I don't think the lab is being run that well and I can't pretend that I'm happy here."

"I don't want you to take this the wrong way, but from what I'm seeing, I don't know if you'd be happy anywhere, Andrew," said Mr. Ferragamo in a kind voice.

"You know what? This is just ridiculous. I quit!" And Andrew stomped out the door.

Questions for Thought and Reflection

1. What can happen when someone like Andrew doesn't want to be part of the work team?
2. What would be the possible consequences for the lab if Andrew had stayed in the job and continued his negative behavior?
3. If Andrew had not quit, do you think Dr. Ferragamo should have fired him? Why or why not?
4. What does Andrew need to do if he is to have a successful future?

Prescription for Success: 17-5 Put It in Words

Write a letter of resignation for a job that you have enjoyed. You are leaving to work in a larger facility where you have been offered a position with more responsibilities at higher pay.

Hitting Rough Waters: What to Do if You're Fired

"Men's best successes come after their disappointments."
—Henry Ward Beecher

Being fired from a job can be like being tossed off a ship into high seas. The water is cold, and the waves are scary. You may

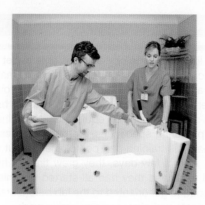

FIGURE 17-5 When you leave a job, offer to train your replacement. A smooth transition will benefit both your employer and the patients or clients. *What are the possible consequences when employees leave without making smooth transitions?* (From Sorrentino S, Remmert L: *Mosby's textbook for nursing assistants,* ed 8, St Louis, 2012, Mosby.)

wonder if you'll survive. Not only can you survive being fired, but you can also use the experience to grow personally and professionally.

Your first concern, however, is to stay afloat. Thrashing about by becoming angry and defensive and lashing out at your supervisor will only make matters worse and put your career in danger of drowning. When you receive the news that you are being fired, it is recommended that you do the following:

- Understand that firing an employee can difficult and uncomfortable for supervisors.
- Ask for an explanation of the reasons for the decision. It is likely that you've already been advised about problems regarding your performance. Ask about anything you don't understand or believe had been corrected.
- Listen carefully and ask for feedback when necessary. This may be difficult under the circumstances, but it is critical for the communication to be as clear as possible.
- Request an opportunity to explain your side of the situation if you believe there has been a misunderstanding. Don't insist, however, if you are told that the decision is final. It will only hurt your case to argue, yell, or use abusive language.
- Ask your supervisor for suggestions about what you can do to prevent this from happening at a future job.
- Don't bring out your list of what is wrong with the workplace, supervisor, coworkers, and so on. This gives the appearance of making excuses and acting defensively. Keep focused on learning why this decision was made about you.

Be aware that in today's legal climate, many employers have dismissal policies that may seem harsh. For example, your supervisor may not be allowed to give you details about how the decision to dismiss you was made. You may be asked to gather your things, under supervision, and leave the workplace immediately. Keep in mind that these policies apply to all employees who are dismissed, not just you. Don't feel that you have been targeted or are necessarily considered to be

dishonest. Do your best to maintain your composure and do not make an already difficult situation worse.

Downsizing

Downsizing means reducing the number of employees. Companies sometimes let some employees go to control costs or to survive as a business. For example, a medical laboratory may be losing money because of competition and therefore not able to afford the cost of its current staff. Or an economic slowdown can reduce the amount of business. Downsizing also can occur when companies merge. If two clinics are combined as a result of one company buying another, there may be duplications in the staff.

The decision about who to keep and who to let go is not easy for managers. Frequently, downsizing requires cuts to be made at all levels, so the managers themselves may lose their jobs. If you are ever let go because of downsizing, try your best not to take it personally. You are not being fired for poor performance; rather, you are a victim of circumstances beyond your control. Future potential employers are likely to understand your situation.

Getting to Shore

"Success seems to be largely a matter of hanging on after others have let go."
—William Feather

Life preservers come in many forms: friends, family, mentors, instructors, and other school personnel. Use them wisely. Their role is to provide encouragement, emotional support, and honest feedback; it is not to listen to endless complaints and harrowing stories about the job and how you were mistreated.

Bring your personal resources to the rescue efforts. Rebuild your confidence by reviewing your strengths, achievements, and positive traits. Losing a job need not drown your chances for long-term success. You can get to shore by deciding to learn from the experience and by taking the actions necessary to move on with your career.

Start the process by looking at yourself honestly. Recognizing the need for self-improvement is empowering because then you can take responsibility for making changes to improve your future. Blaming others, or denying that you are at fault in any way, puts change out of your control. It's like saying, "I'm doomed, because I have to depend on others to save me. There's nothing I can do."

Accepting responsibility means asking some hard questions to help you learn from the experience of being fired. This is the first step to prevent it from happening again. Whatever the problems, you must be willing to face them and commit to finding solutions. Table 17-2 contains examples of questions and actions for dealing with specific problems.

Note: If, after conducting your self-evaluation, you sincerely believe that your dismissal was unjust, unfair, and/or based on factors that were not related to your job performance (discrimination), you may decide to seek legal advice. You must be prepared to demonstrate and document that your performance was satisfactory and to prove that you were treated unfairly.

TABLE 17-2

Learning from Experience

Reason Given for Dismissal	Types of Questions to Ask Yourself	Suggested Actions
Poor work performance	Do I lack the skills? Am I simply careless? Do I work too quickly? Do I care about the quality of my work? Am I aware of my poor performance? Do I ask for help when I'm not sure about something? Am I willing to work on improving my skills?	Contact your school for possible refresher training. Review textbooks, notes, and tests. In the future, ask your supervisor for help when you are having difficulty. Don't ignore problems. Never try to cover up poor performance. It will become obvious and is not fair to those who depend on your work.
Excessive absences	Am I failing to make work a top priority? Am I practicing good health habits? Getting enough rest? Are there health problems I need to take care of? Do I need to improve my personal organization skills to prevent frequent personal "emergencies"?	Commit to making work a top priority. Develop good health habits and seek professional help if necessary. Develop backup plans for childcare, transportation, etc. Redefine "emergency." Work to become accident-proof rather than accident-prone. Seek help in resolving personal and/or family problems.
Violation of facility rules and/or failure to follow directions	Do I know the rules but choose to disregard them? Why? Do I misunderstand directions? How can I learn what rules are in force?	Review the importance of following rules for maintaining personal and patient safety and fulfilling legal and regulatory requirements. Ask for explanations of rules or directions you don't understand. Read policy and procedure manuals and any other sources of facility rules.
Inability to get along with others; poor interpersonal skills	Is there a pattern to my relationships with others? Do I fail to listen? Do I insist on being right and/or having my own way? Am I willing to do my share of the work? Do I gossip at work and talk about people behind their backs? Do I get involved in disputes and take sides?	Review the principles of good communication. Take a communications and/or interpersonal relations class. Request honest feedback from someone you trust. Seek counseling to help you examine and improve your relationships with others.
Poor attitude, lack of professionalism	In what ways is my behavior unprofessional? Is my concept of "professionalism" different from the employer's? Am I willing to change? Can I put patient and employer needs before my own preferences? What contributes to my poor attitude? Am I willing to change? What can I do to change?	Think about your reasons for choosing a career in health care to see whether your conduct is in alignment with them. Review the purpose and components of professionalism. Observe successful health care professionals. Seek help from a mentor.
Failure to follow safe techniques	Do I know the proper techniques? Do I understand the importance of using safe techniques? Do I understand the negative consequences of using improper techniques?	Review textbooks and notes from class and skills lab. Take refresher courses that include skills training.

Getting Back on Course

"Turn your stumbling blocks into stepping stones."

—Anonymous

When looking for another job, you may worry about telling potential employers you were fired from your last one. First of all, you don't have to volunteer this information if you are not asked. But if you are, be truthful. State that it didn't work out and that you were let go. It's not necessary to explain the situation in detail. Do not blame or criticize your previous employer. Do explain what you have learned from the situation and what you have done to ensure that it won't happen again. This demonstrates your honesty and ability to learn from mistakes, important qualities in the workplace. Let the employer know you are committed to getting your career back on course and want to begin by making a positive contribution to his or her organization. Once you are reemployed, there are ways you can avoid getting back into rough waters, such as the following:

- Do your best to keep communication lines open with your new supervisor.
- Learn to recognize warning signs and address problems immediately. Don't try to deny or cover them up. This only makes the situation worse.
- Ask for help before you get into trouble.
- Request regular feedback from your supervisor about your performance.
- Be conscientious about performing regular self-evaluations.

Many people who lose their jobs manage to bounce back and achieve career success. You can, too, if you use the experience as an opportunity to learn and grow, not as an excuse for future failure.

Enriching Your Career

The health care field offers many employment opportunities. There are dozens of ways to add interest and variety to your career. Your training may qualify you to work in a variety of settings. For example, the following are just some of the environments in which health care professionals work:

1. Hospitals
2. Long-term care facilities
3. Schools
4. Prisons
5. Homeless shelters
6. Mobile vans that provide medical care to migrant farm workers
7. Private homes
8. International settings, such as the Peace Corps or religious missions

Some professions offer great flexibility in locations and schedules. Certain occupational areas allow you to choose between working for one employer or for an agency that sends you on a variety of assignments that range from one day to six months or longer. If you enjoy a change of scenery and even a bit of adventure, you can look for short-term assignments at locations around the country—or even around the world.

The nature of health care delivery today enables professionals to apply their skills in a variety of ways. Your profession may allow you to accept new challenges and gain enriching experiences. Let's look at a few types of jobs available for health care professionals who have the necessary qualifications:

- Direct patient care in many specialty areas
- Education of both patients and other health care personnel
- Management and administration
- Quality review (checking patient records for accuracy and completeness of documentation and treatment outcomes)
- Oversight of performance improvement (comparing a facility's performance in specific areas, such as infection control, with health care industry standards)

Prescription for Success: 17-6
Find Out More

Research the work settings and types of jobs available in your occupational area.
1. How many can you find? List five here.
2. What qualifications are necessary for each?
3. Which ones seem most interesting to you?

Career Laddering

The concept of career laddering was introduced in Chapter 1. A career ladder consists of all the job titles within an occupational area that require various levels of education, skills, and responsibility. Figure 17-6 contains three health care examples. (See also Figure 17-7.)

Being successful does not necessarily mean climbing the ladder. In fact, aiming to do your best at your chosen level is a worthy goal. Gaining experience, perfecting your skills, and staying current are activities that can provide long-term satisfaction.

It is important to understand that the nature of the work varies among the levels. What is most appealing to you may not be found at higher-level jobs. For example, in the field of occupational therapy, a certified occupational therapist assistant generally spends more time working with patients than does the therapist, who often spends more time performing patient assessments, writing treatment plans, and performing administrative tasks. The conditions under which you work and the nature of the tasks may be different as well. In another example, a dental assistant works closely with the dentist, helping with a variety of procedures. A hygienist, on the other hand, works primarily alone with patients and performs similar work with each one.

Positions that have more supervisory responsibilities may limit the time spent performing lab tests, getting to know patients, giving treatments, or doing other tasks you enjoy. Before deciding to pursue additional training to move up the ladder, thoroughly investigate a job title that interests you by doing the following:

- Observe people at work who have the position.
- Interview them about their duties and responsibilities.
- If you are not working closely with professionals at the targeted level, ask permission to **job shadow** in another department or facility.
- Read about the job duties (see the Occupational Outlook Handbook at www.bls.gov/ooh).
- Request information from the appropriate professional organization.
- Review a sample curriculum and course descriptions.
- Obtain job descriptions.

Some schools have **step-up programs** so students can apply the courses they took for one occupational level to the next level. For example, there are programs that grant academic credits and waive certain courses for licensed practical nurses and licensed vocational nurses who enroll in registered nurse programs. Step-up programs are not available at all schools. They may also be selective about the schools from which they accept credits. Be sure to inquire about the transfer of credit policy when deciding where to pursue advanced training.

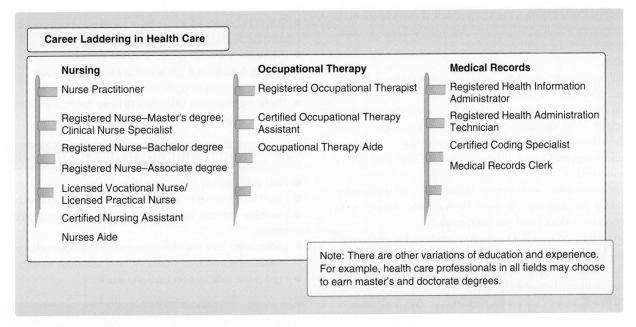

FIGURE 17-6 Examples of career laddering in health care. *What does the career ladder for your occupation look like?*

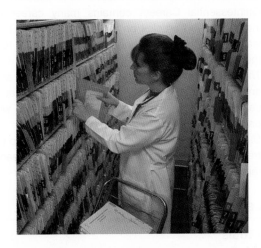

FIGURE 17-7 After gaining work experience, a medical records clerk may decide to pursue further training and become a coder or even a health information administrator. At the same time, she may find her current job satisfying. *Should all health care workers aim for higher levels in their occupations? Why or why not?* (From Bonewit-West K, Hunt S, Applegate E: *Today's medical assistant: Clinical and administrative procedures,* ed 2, St Louis, 2013, Saunders.)

Prescription for Success: 17-7
Your Career Ladder

Investigate the career ladder(s) in your occupational field.
1. What are the specific job titles on each rung of the ladder?
2. What are the educational requirements for each?
3. What are the licensing requirements for each?
4. Describe the differences in skill levels and responsibility among the levels.
5. How are the tasks different?

Developing a New Career

Many health care professionals have skills they can transfer from one occupational area to another. After acquiring work experience, you may decide to choose another type of work in which you use your health care background. Additional training or self-directed learning may be necessary to supplement your knowledge and skills.

The following examples illustrate careers open to people with health care backgrounds:
- Sales: Medical and pharmaceutical products
- Instructor or program director: Vocational schools, colleges, and universities
- Legal assistant: For attorneys who specialize in health care cases
- Consultant: Providing advice to individuals and organizations in your areas of expertise
- Writer: Reports, articles, proposals, textbooks, and patient education materials

The Health Care Entrepreneur

An **entrepreneur** is someone who organizes and manages a business. Starting a business or working on your own may appeal to you. Being the boss is an attractive idea: setting your own schedule, being accountable only to yourself, and enjoying the benefits of your work. There is another side to this, of course: having to work many hours, doing all the work yourself, and assuming responsibility for any financial losses. Not everyone is cut out for self-employment. Certain characteristics have been identified as desirable for successful entrepreneurs. Ask yourself if you have the following qualities:
- Competitive. Do you see yourself as a winner? Are you willing to put in the necessary effort to be one?

- Professionally competent. Are you skilled and experienced in the area you wish to pursue? Are your skills up-to-date?
- Persistent. Can you keep trying, even after experiencing failure?
- Willing to take risks. Are you comfortable taking a chance with your time? Your income?
- Self-disciplined. Do you stay with tasks until they are completed? Meet deadlines? Can you stay focused on work when there is something else you want to do?
- Self-confident. Do you believe in yourself and your ability to succeed?
- A problem solver and decision maker. Are you comfortable making decisions on your own? Do you follow through with action once decisions have been made?
- Financially prepared. Do you have enough money to support yourself until you develop an income?
- Organized. Do you organize your time well? Can you attend to more than one thing at a time?
- Informed about laws and regulations. Are you familiar with the laws that affect the area of health care in which you work? Do you understand the tax implications for people who work for themselves?

Health care lends itself to a number of home-based and small businesses. The following are just a few examples:
- Health care and nutritional product sales
- Medical report transcription
- Coding and billing services
- Consulting
- Provision of residential care

A key success factor is choosing a product or service for which there is a market. Even a good idea will fail if there aren't enough customers. Conducting market research is the first step when considering a business idea.

There are many sources of assistance for those who are interested in starting a small business or working on their own. Local Chambers of Commerce, the Small Business Administration, local government agencies, and SCORE, a volunteer group of retired business people, offer a variety of services ranging from free advice to reasonably priced classes to market research data. Colleges, universities, and adult education programs offer useful classes. Learn all you can before making the decision to venture out on your own.

Smooth Sailing

Managed wisely, your career can be a continual source of satisfaction. Choosing to work in health care ensures that what you do each day will benefit others. Monitor your performance, watch for opportunities, and enjoy the gratification that comes from staying on course and arriving at your planned career destination.

Summary of Key Ideas

- Careers must be managed to stay on course.
- Take responsibility for your performance evaluations.

- Staying connected and current increases both your career success and your enjoyment of work.
- Promotions are not given; they are earned.
- Getting fired from a job is not the end of a career.
- Never burn your bridges when leaving a job.
- There are many opportunities to keep your career interesting and engaging.

Positive Self-Talk for This Chapter

- I am successfully managing my career.
- I continually strive to improve my work and stay on course.
- I am able to make wise decisions about the direction of my career.
- I effectively use self-management tools like performance evaluations, decision matrices, and self-questioning.
- I get great satisfaction from my work.

Internet Activities

For active web links to the web sites needed to complete these activities, visit http://evolve.elsevier.com/Haroun/career/.
1. Quintessential Careers contains many career tools, including short articles on job-related issues. Read at least five of the articles and prepare a list of 10 recommendations for achieving workplace success.
2. The Wall Street Journal's career website has articles and corresponding quizzes to help readers achieve career success. Choose an article to read and write a paragraph describing what you have learned.
3. U.S. News and World Report can help you keep up on trends in health care. Choose two articles to read and report on.

To Learn More

Mind Tools

www.mindtools.com

This career-success website has articles on many topics including leadership and decision-making.

Occupational Outlook Handbook

U.S. Department of Labor

www.bls.gov/ooh

This is a source of detailed information about hundreds of careers, including typical job descriptions, educational requirements, and average salaries. It is updated every two years. It is a good source to explore career laddering, careers that are related, and possible work settings for various occupations.

Quintessential Careers

www.quintcareers.com/workplace_resources.html

The "Workplace Resources for Dealing With Your Current Job/Employer" page has links to dozens of helpful articles.

Professional Organizations for Health Care Occupations

Occupation	Organization	Contact Information
Cardiovascular Technologist	Alliance of Cardiovascular Professionals	P.O. Box 2007 Midlothian, VA 23113 (804) 632-0078 www.acp-online.org
Dental Assistant	American Dental Assistants Association	35 E. Wacker Drive Suite 1730 Chicago, IL 60601 (312) 541-1550 www.dentalassistant.org
Dental Hygienist	American Dental Hygienists' Association	444 N. Michigan Avenue, Suite 3400 Chicago, IL 60611 (312) 440-8900 www.adha.org
Dental Laboratory Technician	National Association of Dental Laboratories	325 John Knox Road # L103 Tallahassee, FL 32303 (800) 950-1150 www.nadl.org
Diagnostic Medical Sonographer	Society of Diagnostic Medical Sonographers	2745 Dallas Parkway Suite 350 Plano, TX 75093 (800) 229-9506 (214) 473-8057 www.sdms.org
Dietary Technician	Academy of Nutrition and Dietetics	120 South Riverside Plaza, Suite 2000 Chicago, IL 60606 (312) 899-0040 ext. 5400 www.eatright.org
	Society for Nutrition Education	9100 Purdue Road Suite 200 Indianapolis, IN 46268 (800) 235-6690 (317) 328-4627 www.sne.org
ECG Technician (Electrocardiographic Technician)	Alliance of Cardiovascular Professionals	P.O. Box 2007 Midlothian, VA 23113 (804) 632-0078 www.acp-online.org

Continued

Occupation	Organization	Contact Information
EEG Technician (Electroneu-rodiagnostic Technician or Technologist)	The Neurodiagnostic Society	402 East Bannister Road Suite A Kansas City, MO 64131 (816) 931-1120 www.aset.org
Emergency Medical Technician	National Association of Emergency Medical Technicians	P.O. Box 1400 Clinton, MS 39060 (800) 346-2368 www.naemt.org
Health Information Technician	American Health Information Management Association	233 N. Michigan Avenue 21st Floor Chicago, IL 60601 (312) 233-1100 www.ahima.org
Home Health Aide	National Network of Career Nursing Assistants	3577 Easton Road Norton, OH 44203 (330) 825-9342 www.cna-network.org
Massage Therapist	American Massage Therapy Association	500 Davis Street Suite 900 Evanston, IL 60201 (877) 905-0577 www.amtamassage.org
	Associated Bodywork and Massage Professionals	25188 Genesee Trail Road Suite 200 Golden, CO 80401 (800) 458-2267 www.abmp.com
Medical Assistant	American Association of Medical Assistants	20 N. Wacker Drive Suite 1575 Chicago, IL 60606 (312) 899-1500 www.aama-ntl.org
	American Medical Technologists	10700 West Higgins Road Suite 150 Rosemont, IL 60018 (847) 823-5169 www.americanmedtech.org
Medical Biller	Medical Association of Billers	2620 Regatta Drive Suite 102 Las Vegas, NV 89128 (702) 240-8519 www.physicianswebsites.com
Medical Insurance Coder	American Academy of Procedural Coders	2480 South 3850 West Suite B Salt Lake City, UT 84120 (800) 626-2633 www.aapc.com
	American Health Information Management Association	233 N. Michigan Avenue, 21st Floor Chicago, IL 60601 (312) 233-1100 www.ahima.org
Medical Laboratory Assistant or Medical Laboratory Technician	American Medical Technologists	10700 West Higgins Road Suite 150 Rosemont, IL 60018 (847) 823-5169 www.americanmedtech.org

Occupation	Organization	Contact Information
	The American Society for Clinical Laboratory Science	1861 International Drive Suite 200 McLean, VA 22102 (571) 748-3770 www.ascls.org
Medical Transcriptionist	Association for Healthcare Documentation Integrity	4230 Kiernan Avenue Suite 120 Modesto, CA 95356 (800) 982-2182 www.ahdionline.org
Nursing Assistant	National Network of Career Nursing Assistants	3577 Easton Road Norton, OH 44203 (330) 825-9342 www.cna-network.org
Occupational Therapy Assistant	American Occupational Therapy Association	4720 Montgomery Lane Suite 200 Bethesda, MD 20814 (301) 652-6611 www.aota.org
Ophthalmic Laboratory Technician	Opticians Association of America	3740 Canada Road Lakeland, TN 38002 (901) 388-2423 www.oaa.org
Ophthalmic Medical Assistant	Association of Technical Personnel in Ophthalmology	2025 Woodlane Drive St Paul, MN 55125 (800) 482-4858 www.atpo.org
Optician	Opticians Association of America	3740 Canada Road Lakeland, TN 38002 (901) 388-2423 www.oaa.org
	National Academy of Opticianry	8401 Corporate Drive Suite 605 Landover, MD 20785 (800) 229-4828 www.nao.org
Optometric Technician	American Optometric Association	1505 Prince Street Suite 300 Alexandria, VA 22314 and 243 North Lindbergh Boulevard Floor 1 St Louis, MO 63141 (800) 365-2219 www.aoa.org
Pharmacy Assistant or Technician	National Pharmacy Technician Association	P.O. Box 683148 Houston, TX 77268 (888) 247-8700 www.pharmacytechnician.org
	American Pharmacists Association	2215 Constitution Avenue NW Washington, DC 20037 (202) 628-4410 www.pharmacist.com
Phlebotomist	American Medical Technologists	10700 West Higgins Road Suite 150 Rosemont, IL 60018 (847) 823-5169 www.americanmedtech.org

Continued

Occupation	Organization	Contact Information
Physical Therapist Assistant	American Physical Therapy Association	1111 North Fairfax Street Alexandria, VA 22314 (703) 684-2782 (800) 999-2782 www.apta.org
Physician Assistant	American Academy of Physician Assistants	2318 Mill Road Suite 1300 Alexandria, VA 22314 (703) 836-2272 www.aapa.org
Practical or Vocational Nurse	National Association for Practical Nurse Education and Service	1940 Duke Street Suite 200 Alexandria, VA 22314 (703) 933-1003 www.napnes.org
Psychiatric or Mental Health Technician	American Association of Psychiatric Technicians	1220 S Street Suite 100 Sacramento, CA 95811 (800) 391-7589 www.psychtechs.org
Radiographer or Radiologic Technologist	American Society of Radiologic Technologists	15000 Central Avenue SE Albuquerque, NM 87123 (800) 444-2778 (505) 298-4500 www.asrt.org
Registered Nurse	National League for Nursing	The Watergate 2600 Virginia Avenue, NW Eighth Floor Washington, DC 20037 (800) 669-1656 www.nln.org
	American Nurses Association	8515 Georgia Avenue Suite 400 Silver Spring, MD 20910 (800) 274-4262 www.nursingworld.org
Respiratory Therapist	American Association for Respiratory Care	9425 N. MacArthur Boulevard Suite 100 Irving, TX 75063 (972) 243-2272 www.aarc.org
Surgical Technologist	Association of Surgical Technologists	6 West Dry Creek Circle Suite 200 Littleton, CO 80120 (800) 637-7433 www.ast.org
Veterinary Technician	National Association of Veterinary Technicians in America	P.O. Box 1227 Albert Lea, MN 56007 (888) 996-2882 www.navta.net

Useful Spanish Phrases

How to Use the Pronunciation Guides

1. Stress the syllables (parts of words) that are in capital letters.
2. "oh" is pronounced as in "toe."
3. "ah" is pronounced as in "father."
4. "ay" is pronounced as in "say."
5. "oo" is pronounced as in "moon."
6. "s" is always pronounced as in "set."
7. The letter "h" is always silent in Spanish.
8. When there is an English word given as a syllable, pronounce it as you would the word by itself. If letters in the word are silent in English, do not pronounce them. In "comb," for example, don't pronounce the "b." Just say the word.

Note: The "official" phonetic alphabet is not used here because many people who have not studied languages are not familiar with the special markings.

General Spanish Phrases

English	Spanish
Hello, hi.	Hola. (OH-lah)
Good morning.	Buenos días. (bway-nohs DEE-ahs)
Good afternoon.	Buenas tardes. (bway-nahs TAR-dace)
Good evening, good night.	Buenas noches. (bway-nahs NO-chase)
Please.	Por favor. (por fah-VOR)
Thank you.	Gracias. (GRAH-see-ahs)
You're welcome.	De nada. (day NAH-dah)
Yes.	Sí. (see)
No.	No (no)
My name is _____.	Me llamo _____ (may YAH-mo) *or* Mi nombre es_____ (me NOHM-bray ace)
What is your name?	¿Cómo se llama usted? (COMB-oh say YA-mah oo-sted)
Nice to meet you.	Mucho gusto. (MOO-choh GOO-stoh)
Do you speak English?	¿Habla usted inglés? (AH-blah oo-STED eeng-GLACE)
Do you understand English?	¿Comprende usted inglés? (comb-PREN-day oo-STED eeng-GLACE)
Do you understand me?	¿Me comprende usted? (may comb-PREN-day oo-STED)
Repeat, please.	Repita usted, por favor. (ray-PEE-tah oo-STED por fah-VOR)
I don't understand Spanish very well.	No comprendo el español muy bien. (no comb-PREN-doh el es-pahn-NYOL moo-ee bee-EN)
How do you feel?	¿Cómo se siente? (COMB-moh say see-EN-tay)
Good.	Bien. (bee-EN)
Fair.	Así, así (ah-SEE, ah-SEE) *or* Regular (ray-goo-LAHR)
Bad.	Mal. (mahl)
What is wrong?	¿Cuál es el problema? (kwal es el pro-BLAY-mah) *or* ¿Qué le pasa? (kay lay pah-sah)
Do you have pain?	¿Siente usted dolor? (see-EN-tay oo-STED doh-LOR)
Where?	¿Dónde? (DOHN-day)
Show me.	Enséñeme. (en-SEN-yay-may)

Continued

English	Spanish
Are you comfortable?	¿Está usted cómodo? (es-TAH oo-STED COMB-oh-doe)
It is important.	Es importante. (es eem-por-TAHN-tay)
Be calm, please.	Cálmese usted, por favor. (CALL-may-say oo-STED, por fah-VOR)
Don't be frightened.	No tenga usted miedo. (no TANG-gah oo-STED mee-AY-doh)
We are here to help you.	Estamos aquí para ayudarle. (eh-STAH-mohs ah-KEY pah-rah ah-you-DAR-lay)
Please come with me.	Acompáñeme usted, por favor. (ah-comb-PAWN-yay-may oo-STED por fah-VOR) *or* Por favor, venga usted conmigo. (por fah-VOR VEN-gah oo-STED cone-ME-go)
Go to the hospital.	Vaya usted al hospital. (VA-yah oo-STED ahl oh-spee-TAHL)

Basic Emergency Admission Questions

Allergies	Alergias (ah-LAIR-hee-ahs)
Antibiotics? Which ones?	¿Antibióticas? ¿Cuáles? (ahn-tee-bee-OH-tee-cahs. KWAH-lace)
Aspirin?	¿Aspirina? (Ah-spee-REE-nah)
Sulfa drugs?	¿Drogas de azufre? (DROH-gahs day ah-SOO-fray)
Pain medications? Which ones?	¿Pastillas para dolor? ¿Cuáles? (paw-STEE-yahs PAH-rah doe-LORE. KWAH-lace)
Others?	¿Otras? (OH-trahs)
Required medications	Medicinas requiridas (meh-dee-SEE-nahs ray-care-EE-dahs)
Medical problems	Problemas médicos (pro-BLAY-mahs MEH-dee-cohs)
Blood type	Grupo sanguineo (GROO-poh sahn-GEE-nay-oh)
Religion	Religión (ray-lee-hee-OHN)
Referral physician	Médico que lo mandó (MEH-dee-coh kay low mahn-DOE) [Patient is male] Médico que la mandó (MEH-dee-coh kay lah mahn-DOE) [Patient is female]
What type of medical insurance do you have?	¿Qué tipo de seguro médico tiene usted? (kay tee-poh day say-GOO-roh tee-EN-ay oo-STED)
What is your Blue Cross number? Kaiser?	¿Cuál es su número de Blue Cross? ¿De Kaiser? (kwal es sue NEW-meh-row day Blue Cross? Day Kaiser?)
Do you have a Medicare card?	¿Tiene usted tarjeta de Medicare? (tee-EN-ay oo-STED tar-HEY-tah day Medicare)
Fill out this form, please.	Llene usted esta forma (*or* planilla), por favor. (YEAH-nay oo-STED ES-ta FOR-mah, por fah-VOR)
Sign here, please.	Firme usted aquí, por favor. (fear-may oo-STED ah-KEY, por fah-VOR)
This is an authorization form. Please read it and sign here.	Esta es una forma de autorización (*or* forma de permiso). Favor de leerla y firmarla aquí. (ES-tah es OO-nah FOR-mah day ow-tore-ee-sah-see-OWN (FOR-mah day pair-MEE-so). Fah-VOR day lay-ERR-lah ee FEAR-mar-lah ah-KEY.

Note: Page numbers followed by *b* indicate boxes, *f* indicate figures, and *t* indicate tables.

Retention, success tips for improving, 53
Reviewing
    in note-taking, 97–98
    in reading, 104–106, 104t
Role play, 140, 141f

S

Safety
    laboratory skill development and, 141
    and Occupational Safety and Health Act
        (OSHA), 311
Salary discussion, after interview, 285
Salary expectation, Q&A on, 30b
Sample, in statistics, 156
Satisfaction, in work, 313–314, 314b
Saturated fats, definition of, 35
Scan, 67, 73
SCANS report, 9–10, 10b
    competency development, 300–310
        adapting to changing conditions, 308–309,
            309f, 309b
        avoiding burnout, 309–310, 310b
        confidentiality, 302–303, 302b–303b
        cost control, 307
        cross-training, 309, 309b
        ethics, 301, 301b
        integrity and honesty, 301–303
        loyalty, 301
        management styles, 304, 305t, 306b, 312
        morale, 301, 312
        problem solving and, 306
        responsible behavior, 303, 303b
        self-management, 308, 308b
        self-worth, 300–301, 300b
        work ethic, 301
        working with supervisor, 304–306, 305f,
            312
Scheduling, 3
    in job search, 220
    for time management, 42
School
    applying life experience in, 59t
    career services, 223–225, 224b, 225f
    catalog, 6
    combining work and, 64–65
    connecting career and, 2–4
    resources, taking advantage of, 6
        prescription for success for, 6b
    step-up programs in, 330
Scope of practice, 295, 309, 309b, 312
Self-advocacy, 77, 85
Self-assessment, prescription for success for,
    10b
Self-awareness, performance reviews and, 316
Self-esteem
    definition of, 2
    of patient, 11
Self-evaluation
    after being fired, 328, 329t
    after interview, 282b
Self-fulfilling prophecy, 19, 20f
Self-improvement, after being fired, 328
Self-management, developing competencies, 308,
    308b
Self-worth
    developing competencies, 300–301, 300b
    in self-assessment, 10b
Sense of humor, for handling stress, 46
Sensory impairments, communication to, 211
Sentence, common ailments, 122t
Sexual harassment, 310
Short-answer questions, 133–134
Short-term goals, 38
Simulated externships, 149–150
    success tips for, 149

Situational questions, in interview, 261, 265,
    265b
Skim, 67, 73
SMART goals, 323b
Social support, types of, 64
Soft skills, definition of, 201–202
Sounds, combining, in English, 72–73, 73b
Spanish languages. *see also* English-as-a-second-
        language students
    English-as-a-second-language students,
        68
    medical word and everyday, 68t
    phrases, benefits of knowing, 28–29
Speaking, 183–184, 183t, 184f
    improving, 69, 69f, 71b
    tips for sending effective messages, 184
Special skills, as resume building blocks, 27, 27f,
    28b, 239, 239b
Specific to general learning
    examples of, 50t
    versus general to specific, 50t
Spelling, 124b
    commonly confused words, 127t–128t
    commonly misspelled words, 126t
    first aid for, 124
    improving, 73–74
    rules for, 125t
    success tips for, 124–126
Spiritual practices, beliefs and, 179t–180t
Standard precautions, 2, 16, 141, 295, 311
STAR approach, 265
Step-up programs, 315, 330
Stereotypes
    definition of, 175
    understanding and, 178
Sterile technique, 2, 16
Stress, 45–47, 47b
    avoiding burnout, 309–310, 310b
    definition of, 35
    on the job, 47b
    management, behavioral interview questions
        regarding, 264t
    sources of, 45–46
    success tips for handling, 46–47, 46f, 46b
Student
    responsibilities of, 7, 7b, 9b
    rights of, 5–6, 6b–7b
Study
    habits, effective, developing, 52–53, 52b
    learning to, 135b
    skills, 2, 57, 65
        prescription for success for, 5b
Study groups, 57, 65, 67, 69, 77
    teamwork skills in, 193
Success
    cultural beliefs and, 179t–180t
    first step to, 2, 2f
    planning for career, 9
    skills for, 5b
Suffixes, 77, 83t, 109
Supervisor
    becoming, 322–323, 322f, 322b
    in giving performance reviews, 316
    working with, 304–306, 305f, 312
Support group, 59
    definition of, 57
    for handling stress, 46
Support system
    during job search, 222, 222b
    social, 64
Support team, 64b
Supporting goals, 38
Syllabi, 19, 25
Syllable, 67, 72, 73t, 77, 109
Symbols, and abbreviations in note-taking,
    95–96, 95b–96b, 95t, 96f

T

Targeted objective, 237, 237b
Team members
    differences among, 194
    tips for effective, 194–195
Teamwork, definition of, 175, 193
Teamwork skills, developing, 193–195, 194f,
    194b–195b
Technical manuals, 300
Technical skills, mastery of, 214, 214b
Technology, for getting organized, 45
Telephone, 220
Temperature, measurement for, 157t, 158f
Terminally ill patients, communication with,
    211
Test taking, skills for, 4, 4f
Tests, 126–136, 126t, 128f, 129b
    after taking, 134–136
    for anxiety, 130–131
    day before, 131
    day of, 131–132
    on the job, 130b
    for learning disabled students, 84t
    preparing effectively for, 130, 130b
    problems in, 134t
    procrastination and, 131
    professional exams and, 136
    realities about, 129–130
    techniques for, 132–134
        essay questions, 134
        fill-in-the-blank questions, 133
        matching questions, 133
        multiple choice questions, 132–133
        short-answer questions, 133–134
        true-false questions, 132
    use of, to advantage, 128–129, 130b
    what they are and are not, 129–130
Text, 114
    definition of, 109
Textbook, anatomy of, 102–103, 103b
Thank-you letter, 283–284, 283f, 284b
Thank-you-plus letter, 284, 284b, 285f
Theory, 140
Therapeutic communication, 206–211
    to special situations, 211
    techniques, 209t
Thoughts, tripped up by your, 41
Time, cultural beliefs and, 179t–180t
Time management, 41–44
    efficiency for, 41
    and family, 60, 60f, 60b
    in handling stress, 46
    on the job, 43b
    in job search, 220
    prescription for success, 42b–43b
    prioritizing and, 41, 60, 60f
    skills for, 2, 3t
    for students with learning disabilities, 84t
    success tips for, 42–44, 42b–43b
Toxic
    definition of, 295
    Occupational Safety and Health Act (OSHA),
        311
Traditional questions, in interview, 263,
    263b
Trans fat, definition of, 35
Transferable skills
    definition of, 19
    in resume, 25, 26f
True-false questions, 132
Tutor, 57, 58t, 77

U

Universal precautions, 141